DIMENSIONS OF COMMUNITY MENTAL HEALTH CARE

DIMENSIONS OF COMMUNITY MENTAL HEALTH CARE

edited by

M.P.I. Weller

MA (Cantab.) MB,BS, FRC Psych., C.Psychol., FBPsS
Consultant Psychiatrist,
St Ann's, Whittington and Royal Northern Hospitals,

Honorary Senior Lecturer
The Royal Free Hospital
School of Medicine
London

and

M. Muijen

MSc, MD, PhD, MRCPsych
Director, Research and
Development for Psychiatry,
London

W.B. Saunders Company Ltd
London   Philadelphia   Toronto
Sydney   Tokyo

W.B. Saunders Company Ltd	24–28 Oval Road London NW1 7DX, UK

Baillière Tindall

The Curtis Center
Independence Square West
Philadelphia, PA 19106–3399, USA

55 Horner Avenue
Toronto, Ontario M8Z 4X6, Canada

Harcourt Brace & Company
(Australia) Pty Ltd
30–52 Smidmore Street
Marrickville, NSW 2204, Australia

Harcourt Brace Japan Inc.
Ichibancho Central Building
22–1 Ichibancho
Chiyoda-ku, Tokyo 102, Japan

A catalogue record for this book is available from the
British Library

ISBN 0–7020–1612–8

This book is printed on acid-free paper

Typeset by J&L Composition Ltd, Filey, North Yorkshire
Printed and bound in Great Britain by Mackays of Chatham PLC, Chatham, Kent

CONTENTS

vi   CONTENTS

CONTRIBUTORS

D. Abrahamson
Consultant Psychiatrist, Goodmayes Hospital, Ilford, Essex

D. Bhugra
Senior Lecturer, MRC Social and Community Psychiatry Unit,
Institute of Psychiatry, Denmark Hill, London

P. Campbell
Camden Mental Health Consortium, Camden, London

J. Carson
Lecturer in Clinical Psychiatry, Institute of Psychiatry,
Denmark Hill, London

D.J. El-Kabir
Principal and Chairman of the Trustees, Wytham Hall,
Physician-in-charge, Great Chapel Street Medical Centre, London

T. Glynn
Project Manager, Tomswood Hill Project, Claybury Hospital,
Woodford Green, Essex

J. Gopaulen
Area Nurse Manager, Claybury Hospital, Woodford Green, Essex

C. Kirk
Formerly: Administrator, Friern Hospital, London

G. McNamee
Senior Manager, Community Mental Health and ALD Services,
West Lambeth Community Care (NHS) Trust, London

N. Mills
Clinical Psychologist, Department of Psychology,
Fulbourn Hospital, Cambridge

I. Morris
Head of Clinical Psychology, Guy's and St Thomas' NHS Trust,
London

M. Muijen
Director, Research and Development for Psychiatry, Borough,
London

A. Neeter
Camden Mental Health Consortium, Camden, London

D. Ross
Camden Mental Health Consortium, Camden, London

P. Ryan
Project Manager RDP Case Management Project, Research and
Development for Psychiatry, Borough, London

G. Shepherd
Consultant Clinical Psychologist and Head of Department,
Department of Psychology, Fulbourn Hospital, Cambridge

K. Singh
Clinical Psychologist, Department of Psychology,
Fulbourn Hospital, Cambridge

G. Strathdee
Consultant Community Psychiatrist, Maudsley Hospital,
Denmark Hill, London

E.F. Torrey
Clinical Research Psychiatrist, Department of Health and Human
Services, National Institute of Mental Health, St Elizabeth's
Hospital, Washington DC, USA

M.P.I. Weller
Consultant Psychiatrist, St Ann's, Whittington and Royal Northern
Hospitals, Honorary Senior Lecturer Royal Free Hospital Medical
School, London

PREFACE

We invited the contributing professionals to write from their own perspectives, expressing their own viewpoints. We realized that such a policy would inevitably generate some contradictions. Initially, we tried to reconcile some of these, but we came to feel that this was inappropriate. Instead we saw this book as an opportunity to explore independent, diverging developments. With a crystallizing service, as we now have in the UK, it is inevitable that people starting from different positions may have a different emphasis in the way they would prefer to see the service develop. We saw our task as facilitating further dialogue and discussion, to help draw some of these viewpoints together in planning a comprehensive and integrated service.

As testimony to the fruitfulness of such an approach, the editors themselves did not start from completely coincidental standpoints, but have found that in planning and developing this book their views and aspirations have drawn closer together. It is our hope that readers may have a similar experience and be able themselves to see ways of reconciling some of the remaining differences, which are inevitable in a multi-author work.

The restructuring and reorganization of a traditional service is an awesome task, fraught with difficulties. Even if the way forward is clear the means to achieve appropriate change is often uncertain. We are often faced by awkward decisions and execution of general policies is often difficult. It is easier to paint with broad brush strokes than to focus on detail. An anecdote illustrates the problem. The millipede had difficulty getting his football boots on in time to play in the match. This recurrent frustration led him to consult the wise owl. The owl listened patiently and then gave the millipede his considered advice: 'change into a rabbit', he pronounced. The millipede left with a glad heart, believing that his problems were over, but then came back bewildered. 'How do I change into a rabbit?' he asked tentatively. 'Ah', the wise owl responded, 'I give advice on policy, not on execution'.

When all is said, what struck us most forcefully, in assembling this book, is not that there should be differences of opinion, but that these should be so few and that a broad consensus and coincidence of viewpoints has emerged without any attempt to direct the individual authors or to attempt to shape their contributions. We found this encouraging for the future of a developing service. With such a broad agreement, more than further debate, we now need the means to realize these new dimensions of care.

Malcolm P.I. Weller
Matthijs Muijen

1 WHERE WE CAME FROM: RECENT HISTORY OF COMMUNITY PROVISION

M.P.I. Weller

REASONS FOR CHANGE

The original impetus to close psychiatric hospitals in the UK originated in a dubious extrapolation of hospital discharge figures, in a paper that drew methodological criticisms (Tooth and Brooke, 1961). The paper appeared in the same year and in the same journal (the *Lancet*) as two others discussing general hospital closures, and was published in the same year as Goffman's influential polemic *Asylums*. The Tooth and Brooke paper predicted that the long-stay population was declining at such a rate that it would be eliminated in about 16 years. Replacement would generate an estimated need for 890 long-stay beds per million of the population and an overall figure of 1800 beds per million for all types of care. These predictions were discussed in a subsequent Editorial in the *Lancet* (1961), which stated 'all share the Minister of Health's hope that the number of beds in mental hospitals can be safely reduced'. Quite apart from the illogicality of extrapolating an alleged linear trend to extinction, the tapering figures cited by Dr Tooth and Miss Brooke did not seem to justify the assumed linear trend of decline:

Long-stay patients in hospital on 31 December	1954	112 113
Deaths and discharges	1955	8 163
	1956	7 432
	1957	6 608
	1958	6 249
	1959	5 953

The paper by Tooth and Brooke (1961) and the Editorial in the *Lancet* (1961) were based partly on subjective assessments which, as one critical correspondent pointed out, 'are still matters of opinion, even when expressed as percentages to the first decimal place' (Waind, 1961). Nonetheless, even if closures are not to take place by the sustained rate of discharge of long-stay patients, with an inconsequential build-up of 'new' long-stay patients, the objective of psychiatric hospital closures is still being actively pursued with enthusiasm and goodwill (*The Health of the Nation*, 1991).

The prescient words of Egan (1961), discussing the contentious Tooth and Brooke extrapolation of bed reductions, seem apposite: 'Areas like Burnley and Oldham would seem tailor made for a planned investigation into the effects on family life of keeping chronic psychotics and other permanent invalids at home. . . . It may show that psychotics find hospital treatment outside of their home areas.' The American experiences of a drift of the mentally ill to the decaying city centres (Farris and Dunham, 1939; Hollingshead and Redlich, 1958; see also Chapter 15) confirm these suspicions, to which must be added the drift of drug addicts, alcoholics, and schizophrenics into London (Royal College of General Practitioners, 1981; Weller *et al.*, 1987, 1989).

HOSPITAL PLAN FOR ENGLAND AND WALES 1962

Tooth and Brooke's conclusions struck a responsive chord, sitting easily with a growing concern for civil liberties. The simple extrapolation was stripped of all caveats and incorporated as policy objectives into the *Hospital Plan for England and Wales* by Enoch Powell, the Minister of Health, who presented his deliberations to Parliament in 1962. The considerable local variations in bed

1985 (□) 1986 (○) 1987 (⬠) 1988 (◇) and 1989 (▭)

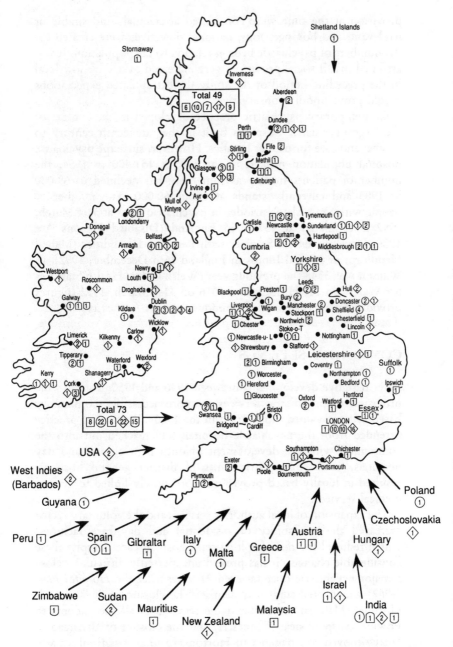

Figure 1 Places of birth of 175 destitute people interviewed in London.

provision at the time were considered artefactual, undesirable or irrelevant, and homogeneous, national objectives were created for the numbers of psychiatric beds in relation to the population. It was assumed that if social provision were increased over their low level in the preceding period of the study the extrapolated expectations would prove unduly conservative!

Contemporary psychiatric practice developed in the context of the large psychiatric hospitals built in the nineteenth century to protect and care for pauper lunatics. However, since the psychiatric hospital population peaked in the UK at 151 400 in 1954, the number of patients finding asylum there has declined to 69 000 in 1983 and currently stands at about 60 000. The number of people with unfinished episodes in psychiatric units at 31st March, 1992 is estimated at 45 000 in England (Disabled Persons Act 1986; Development of Services with Learning Disabilities (Mental Handicap) or Mental Illness in England 16th December, 1992). In Wales it was 3348 the previous year (Welsh Office Health Statistics for Wales No 11, HMSO) and 3016 on 31st March, 1992 (figures provided by Welsh Health Commons Services Authority).

COMMUNITY SETTINGS

After tentative developments between 1930 and 1950, a shift in the provision of psychiatric services to more accessible, community based settings gained momentum in the 1960s. Psychiatric practice extended from the psychiatric hospitals and reached out into the community with the development of outpatient clinics, and day hospitals, whilst psychiatric units in district general hospitals resulted in locally based provision, more closely linked to general medical services.

The expansion of local authority services and the voluntary sector increased the availability of residential and day care facilities, which reduced the need for long-term hospital care. Despite these considerable changes, it has proved unexpectedly difficult to close a major psychiatric hospital even 21 years after the *Hospital Plan* (1962) which predicted their demise. The closure of St Wulstan's Hospital, Malvern, necessitated the removal of all the patients to Powick Hospital near Worcester, and the closure of Banstead in Surrey moved 380 patients to Horton Hospital seven miles away and over 140 patients to other hospitals, St Mary Abbots, St Charles and the Gordon, in London, and others to a home for the elderly, mentally infirm. The long-stay patients at Friern Hospital, after ten years of closure plans, will move 'temporarily' to St Annes' Hospital (at a cost of £70 million).

Although some district general hospitals have increasingly operated independently of large psychiatric hospitals outside their catchment area, most have continued to rely on psychiatric hospitals for back-up services, particularly for the more chronic, severely disabled patients. However, we are now entering a more radical period of deinstitutionalization with the Minister of Health and the regional health authorities pressing for hospital closures within specified time-limits.

ENDS AND MEANS

This book will examine how services provided by psychiatric hospitals can be replaced by suitable alternatives and identify the facilities necessary to provide a comprehensive district based service reducing reliance on hospital facilities and providing a flexible range of services.

There is intense public awareness of this process of transferring the centre of gravity of care away from the hospitals and a potential willingness to accept community based projects. However, as the Report of the Select Committee of the House of Commons (1985) stated, 'Beyond a general recognition that the days of the largest hospitals are over, there is no consensus on community care.' Hawks (1975), in an analysis of the assumptions underlying community care, commented, 'To return a patient to the bosom of the community has a certain moral imperativeness which recommends its uncritical acceptance, as does the rejection of all forms of institutional care.' Heginbotham (1985), a past director of Mind wrote, '. . . segregation in institutions implies and strengthens differentness (sic) rather than sameness or wholeness . . . .' Similar ideas were pungently expressed by the pioneer Franco Basaglia who, however, argued, 'There is a danger then that community care is a somewhat empty slogan fuelled by criticism of the mental hospitals yet failing to articulate in a clear way the nature of alternative provision'. Such alternatives and facilitating arrangements form the major portion of this book. Some framework and guiding principles first need to be established.

Attempts have been made to clarify what is meant by the term community care and to define it more precisely. Bennett and Morris (1983) have suggested that four principles can be discerned underlying the concept.

Firstly, and perhaps most prominently, they comment that, 'The social aim of the community care movement is one that advocates that the environments of handicapped people should, as far as possible, reflect normal community life, and that forms of institutional care that segregate them from society are unacceptable'. This means that the patient's local community, and not the institution, must provide the context for treatment, rehabilitation, support and long-term management.

Secondly, they suggest that merely changing the *locus* of care from hospital to community is not a panacea. Sheltered community based settings have been shown in the past to develop some of the institutional practices previously associated with the psychiatric hospital (Apte, 1968; Carter and Evans, 1978). Care and expertise must therefore be available to ensure that community facilities provide a social milieu which is accepting and enabling, and certainly does not reject those with the most severe impairments.

Thirdly, an active approach to rehabilitation and support is necessary to ensure that the needs of patients are regularly reviewed and all reasonable steps are taken to maximize their functioning, minimizing the effects of long-term mental illness in as normal a setting as possible.

Fourthly, they suggest that the role of the hospital needs reconsideration. Sometimes community care has masqueraded as a rejection of the medical model in favour of a definition of mental illness as social distress. However, severe mental illness is a complex phenomenon with diverse causes and consequences. Several agencies must act together in concert to meet comprehensively the needs of mentally ill people. Medical services and hospital admission are not *alternatives* to community care, but one aspect of a network of service all relevant to the provision of adequate locally based care.

The Select Committee of the House of Commons, 1985, also tried to elucidate general principles, which they felt formed the basis for defining community care. These included:

1. A preference for home life over 'institutional' care.
2. The pursuit of the ideal of normalization and integration and avoidance as far as possible of separate provision, segregation and restriction (i.e. the least restrictive alternatives).
3. A preference for small over large.
4. A preference for local services over distant ones.

An articulated set of principles, such as the above, translated into aims and objectives, provide guidance in designing a community based service to meet the needs, comprehensively, of mentally ill people in a flexible way.

DEVELOPING IDEAS

As our understanding of the meaning of community care has developed, so some of the earlier ideas which influenced the move towards the community have been reconsidered. The momentum of the community care movement in the 1960s was influenced by a desire for radical social change and prevailing optimism in psychiatry. The introduction of the 'major tranquillizers' and their widespread use by the late 1950s, the relaxation of institutional life, plus the success of earlier methods of rehabilitation and resettlement outside hospital, resulted in an open and optimistic attitude in British psychiatry. Wing (1978) commented of this period, 'It was assumed that if significant attention were to be given to the acute stages, chronic disabilities would be prevented'. Thus the optimistic predictions of the *Hospital Plan* (1962) assumed that the contribution of medical services could be limited to acute psychiatry, any problems of residual disability being addressed by local authority support services. Cynics have felt that these ideas have been impelled by financial considerations and note that the services focused on chronic problems (mental illness, mental handicap and the elderly) were omitted from the early plans for the NHS. They were only included in the National Health Service Act of 1946 for England and Wales (extended to Scotland the following year) after energetic lobbying by the Royal Medical Psychiatric Association, which expressed its concern for an estimated four million psychiatric casualties if there were intensive bombing.

DIFFICULTIES TO BE RESOLVED

As we have seen, Tooth and Brooke's figures did not entirely support the linear trend on which their predictions were based but the eloquent predictions of the Minister of Health, based on a simplified model assuming the best possible scenario (*if* the trend continued, *if* we did not have an ageing population, *if* the public developed sufficient tolerance), were extremely influential and his words continue to be cited today.

Baldwin and Hall (1967), Rollin (1969) and later Hailey (1971) all drew attention to the curvilinear decline of the long-stay population. They suggested that, as the less impaired patients responded to programmes of rehabilitation, the residual population comprised a group of much more disabled patients, who were less responsive to the methods of rehabilitation then available. This group, sometimes referred to as the 'old' long-stay, has been described in many publications (e.g. Baldwin and Hall, 1967; Fottrell *et al.*, 1975; Erbinger and Christie-Brown, 1975). They are highly dependent on nursing staff for their basic needs, and often display behavioural problems which exclude them from most residential facilities.

A recent survey from one health district conducted by consultant staff, including this author (Friern Hospital survey, 1985 (unpublished); Campbell *et al.*, 1990), revealed that 83% of the high dependency patients had been in hospital for more than 15 years. Despite the fact that over half were more than 70 years of age, over 60% displayed behavioural problems, such as verbal abuse with occasional physical aggression, fire risk, and frequent fluctuations in their mental state; 34% of the patients had caused one or more episodes of acute disturbance during the year preceding the survey. This group of patients is, therefore, far from 'burnt out' and consists of people who are elderly, fragile and severely handicapped by their psychiatric problems. To meet their needs effectively they require a high staff–patient ratio, with staff who are experienced in dealing with relatively frequent disturbances. Drug and alcohol abuse, aggression and severe psychosis also create difficulties in community support.

STAFF SUITABILITY

The availability of nursing staff continues to decrease. There is a national shortage, most severe in London, and psychiatric nursing is less popular than general nursing. Care assistants are basically untrained and seldom stay in post longer than six months. Compounding staffing inadequacies, the move towards community care is initially unsettling because hospital closure plans have preceded the creation of community facilities, inducing many of the better nurses to seek more secure employment, whilst recruitment has suffered.

Because of the increasing psychiatric morbidity of the residual long-stay patients, the sustained discharge of long-stay patients is unlikely, in itself, to lead to hospital closures. A study of the population of three large hospitals shows a decelerating decline that forms a plateau around 700 patients (J. Leff, personal communication).

This is not to suggest that it is not possible, or desirable, to care for more dependent and disturbed patients in the community. However, it does point to the need for residential settings with better staffing levels and greater expertise than before. Such an endeavour will need a substantial investment in resources and staff training, tenacity of purpose amongst the staff, with flexible and innovative approaches, if it is to result in an improvement in standards of care.

However, it can be argued, that the 'old' long-stay represent a legacy from the past. The 'new' long-stay are perhaps a more pertinent challenge to current optimism concerning the effectiveness of psychiatric rehabilitation, and the viability of care in the community for all of those experiencing severe and chronic psychiatric disability. These are seriously impaired patients, who have continued to accumulate as long-stay residents in psychiatric hospitals *despite* the development of alternative facilities in the community and more active attempts to prevent long-term hospitalization.

One comprehensive survey (Mann and Cree, 1976) studied 'new' long-stay patients who had accumulated in English psychiatric hospitals during the preceding three years. One hospital from each of the 15 regional health authorities in England was sampled. The research team made judgements concerning the need for continuing hospital care and concluded that one-third of the 400 patients surveyed would continue to need hospital care even if improved community facilities were available.

A subsequent Scottish study (McCreadie *et al.*, 1983) surveyed patients who had been in hospital between one and six years. They used slightly different criteria to Mann and Cree and concluded that 38% of the population which they examined could have lived outside hospital had community services been adequately developed. However, this left 62% of their sample who were considered to be appropriately placed in hospital or who would need a level of care then rarely available outside a hospital setting. They suggested that the local authorities had not made much progress in providing facilities which could cope with those more severely handicapped in the ten years since the Mann and Cree study was conducted, concluding that the Health Service might need to continue to provide some residential settings for this group of patients.

The size of the 'new' long-stay group and the rate of its accumulation will, to some degree, depend on local factors. The measures by which community care policies are actively pursued, the number and range of community facilities available, the organization and expertise of services providing care for those with chronic psychiatric handicaps, and demographic variables, all of these will influence the extent to which hospitals continue to be needed for long-term asylum.

DEMOGRAPHIC VARIABLES AND PROBLEM AREAS

Some variations in the size of the 'new' long-stay can be discerned from services which maintain a case register. This method of monitoring contacts with a local psychiatric service can demonstrate the use being made of different elements in the service. Data from eight case registers throughout the country (Wing, 1989) indicate that the size of the 'new' long-stay population will vary considerably. Fewest patients continue to accumulate in rural areas, more accumulate in small towns but the most significant numbers can be found in the large urban areas. Two hypotheses have been put forward to account for this finding. There is some tendency for those with psychiatric illness to drift to the inner cities where they lack roots and supportive social networks that might ameliorate the impact of severe psychiatric problems, a trend identified in several recent surveys (Freeman and Alpert, 1986; Freeman, 1988; Campbell *et al.*, 1990; Royal College of General Practitioners, 1981; Weller *et al.*, 1987). Secondly, psychiatric difficulties might be exacerbated by the social deprivation likely to be more prevalent in inner city areas. Both these factors contribute to social disadvantages which will intensify the degree of handicap.

Many patients living outside hospital, therefore, require long-term support and appropriate rehabilitation services. They cannot be defined by their length of stay but they are sometimes referred to as the 'new' long-term, 'young adult chronic patients' (Lamb and Grant, 1982), or 'high-contact patients' (Wing, 1962). These terms refer to those with severe and chronic psychiatric disability, who have not necessarily experienced long hospital admission but who, nevertheless, require a network of services to enable them to survive with dignity and personal satisfaction in the community. They have been referred to as an 'uninstitutionalized generation' (Pepper, 1985). While the problems of prolonged institutionalization are therefore reduced, other difficulties have emerged. Bachrach (1982) emphasizes that this is a heterogeneous group: 'They constitute neither a uniform diagnostic entity nor a group with fixed and predictable symptomatology.'

Sheets *et al.* (1982) suggest these patients present with problems which can be divided into three categories.

One group consists of patients with predominantly negative features, with problems of motivation and passivity, readily deteriorating into a life of dependency.

A further group, who function well between more disturbed episodes, nevertheless, are seriously socially disabled. Bachrach (1982) describes them as '. . . isolated individuals with limited social supports and little hope of lasting success despite their aspirations'.

Sheets' third category includes those described as '. . . aggressive and basically noncompliant persons who have low tolerance for frustration', resulting in impulsive, antisocial behaviour, which frequently falls foul of the law.

It seems inherently unlikely that all these categories will be readily contained within existing social service provisions; certainly this is not the case at present. There is an incentive, which the Audit Commission investigation in 1986 described as 'perverse'

(Audit Commission, 1986), for local government to offload their responsibilities onto institutions and it is difficult to believe that increasing the area of responsibility will overcome the problem. Hospitals do not have a responsibility to take all patients, and they sometimes fail to accept prisoners and those on remand (Coid, 1988) who, in the past, would have seemed eminently suitable for hospital admission. Nevertheless they have a laudable record in this regard when compared to local authorities, who already have heavy responsibilities that they have done little to discharge since the obligations were created in the 1959 Mental Health Act to provide residential and training centres and to attend to rehabilitation, shelter and supervision. Overlapping obligations were also expressed, successively, in the National Assistance Act 1948, the Housing Act 1967, and the Homeless Persons Act 1976. This manifest failure does not inspire confidence in the new community care legislation channelling money into local government, encouraging it to seek the cheapest available forms of 'appropriate' care.

Neglect in hospitals must not be replaced by neglect in the community. The ultimate success of our policies will be judged by this criterion. Nevertheless, we live in exciting times. The movement towards community care is gathering impetus and innovation and enthusiasm are widely apparent. New developments are occurring almost daily to change the pattern of care from a system which has been in place since the Victorian era. The old style hospitals are now decaying and crumbling away, they are a third to a half empty, and often occupy valuable sites as cities have grown up around them.

The will to produce change has never been more apparent, and an alliance has developed between psychiatry and other groupings to deliver psychiatric care in a more enterprising and appealing way, as described in many chapters in this book.

The general feelings of optimism are tempered only by the realization that there are some gaps in the framework of provision, which have long been with us and which are difficult to address. Another source of unease is whether finance will be adequate to drive these exciting changes to a universally successful conclusion.

Finally, there is the concern that as enthusiasm wanes, humdrum but serious needs will be neglected, while recruitment into service provision will prove difficult. The development of the present attitudes has been punctuated by tensions between various professional groupings and accusations that psychiatrists are self-seeking and reactionary. This criticism fails to encompass the certainty that there will be a residual need for asylum (haven or sanctuary) for some patients and for an efficient and adequate acute psychiatric service with appropriate inpatient facilities.

ACUTE SERVICES

The impetus to press on with discharging long-stay patients has perhaps failed to incorporate fully the probable need for expanding acute facilities. It is hoped that by energetic and prescient intervention some of the long-term psychiatric morbidity will be checked at an incipient phase and some of the acute psychiatric admissions and chronic casualties will be avoided. Against this it has to be recognized that the long-stay patients who are discharged are an especially vulnerable population, and a proportion will need readmissions from time to time (about one in seven per annum in the careful Friern placements). Such readmissions can be difficult to put into reverse because the disturbance which led to the admission prejudice the community care arrangements. These problems can be tackled by more acute beds and better training and staffing in residential units, particularly at night, and should not deflect our vision of a comprehensive, community based service.

PROBLEM AREAS

Evidence of policy failure and patient neglect is readily apparent in the community in day-to-day psychiatric practice. Johnstone et al. (1984) followed up 94 schizophrenic patients discharged from an English hospital five to nine years previously, out of an original cohort of 120; more than 50% of those discharged had definite psychotic symptoms, when those currently readmitted were excluded, 'and by all available accounts, many were consistently and severely impaired'. Despite this, 27% had no contact with medical or social services and 'severe emotional, social and financial difficulties were commonplace . . .'. The authors commented that 'the standard of care in the community was . . . far from optimal'.

The situation is even worse in Scotland (McCreadie *et al.*, 1985) where 40% of those discharged had no contact with aftercare services, a figure that rose to 75% among discharged first admissions out of 571 'new chronic inpatients', from many different hospitals, aged between 18 and 64 years who had spent more than one but less than six years in hospital.

McCreadie's rural figures belie wide differences. The point prevalence is about 2 schizophrenic sufferers per 1000 of the general Nithsdale population. In the inner London district of Camden, the point prevalence of schizophrenia is over 8.5 per 1000 and the lifestyle is dismal if not dangerous (Campbell *et al.*, 1990). A similarly high prevalence figure was recorded in Salford (Freeman and Alpert, 1986; Freeman, 1988), possibly because of a shifting population, as patients drift away, moving from districts where they were known (Johnstone *et al.*, 1985; Weller *et al.*, 1987) to anomic city centres (Faris and Dunham, 1939; Hollingshead and Redlich, 1958; Weller *et al.*, 1989). Similar problems of patients failing to attend for follow-up on discharge and disappearing from the area have been experienced at Powick Hospital, the first hospital in England to be closed, and where additional finances were provided early to promote a successful outcome (personal communication of staff). At least some schizophrenic sufferers migrate (Ødergaard, 1932; Jauhar and Weller, 1982; Weller and Jauhar, 1987), and thereby prejudice follow-up. A suitable comprehensive register, tracing patients via social security claims and prisons could clarify the situation. The migration tendencies may be only relocation in an adjacent local authority, but this may lead to irreconcilable border disputes that prevent the patient receiving day care, social work support, or even the statutory approved social worker's consideration of medical recommendations for compulsory admission (Brahams and Weller, 1985).

On street surveys we have found actively hallucinating destitute men who had never received any treatment, many not claiming any benefits of any kind. These men had no friends or family support, and generally lacked medical or dental care (Weller *et al.*, 1989). One man with tuberculosis was sleeping under the arches of Charing Cross station on Christmas Eve without his medication. It is this group, whose needs are not being met at all, on whom our planning should focus, as a matter of the most pressing priority.

'The problem is complicated by the resistance which many

patients show to anything "psychiatric", and regard the outpatient department as the door to the "asylum". Any recommendation for psychiatric treatment may provoke hostility and resentment from which the practitioner may retreat.' (MacCalman, 1951, cited Heimler, 1967, p. 140). We may hope that the change in direction away from traditional, rather ominous venues and types of psychiatric care will weaken this attitude. However, there remain the vexed questions of finance and employment prospects for patients with psychiatric histories or, worse, psychiatric histories and residual symptoms.

ECONOMIC FACTORS

Economic factors are important determinants of outcome, both in terms of the provision of sufficient finance for caring arrangements and in the opportunities for gainful employment for those who have suffered mental illness, particularly those with residual symptoms (Warner, 1985, 1988). Regrettably, both these are areas of difficulty. By this token one is suspicious that 'normalization', i.e. leading as normal a life as possible, will come to imply that nothing special need be created. The old psychiatric hospitals responded to the criticisms that too little was expected of the patients who, it was wrongly imagined, were insensitive to expectations. Initiatives were energetically pursued to commence socially based treatment schedules, but the costs, particularly the staffing costs, rose considerably. At the end of the day it was decided by the North East Thames Region to close Friern and Claybury Hospitals because they were particularly expensive, despite the fact that they were the inheritors of a generation of financial neglect. (At that time (1982) patients, including acute patients, were costing £13 000 per annum.)

A central tenet of current thinking is a preference for small over large, which necessarily eliminates the economies of scale inherent in the old system of institutional care. To the seemingly inevitable increase in operating costs arising from this factor must be added the peripatetic costs of care delivery and the double running costs during a transition period. NE Thames Regional Health Authority designated provider groups to cost community provisions for the four districts served by Friern Hospital to replace the hospital.

Some £20 million were projected, compared to the hospital budget of £14 million. The region then specified a total budget allocation for this priority service of £9 million (NE Thames Regional Health Authority, 1983). These are small sums compared with the £70 million spent on capital projects or the £17 billion of backlog NHS repairs and maintenance. The figures illustrate the visible costs to the health authority but not the costs of additional social service funding flowing to discharged patients. Recent financial constraints will impede the repetition of earlier successes.

Apart from financial considerations, any change in practice, particularly shifting the locus of care to a more accessible Community base, has to be handled sensitively so that morale can be maintained. The most crucial period, which may last for ten or more years, lies between the initial announcement of hospital closure and new facilities coming on stream. It should be obvious that precious staff have to have their futures assured when a hospital is nominated for closure, but they may be left unnecessarily doubtful and uncertain for want of attention to these obvious considerations, and maintaining and recruiting staff during this twilight period is extremely difficult.

We must set our sights on creative ways to overcome these obstacles and incorporate an expansion of outreach clinics and the development of court facilities to deflect the mentally ill out of custody. Professionals must join hands with lay helpers and both must participate in the creation of facilities as well as the delivery of care. Yet despite the best of wills, and despite arguments to the contrary, it is difficult to see an alternative, comprehensive and flexible service arising from the ashes of the old psychiatric hospitals without generous finance.

REFERENCES

Apte, R.Z. (1968) *Halfway Houses*. Occasional Papers of social administration, no. 27. Bell, London.

Audit Commission (1986) HMSO, London, p. 4.

Bachrach, L.L. (1982) Assessment of outcomes in community support systems: results, problems and limitations. *Schizophrenia Bulletin*, 8 (1), 39–61.

Baldwin, J.A. and Hall, D.J. (1967) Estimation of the outcome of a standing mental hospital population. *British Journal of Preventive and Social Medicine*, **21**, 56–65.

Bennett, D.H. and Morris, I. (1983) Deinstitutionalisation in the United Kingdom. *International Journal of Mental Health*, **11** (4), 5–23.

Brahams, D. and Weller, M.P.I. (1985) Crime and homelessness among the mentally ill. *New Law Journal*, **135**, pt 1 626–629, pt 2 761–763. (Reprinted with added appendix, *Medico-legal Journal* (1985) **54** (1), 42–53.)

Campbell, P.C., Taylor, J., Pantelis, C. and Harvey, C. (1990) Studies of schizophrenia in a large mental hospital proposed for closure, and in two halves of an inner London borough served by the hospital. In: *International Perspectives in Schizophrenia* (I. Weller, ed.). John Libbey, London.

Carter, J, and Evans, T.N. (1978) Intentions and achievements in admissions of the elderly to residential care. *Clearing House for Local Authority Social Services Research*, no. 9, pp. 71–99.

Cuid, J.W. (1988) Mentally abnormal prisoners on remand: 1—Rejected or accepted by the NHS? *British Medical Journal*, **296**, 1779–1782.

Editorial (1961) *Lancet*, 27 May, 1151.

Egan, G.P. (1961) Needs and beds. *Lancet*, **i**, 1284–1285.

Erbinger, L. and Christie-Brown, J.R. (1975) Social deprivation amongst short stay psychiatric patients. *British Journal Psychiatry*, **1980**, 136, 46–52.

Faris, R.E.L. and Dunham, H.W. (1939) *Mental Disorder in Urban Areas*. University of Chicago Press, Chicago.

Fottrell, E., Peermohamed, R. and Kothari, R. (1975). Identification and definition of long-stay mental hospital population. *British Medical Journal*, **iv**, 675–677.

Freeman, H.L. (1988) *Mental Health and the Environment*. Churchill Livingstone, London.

Freeman, H. and Alpert, M. (1986) Prevalence of schizophrenia in an urban population. *British Journal of Psychiatry*, **149**, 603–611.

Goffman, E. (1961) *Asylums*. Anchor Books/Doubleday, New York.

Hailey, A.M. (1971) Long-stay psychiatric in-patients: a study based on the Camberwell Register. *Psychological Medicine*, **1**, 128–142.

Hawks, D. (1975) Community care on analysis of assumptions. *British Journal of Psychiatry*, **127**, 276–285.

Heginbotham, C. (1985) Consumer choice: change and conflict in community care. Oldham AMA Conference, 27th September.

Heimler, E. (1967) *Mental Illness and Social Work*. Penguin, Harmondsworth and Victoria.

Hollingshead, A.B. and Redlich, F.C. (1958) *Social Class and Mental Illness: A Community Study*. John Wiley & Sons, New York.

Jauhar, R. and Weller, M.P.I. (1982). Psychiatric morbidity and time zone changes. A study of patients from Heathrow Airport. *British Journal of Psychiatry*, **140**, 231–235.

Johnstone, E.C., Owens, D.G.C., Gold, A., Crow, T.J. and MacMillan, J.F. (1984) Schizophrenic patients discharged from hospital—a follow-up study. *British Journal of Psychiatry*, **145**, 586–590.

Johnstone, E.C., Owens, D.G.C., Frith, C.D. and Calvert, L.M. (1985) Institutionalization and the outcome of functional psychoses. *British Journal of Psychiatry*, **146**, 36–44.

Lamo, H.R. and Grant, R.W. (1982) The mentally ill in a county jail, *Archives of General Psychiatry*, **39**, 17–22.

Mann, S. and Cree, W. (1976). New long-stay psychiatric patients: a national survey of fifteen mental hospitals in England and Wales 1972/3. *Psychological Medicine*, **6**, 606–616.

McCreadie, R.G., Oliver, A., Wilson, A. and Burton, L.L. (1983) The Scottish survey of new chronic inpatients. *British Journal of Psychiatry*, **143**, 564–571.

McCreadie, R.G., Robinson, A.D.T. and Wilson, A.O.A. (1985) The Scottish survey of new chronic in-patients: Two year follow-up. *British Journal of Psychiatry*, **147**, 637–640.

NE Thames Regional Health Authority (1983) *Report on Feasibility Studies*, July, Appendix D.4.

Ødegaard, O. (1932) Emigration and insanity. *Acta Psychiatrica Scandinavica* Suppl. 4.

Pepper, B. (1985). The young adult chronic patient: population overview. *Journal of Clinical Psychopharmacology*, 3 (3 suppl.), 35–75.

Rollin, H.R. (1969) *The Mentally Abnormal Offender and the Law*. Pergamon Press, London.

Royal College of General Practitioners (1981) *Survey of Primary Care in London*. Occasional Paper 16.

Sheets, J.L., Prevost, J.A. and Reihman, J. (1982) Young adult chronic patients: Three hypothesised sub-groups. *Hospital and Community Psychiatry*, **33** (3), 197–203.

The Health of the Nation (1991) Cm 1523. HMSO, London.

Social Services Committee of the House of Commons (1985) *Community Care with Special Reference to Adult Mentally Ill and Mentally Handicapped*. Second report of the Committee. London: HMSO.

Tooth, G.C. and Brooke, E.M. (1961) Trends in the mental hospital population and their effect on future planning. *Lancet*, **i**, 710–713.

Waind, A.P.B. (1961) *Lancet*, 22 April, 884 (letter).

Warner, R. (1985) *Recovery from Schizophrenia: Psychiatry and Political Economy*. Routledge and Kegan Paul, London.

Weller, M.P.I. and Jauhar, P. (1987) Wandering at Heathrow airport. *Medicine Science and Law*, **27**, 37–39.

Weller, B.G.A., Weller, M.P.I., Cocker, E. and Mohamed, S. (1987). Crisis at Christmas 1987. *Lancet*, March 7, 553–554.

Weller, M.P.I., Tobiansky, R.I., Hollander, D. and Ibrahimi, S. (1989) Psychosis and destitution at Christmas 1985–88. *Lancet*, **ii**, 1509–1511. (Reprinted in: *A Yearbook Guide to Clinical Medicine*. (1991) Ed. J.A. Talbot. Mosby-Year Book, Chicago.

Wing, J.K. (1962) Institutionalism in mental hospitals. *British Journal of Social and Clinical Psychology*, **1**, 38.

Wing, J.K. (1978) Long-term community care: experience in a London borough. *Psychological Medicine*, Suppl. No. 2.

Wing, J.K. (ed.) (1989) *Health Services Planning and Research. Contributions from Psychiatric Case Registers*. Gaskell, London.

2 WHERE WE ARE GOING

M.P.I. Weller

LONG-TERM SUPPORT AND REHABILITATION SERVICES: RESOURCE IMPLICATIONS AND LEGAL LOOPHOLES

In planning for a reorientation of services we must anticipate a period of double running costs and considerable capital expenditure to provide suitable community venues for care provision. Financial constraints limit a smooth transition. Pressures on local authorities are considerable. A burden of historic debt often coexists with restraints on raising local Government charges. Local social services are focused on child care, deflecting the attention of diminishing numbers of field workers from mental health issues. The small proportion of the mental health budget currently spent on community placements ignores the fact that some 90% of psychiatric morbidity is treated by GPs.

Psychiatric hospitals may be conceived as pots of gold which, by their closure, will overcome financial difficulties. Apart from the need to reprovide for an acute sector, this may be an illusion.

Much of the planning for UK community care envisages selling land and existing buildings and moving health service income to local authorities or voluntary bodies. The sums do not add up. The cost of closing a hospital can absorb the greater part of the capital. After 10 years of the realization of closure plans, Friern Hospital has spent £70 million on reprovision facilities. Because fixed costs run on inexorably, even though the number of patients cared for decreases, the cost per inpatient has risen from £13 000 per annum to nearly £20 000 over the period, and some of the most able patients are now being treated in community placements at a cost of £35 000 per annum.

TRAINING

Uncertain finance apart, one is concerned that the personnel in local authority employ have neither the training nor skills to provide for the range of psychopathology at present being treated in hospitals.

The confident aspirations of British local authorities to provide a standard of care exceeding that obtainable in psychiatric hospitals are suspect. Social workers lack training and experience (Barclay, 1982). Since 1971, social services have had responsibility for community based services. There has been a steady discharge of long-stay patients at a rate of 2000–3000 per annum, amounting to some 100 000 since 1952, yet only 6800 are residing in local authority provision, according to the Audit Commission, a higher figure than the previous DHSS one of 4000; but the increase has been accompanied by a reduction in back-up services, such as meals on wheels and home helps (Andrews, 1985). Day centres are few and are failing to increase in line with guidelines issued in 1975 (GLC Health Panel, 1983). Much of the work of social services is discretionary and where statutory obligations towards the mentally ill exist, for example to house the vulnerable homeless, they are subtly evaded (Brahams and Weller, 1985). Recent legal developments, outlined in 'Caring for People' could change this situation either for the better or the worse. Chapter 5 details these developments.

The second Minority Report by Professor R. Pinker, worryingly, yet appropriately, entitled 'An Alternative View' in the Barclay Committee Report (1982) has some sound things to say. Professor Pinker is properly concerned at the continuing dilution of skills and diffusion of effort, and argues persuasively for strong professionalism; this involves, inter alia, clear lines of accountability, a General Social Work Council charged with the maintenance of professional standards and a planned balance between generic abilities and specialist skills. This dissenting view from his 17 colleagues on the Committee and the title of the Report reinforces the concern that the boundaries of social work are too imprecise, as currently constituted, and the statutory obligations insufficient for social workers to be in a strong position to achieve a dominant place in community schemes dealing with fragile, vulnerable people. The problem is perceived as one of psychiatrists dragging their feet and being unduly wedded to traditional hospital based care, but this perception must be in error, since they have already discharged half the long-term patient population and continue to discharge patients. The general impression, however, is that social services have failed to respond adequately to the needs of this group. The problem of care does not end when patients are discharged from hospital.

The problems of chronic mental illness require a life time of support and the concept of rehabilitation must encompass facilities for a continuing process of prompting and encouragement. Those working in hospital settings wish to see the creation of adequate community provisions before the complete closure of the residual long-stay hospital beds. 'Beneath the common sense assumption that this [psychiatry] is par excellence the profession dedicated to the care of the mentally ill, there lies a deeper recognition of the many advances in standards of care that are properly attributable to the work of psychiatrists from the abolition of locked wards to the spread of Day Hospitals. One might speak also of major contributions to aetiological, epidemiological and therapeutic knowledge.' (Pinker in Barclay Report, 1982.)

LEGISLATIVE INADEQUACIES CONCERNING COMMUNITY CARE

There is a school of thought and it is a tempting one to embrace, that *all* one's efforts on behalf of the disadvantaged should be concentrated on bringing about changes in the Law since the handicapped will enjoy a better quality of life only if their rights are safeguarded in law. There is a lot of truth in this. Where provisions are discretionary, or where loopholes are only too visible, one fears that designated providers will not provide.

Most mental health legislation achieved in this century has been concerned principally with the patient's rights regarding compulsory admission and treatment. Admission on a voluntary basis was not possible until the 1930s. The 1959 Mental Health Act was a landmark in its day, and the 1983 Act achieved even more from the point of view of the patient's rights and civil liberties. It is in comparatively recent times that the concept of care and treatment also being a 'right' has come to the fore. The voluntary organizations in the field of mental health are now working towards enshrining such a concept in law.

But it is a mistake to believe that the law changes attitudes. Are we not thus in danger of adopting the fallacy similar to that of institutions causing illness? Laws usually change when society is ready for such changes and this is known as consensus. Indeed, where there is no true consensus, laws, even if passed, are as quickly repealed. An example is the 1978 Act of Parliament which abolished mental hospitals in Italy. There was no true consensus for this. The legislation was achieved on a charismatic platform and was never implemented in the face of stark reality. Much more public education needs, therefore, to be achieved before we can hope for the consensus on care and provision for the mentally disordered which we know to be desirable and necessary.

Enforcement sanctions are lacking even to fulfil the intentions of statutory provisions. The removal of caring responsibility from the NHS (where lack of care can result in claims for negligence) to local authorities, and their social services and housing departments, makes the actual provision of care even more dependent on the patient being in certain geographical 'catchment' areas, intensifying and focusing attention on boundary disputes between 'providers' anxious to be relieved of expensive obligations. This is particularly harmful for mentally ill patients who often wander for reasons beyond their control, and may have very little, if any, allegiance to the community in which they are found at times of crisis in their illness or destitution. This is illustrated in Chapter 9.

Even where the 'catchment' issue has been resolved satisfactorily there is no absolute obligation on local authorities to provide care as the courts have held that where a local authority has insufficient funds to effect its statutory obligations, the courts will not interfere with the exercise of its discretion in allocating priorities. These worrying difficulties are clearly demonstrated by a failure in housing provision where existing legislation is inadequate.

HOUSING

The obligation to house vulnerable homeless people under the Housing (Homeless Persons) Act 1985 expires if a person should 'voluntarily' quit their accommodation and become homeless intentionally. Although in other circumstances, deluded and hallucinated patients may not be held to have testamentary capacity to enter into binding contracts, they are held to be liable in respect of quitting their accommodation, and subsequently cease to be the responsibility of any authority. This despite the fact that their mental disability created their priority need. Added to this problem is the inability of many to claim their entitlements and to fend for themselves. They often need close insightful supervision, but a few showcase units apart, it is extremely difficult to find this entitlement, first created under Part III of the National Assistance Act 1948. This Act laid out the duties of local authorities 'to provide residential accommodation for persons who by reason of age, infirmity or any other circumstances are in need of care and attention which is not otherwise available to them (subsection 1a) . . . In the exercise of their said duty a local authority shall have regard to the welfare of all persons for whom accommodation is provided, and in particular to the need for providing accommodation of different descriptions suited to different descriptions of such persons as are mentioned in the last forgoing subsection' (subsection 2). Despite the clear expectations of the Act, there is no local authority known to the author which made such provision on a permanent basis for people under the age of 65. The situation changed little with the Housing (Homeless Persons) Act 1985, which sought to strengthen entitlements and ostensibly provides for the vulnerable homeless (see R. v. Waveney DC, ex parte Bowers [1983] 1 QB 238 (*infra* p. 42) discussed below) but fails to provide for single drifters and wanderers (see Brahams and Weller, 1985).

Under this current statute further provision is made for the function of local authorities in respect of persons who are homeless or threatened with homelessness. As matters stand at present, 'Homelessness still exists because there are insufficient units of accommodation of decent standard, located in the places which people want or have got to live, and available at prices that even the poorest families can afford.'

The Act provides

> 2–(1) For the purpose of this Act a homeless person or a person threatened with homelessness has a prior. ty need for accommodation when the housing authority are satisfied that he is within one of the following categories:

. . . (c) he or any person who resides or might reasonably be expected
to reside with him is vulnerable as a result of old age, mental illness
or handicap or physical disability or other special reason.

VULNERABILITY

The meaning of 'vulnerable' was judicially considered by the Court
of Appeal in R. v. Waveney DC, ex parte Bowers [1983] 1 QB 238.
The applicant, Bowers, who at the time of the hearing was aged 59,
was an alcoholic and had been an inpatient in hospital from 1971
to 1974. Thereafter he lived in lodgings until he was injured in a
road accident in mid 1980 and suffered a severe head injury that
required six months' hospital treatment. In September 1980 he
was still confused and disorientated for time and place, but was
discharged in December 1980. He returned to his former lodgings,
but was evicted because of excessive drinking. Thereafter he was
homeless, sleeping most nights at the Lowestoft Night Centre. The
housing welfare report revealed that the hospital social worker
thought the applicant was vulnerable because of ill-health, and the
warden at the night centre thought he was a danger to himself. He
had broken his nose three times by falling on his face. The
psychiatrist considered that the applicant had received a serious
head injury, with some persistent disability worsened by drink. The
ideal placement was considered to be a flat on his own with a degree
of shelter.

The housing authority considered that accommodation only had
to be provided for those in substantial need, placing particular
reliance on the words 'substantially disabled mentally or physically'
in the Code of Practice. During argument before the court it was
suggested that the case had to be brought within one or other of
the categories mentioned in s. 2(1)(c).

Waller LJ said (at page 245, H), reversing the decision of
Stephen Brown J in the High Court, that this was not the correct
approach. The first question that had to be considered is whether
or not there is vulnerability. If there is vulnerability, then does it
arise from those matters set out within s. 2(1)(c)? It may not arise
from any single one but it may arise from a combination of those
causes:

The question we have to consider is whether or not the applicant is vulnerable and secondly whether the vulnerability is as a result of old age, mental illness or handicap or physical or other special reason. Dealing first with the meaning of vulnerable, vulnerable literally means 'may be wounded or susceptible of injury' (see the Concise Oxford Dictionary, 6th Edn (1976), p. 1305). In our opinion, however, vulnerable in the context of this legislation means less able to fend for oneself so that injury or detriment will result when a less vulnerable man will be able to cope without harmul effects . . . In this case, the applicant's age was a factor but the brain injury was another important factor.

Whether the brain injury is described as mental handicap or whether it is to be put into the category of other special reason is immaterial. If it had not been for the accident the applicant would not have been a priority need, at any rate until he reached the age of 65, but the accident made . . . the whole difference . . . It is important to draw a distinction between those cases solely due to the problems of drink where the case will normally not come within the provisions of s. 2, and the facts of this case where an accident causing brain damage to a man of 59 has been an important factor.

Other examples of vulnerability offered by the court were a pregnant woman, old age, and being deaf and dumb.

Following the Bowers decision, the mentally ill or handicapped must be regarded as 'vulnerable' and as such, people in priority need. However, in practice, patients from psychiatric hospitals may fail to find accommodation and are highly unlikely to find supervised accommodation as specified under Pt 111, National Assistance Act 1948 and s. 3, Chronically Sick and Disabled Persons Act 1970 (but see R. v. Secretary of State for Social Services, ex p Hincks [1984] *The Lancet*, November 24; [1985] NLJ 48).

Section 117 of the Mental Health Act (1983) goes a considerable way to remedying the situation for patients placed on Section 3 of the Act, but has only recently been properly operated in many instances. Patients who are not subject to Section 3 restrictions (such as patients detained under Section 2) continue to fail to benefit from the requirements of the Housing (Homeless Persons) Act 1985.

There seems to be no decision on whether a mentally ill or unstable schizophrenic patient can form the necessary intention to leave accommodation 'voluntarily' for the purposes of the 1985 Housing Act (part 3 incorporating the 1977 Housing (Homeless Persons) Act). The leading case of Din (Taj) v. Wandsworth London Borough

Council [1983] 1 AC 657 HL (E) and De Falco v. Crawley BC
[1980] QB 460 and Dyson v. Kerrier District Council [1980] 1 WLR
1205, and most recently R. v. Gloucester City Council, ex p Miles
[1985] *The Times* March 6 do not assist. It is submitted that a
mentally unstable patient cannot be considered as legally intending
to become homeless for the purposes of the Act so as to prevent
him from remaining a person in priority need. This would be to
defeat the intention of the purpose of the Act which is to protect
those especially vulnerable.

Schizophrenic patients tend to wander from country to country
(Ødegaard, 1932; Shapiro, 1976; Jauhar and Weller, 1982) and from
one part of the country to another, gravitating to city centres, and
London in particular (Faris and Dunham, 1939; Hollingshead and
Redlich, 1958; Royal College of General Practitioners, 1981; Weller
et al., 1988). For discussion of what factors should be taken into
account in assessing whether an applicant legally has a local
connection with an area, see R. v. Eastleigh BC, ex parte Betts
[1983] 2 WLR 397 HL. There the House of Lords held that the
test to be applied in determining whether a person has a 'local
connection' with an area within the definition of s. 18(1)(*a*) of the
Act was whether the applicant could show, because the onus rested
on him, that he had built up and established by a period of
residence, or by a period of employment, or because of family
associations which had endured in the area, or because of other
special circumstances, that he had a real connection with the area.
Many local authorities have in fact laid down guidelines in an
Agreement on Procedures for referrals of the Homeless entered into
in 1977 which governs agreements between them to share the
burden of housing the homeless. This may create quite artificial
claims. (See also R. v. Barnet LBC, ex parte Nilish Shah [1983] 2
WLR 16, HL.)

The reality is that these wandering patients are poorly equipped
to press for the implementation of their legal rights and it is easy
for local authorities to evade them, even if they accept them, just
by doing nothing for a sufficient time. The urgency of the situation
and the wandering tendencies generally ensure that one way or
another the patient and the problem literally goes away.

It is ironic that next to losing a near relative, moving home is one
of the most stressful events to which most of us are exposed
(Paykel, 1978; Brown and Harris, 1978). In the case of the mentally

ill, those fortunate enough to secure local authority housing are often moved frequently, one of my patients three times in two weeks, after waiting over a year in an acute admission ward for the accommodation. It is still the exception for patients to obtain supervised accommodation that should be provided under Part 111 of the Housing Act 1985 (S.59c).

A serious flaw in the present legislation is the illusion of local authority responsibility for patients returning home on leave whilst on a treatment order under section 117 of the Mental Health Act 1983. Indeed the responsibility that already existed under the National Health Service Act 1977 might have actually been weakened. The local authority is required to provide 'After-care services', which are not specified in the Act. In any event Lord Denning (in Southwark L.B.C. v. Williams [1971] ch. 734 at p. 743) referred to the principle that 'where an Act creates an obligation, and enforces that obligation in a specified manner, we take it to be a general rule that performance cannot be enforced in any other manner'. (See Wyatt v. Hillingdon L.B.C. 76 LGR 727.) Section 124 of the Mental Health Act 1983 provides for the Secretary of State to exercise default powers when a local authority fails in its obligations, and to take over such of the functions of the authority as he deems appropriate. It is unlikely that he would ever feel called upon to do so, but the specific provision makes it more unlikely that an individual would be able to enforce the aftercare provisions of section 117.

Local authorities have the ability to provide 'centres (including training centres and day centres) or other facilities (including domicilary facilities) whether in premises managed by the [local authority] or otherwise, for training or occupation of persons suffering from or who have been suffering from mental disorder'. This ability, conferred by DHSS Circular No. 19/75, is unenforceable, and says no more than the 1977 Act whereby a local authority is *required* to cooperate with the health authority 'in order to advance the health and welfare of the people of England and Wales'. The recent guidelines merely encourage cooperation between health and local authorities. The implementation and quality of care plans varies widely across the country.

One may conclude that in important respects the net effect of the Mental Health Act 1983, introduced as a patients charter, and the DHSS circular has been to weaken the entitlement of patients to local authority provisions, whilst creating a misleading impression that these entitlements have been ensured.

Psychiatric hospitals are scrutinized by local Health Councils, the Commissioners of the Mental Health Act and the Hospital Advisory Board amongst many others; local authority care, on the other hand, remains self-regulating and some external review system should be created.

TREATMENT

A recurrent problem in psychiatric practice is the coincidence of personality problems with psychosis, a frequent combination (so-called co-morbidity) which may lead to intense practical problems. Sufferers are reluctant to cooperate with rules, causing disruption. They intoxicate themselves with drugs and alcohol, exploit other, vulnerable, patients, perhaps stealing from them, intimidating them to supply cigarettes and other favours. Little can be done to alter this pattern in an individual who is not motivated to change.

A further problem is that the psychosis may be poorly controlled because the patient does not comply with prescribed medication and abuses various drugs (Weller et al., 1988). His condition deteriorates to the point where he no longer has insight into his condition, but is still outside the scope of compulsory treatment, causing distress to carers and other patients with whom he may share accommodation. 'It cannot, in my view, be right that an integral part or symptom of some mental illness—an inability to realise that you are ill—should be the cause of people becoming iller than they need' (Norwood, 1991). The reluctance to apply compulsion until late in the day, the exception taken against using emergency powers (section 4), and the reluctance to use treatment orders (section 3); because an observation order (section 2) is 'least restrictive', (but does not entrain useful Sec. 117 procedures discussed earlier), conspire to promote a 'revolving door' of brief admissions for severe states after long periods of deterioration, with increasing difficulty in retaining continuing community care in suitable accommodation.

The problems of ensuring compliance with medical treatment have recently been intensified. It had been believed that there was a legal way to insist on continuing medication for those patients whose severe illnesses had been successfully treated and stabilized under hospital treatment orders (section 3 of the Mental Health Act

1983) and who were allowed to return home for extended periods whilst the hospital orders were periodically renewed. However, R. v. Halstrom, ex parte Waldron R. v. Gardiner and another ex parte [1985] established that this was not lawful and has left a worrisome gap in psychiatrists' ability to treat patients in the community, at precisely the time when the evidence for concern is accumulating. The Mental Health Act Commissioners favour an extension of Guardianship powers to overcome the problem, but local authorities are already reluctant to utilize their existing powers and will be unlikely, readily, to embrace more onerous ones. The British Medical Association cautiously favours a community treatment order in their Annual Report of Council 1988–9 (pp. 47–48), compelling patients to accept medication in the community in the same way as in hospital (under sections 2, 3, 4, 5(ii), 37, and 38), but enforcement of such an order will prove difficult. However, patients could be recalled to hospital and treatment enforced there, a procedure favoured by the Royal College of Psychiatrists. The problem is less the mechanics than an understandable reluctance to enforce continuing medication. This issue is currently being reconsidered.

ADEQUATE FINANCE

The 1983 Mental Health Act had a hurried passage. It seems clear today that the Act created many additional duties that required additional resources, but these did not materialize, and the assumption of the Minister, expressed in the House, that additional facilities were not needed was clearly a mistake. Consider, for example, the sections 30, 35 and 37 whereby those charged or convicted of offences can be transferred to psychiatric hospitals. It is the failure to apply these sections which is at the heart of the difficulty in transferring people from prison to hospital. The administrative burdens entrained by these sections require the hospital to deliver the patient to court at the appointed time, a requirement that it is difficult to induce the court, the police or the probation service to undertake. These additional responsibilities and the encouragement of increased use of Appeal Tribunals, obligatory every six months under the 1983 Act, have generated immense calls on medical resources without additional staffing. (A full analysis of the considerable additional requirements and resource implications of the 1983 Act was prepared by the administrators at Northwick Park Hospital, London, Personal communication, Mr C. Kirk.)

The demands on medical resources will not be lessened by an emphasis on community services, but part of the burden will be transferred to general practitioners. With many initiatives to extend general practice services, time will be at a premium and non-medical time will have to expand. It is important that suitable training schemes embrace these requirements. Care assistants lack coherent training and, typically, stay only a short time in post. They lack a professional body to govern their practice and the issues of confidentiality, transmission of sensitive information and dispensing of medication have still to be addressed.

TRAINING

Care assistants require orientation and information for their difficult task. Their training could reinforce the links that must be forged in the integrated provision of care. The Royal College of Psychiatrists, the Royal College of Nursing, the Clinical Psychology section of the British Psychological Society, the Royal College of General Practitioners and Social Services could amalgamate in setting up and administering suitable training courses. The important contributions should come from those with the greatest hands-on experience of day-to-day patient management.

A feature of such a scheme would require care assistants to rotate around different venues providing various types of psychiatric care and social support, including acute psychiatric wards and long-stay psychiatric wards, while they exist, so that they can quickly gain experience of the more florid aspects of psychopathology with which they might have to deal and to have insight into the wide range of psychopathology and the many facets of its presentation, thus gaining better appreciation of the yardstick to measure changes in severity.

SOME INTERNATIONAL COMPARISONS

The situation in the UK has parallels in other countries and we may profit from their experiences.

United States

The movement towards hospital closure is highly developed in the US, where the old hospitals were seen as repositories of neglected patients and run for the convenience of staff (Goffman, 1961). Efforts were made to replace them, as rapidly as possible, with community mental health centres (CMHCs). The enabling legislation, the Community Mental Health Centers Act, was passed by Congress in 1963 and signed into Law (Public Law 88–164) by President Kennedy in October of that year. Unfortunately, the initial aspirations for these centres were not fully realized and it quickly became apparent that they were incapable of treating and managing the most disturbed patients without a very much greater input of psychiatrists. Less highly trained staff quickly came to rely on the expertise of psychiatrists to a point where their capacity was excessively stretched (Borus, 1984; Donovan, 1982), whilst at the same time the ratio of psychiatrists per CMHC actually diminished, through disenchantment, to less than half between 1970 and 1975 and the proportion of centres with psychiatrists as directors or executive directors fell from 56% in 1973 to 22% in 1977 (Winslow, 1979).

It has been estimated that only 8.4% of the 4.9 million people using specialized mental health services in the US in a given year are treated in CMHCs (Hankin and Oktay, 1979). Inevitably, there was pressure to select patients who could benefit from the new arrangements. A new, and perhaps previously neglected, population was being served by the community health centres, to the detriment of the most severely and chronically ill and the elderly, whilst the traditional services for the most ill were still being conducted in the large psychiatric hospitals (Fink and Weinstein, 1979; Winslow, 1979; Clare, 1980).

In 1990 Los Angeles County Jail daily housed 700 more mentally ill than the largest psychiatric hospital in America, Pilgrim State Hospital in New York and the situation is deteriorating. There is more imprisonment of the seriously mentally ill without criminal charges and less referral to outpatient services (Torrey *et al.*, 1992). In 1987 Mayor Ed Koch ordered the New York City's Police Department to round up the homeless and transport them to Bellevue Hospital. Trumped up charges followed a failure to find beds. Despite a furious backlash from libertarian groups Dr Jack Talbot, a past President of the American Psychiatric Association, considered that 'He (Koch) is the first government official who has truly acknowledged the massive mistakes made by deinstitutionalization'. The situation and the problems are ably reviewed in the chapter by Fuller Torrey (Chapter 15).

Italy

The Italian experience of closing psychiatric hospitals is portrayed differently by different observers, some being eulogistic, but there are many perturbing features. Whatever the alleged merits of the Italian Mental Health Act of 1978 (law no. 180), it has been found defective and has undergone revision, with an extension of compulsory powers, an increase in the number of beds for the acutely ill, with opportunities to transfer to medium-stay units if recovery is delayed and the creation of new long-stay units (Benaim, 1983). The rate of decrease of the number of long-stay patients actually slowed since the passage of law no. 180 (Ramon, 1985), which may therefore be constructed as following rather than leading the reduction in the long-term population, in a similar fashion to the halving of the UK long-stay patient population, sparing only the most disabled, in advance of current policies.

Rome, with a population of 5 million, and a large immigrant population with a disproportionate proportion of mental illness, had three psychiatric units for emergency cases, housed in general hospitals, with a capacity of 15 beds each. This grossly unsatisfactory state of affairs has been partially remedied by increasing the bed numbers from 45 to 60! The hospital stay ranges from one to fourteen days with an average stay of three days according to information provided by the professorial unit. Much of the work of the state hospitals is now undertaken by private hospitals, paid for by the state. This was never the intention of the founders of the change.

Portugal

Purporting to follow the British example, the Portuguese Ministry of Health abruptly announced that the leading psychiatric hospital in Portugal was to close (Lancet 1988 ed.). The hospital, Julio de Matos, consists of a complex of modern buildings and occupies a valuable, extensive site near the centre of Lisbon. It provides care for 700 long-stay patients, an acute service for Lisbon and a back-up service for patients outside the city. It is particularly renowned for its behavioural therapy unit and has a variety of occupational and industrial therapeutic activities on the campus style site.

The effect of prior budget cuts had already been felt by university departments, which were beginning to receive chronic cases previously treated in the hospital. This resulted in a new pressure on acute beds leading to the more rapid discharge of patients, some into precarious social circumstances, in which the stability of their recovery was put in jeopardy.

No firm alternative arrangements to the hospital closure had been proposed for the patients, other than a declared intention to move them to farms in the countryside.

CONCLUSION

We in Britain are striving to develop a system of care that takes as much account of social interactions and meaningful relationships as of medication; that fosters integration into the wider society and does not seek to isolate sufferers from community facilities. Nevertheless, considerable resources are necessary for community schemes to succeed across a broad spectrum of psychopathology, particularly if such schemes are to encompass, adequately, the severe deficits found in chronic schizophrenia, and the behavioural problems found in psychosis and personality disorders. Self-help must not hinder help from others when this is required.

The Health Committee of Parliament has expressed disquiet at the time of going to press (Community Care: Funding from April 1993). The Members express concern at the shift from a demand led system of social security funding to one that is cash limited. The adequacy of the ringfenced transfer of £565 million may prove inadequate. Twenty-six local authorities in England will be facing considerable financial pressures. The government's refusal to guarantee funding to protect drug and alcohol services is viewed with concern.

Complacency, professional selfishness and narrow horizons coexist with vision, initiative and compassion. The rewarding experiences of group sessions, vocational training, counselling and support require suitable premises, training and adequate staffing levels, with back-up for holidays, study leave, emergencies and sickness. Occupational and industrial activities, tailored to the particular needs of patients who find it difficult to work under normal pressures and to sustain concentration, which used to be centred on the hospitals, have to be recreated. They need to have a similar range of facilities to those provided in hospital, but in a more comfortable, friendly and inviting way. Most of all the ideals of community care envisage a living environment that is as close as possible to a normal home.

Against these aspirations, at this moment patients with chronic deficits are still living in lonely bedsitting rooms, chain smoking, eating take-away food or cold food from tin cans, and spending much of the day in bed, partly because they have nothing better to do, and no one to persuade them to the contrary, and partly to keep warm (Weller *et al.*, 1990). This is a bleak alternative to hospital care, but better than being homeless. Too many have slipped through the permeable network of social and medical care and they too, as well as the patients in hospitals, have to be given dignity and fulfilment in a comprehensive community care plan. We can see the promised land, we are eager to proceed but we have to get it right. We are planning for the care of the most vulnerable members of our society, we must not fail them.

REFERENCES

Andrews, K. (1985) Demographic changes and resources for the elderly. *British Medical Journal*, **290**, 1023–1024.

Barclay, P.M. (Chairman) (1982) *Social Workers: Their Role and Tasks*. Bedford Square Press, London.

Benaim, S. (1983) The Italian experience. *Bulletin of the Royal College of Psychiatrists*, **7**, 7–9.

Brahams, D. and Weller, M.P.I. (1985) Crime and homelessness among the mentally ill. *New Law Journal* June and July, **135**, 761–763. Pt. II 135: 626–629 reprinted *Medico-Legal Journal* 1986, **54**, 42–53.

Brown, G.W. and Harris, T. (1978) *Social Origins of Depression.* Tavistock Publications, London.

Clare, A.W. (1980) Community mental health centres. *Journal of the Royal Society of Medicine*, **73**, 75–76.

Community Care: Funding from April 1993 (1993) Report of the Health Committee published by H.M.S.O.

Donovan, C.M. (1982) Problems of psychiatric practice in community mental health centres. *American Journal of Psychiatry*, **139**, 456–460.

Faris, R.E.L. and Dunham, H.W. (1939) *Mental Disorder in Urban Areas.* University of Chicago Press, Chicago.

Fink, P.J. and Weinstein, S.P. (1979) Whatever happened to psychiatry? The deprofessionalization of community mental health centres. *American Journal of Psychiatry*, **136**, 406–409.

GLC Health Panel (1983) *Mental Health Services in London.* Mind.

Goffman, E. (1961) *Asylums.* Anchor Books, Doubleday, New York.

Hankin, J. and Oktay, J.S. (1979) *Mental Disorder and Primary Medical Care.* NIMH, Rockville, Maryland.

Hollingshead, A.B. and Redlich, F.C. (1958) *Social Class and Mental Illness: A Community Study.* John Wiley & Sons, New York.

Jauhar, R. and Weller, M.P.I. (1982). Psychiatric morbidity and time zone changes. A study of patients from Heathrow Airport. *British Journal of Psychiatry*, **140**, 231–235.

Lancet (1988) Portugal: Psychiatric Troubles. (i) 1098 ed, (anon).

Norwood, S. (Judge) (1991) Mental health and the community (editorial). *Medico-Legal Journal*, **59**, 139–140.

Ødegaard, O. (1932) Emigration and insanity. *Acta Psychiatrica Scandinavica* suppl. 4.

Paykel, E.S. (1978) Contribution of life events to causation of psychiatric illness. *Psychological Medicine*, **8**, 245–253.

Ramon, S. (1985) *Psychiatry in Britain: Meaning and Policy.* Croom Helm, Beckenham.

Royal College of General Practitioners (1981) *Survey of Primary Care in London.* Occasional Paper 16.

Shapiro, S. (1976) A study of psychiatric syndromes manifested at an international airport. *Comprehensive Psychiatry*, **17**, 453–456.

Torrey, E.F., Streibein, J., Ezchial, J. *et al.* (1992) A joint report of the National Alliance for the Mentally Ill and Public Citizen's Health Research Group. Forensic Network, 2101 Wilson Boulevard, Suite 302, Arlington, VA, USA.

Weller, M.P.I., Ang, P.C., Latimer-Sayer, D.T. and Zachary, A. (1988) Drug abuse and mental illness. *Lancet*, **i**, 997.

Weller, B.G.A., Weller, M.P.I. and Cheyne, A. (1990) Quality of life after discharge from long-stay wards. *Lancet*, **ii**, 1384–1385.

Winslow, W.W. (1979) The changing role of psychiatrists in the community mental health centres. *American Journal of Psychiatry*, **136**, 24–27.

CASES

De Falco v. Crawley BC [1980] QB 460.

Din (Taj) v. Wandsworth London Borough Council [1983] 1 AC 657 HL (E).

Dyson v. Kerrier District Council [1980] 1 WLR 1205.

R. v. Barnet LBC, ex parte Nilish Shah [1983] 2 WLR 16, HL.

R. v. Eastleigh BC, ex parte Betts [1983] 2 WLR 397 HL.

R. v. Gloucester City Council, ex p Miles [1985] *The Times* March 6.

R. v. Hallstrom ex parte Waldron and Regina v. Gardiner and another ex parte. *The Times* Times Law Report: Detention unlawful for inpatient treatment. Dec. 28th cols. 1–6 (1985).

R. v. Porter *The Times* Jan 22 1985, *Lancet* Feb 2 p. 269; Too few hospital places for mentally abnormal offenders: Plea for action by the Lord Chief Justice.

R. v. Secretary of State for Social Services, ex p Hincks [1984] *Lancet*, November 24; 1985; *New Law Journal* 1985 48.

Southwark L.B.C. v. Williams [1971] ch. 734.

R. v. Waveney DC, ex parte Bowers [1983] 1 QB 238.

Wyatt v. Hillingdon L.B.C. 76 LGR 727.

Some of the legal arguments appeared in Brahams, D. and Weller, M. (1986) Crime and homelessness amongst the mentally ill. *Medico Legal Journal* **54**, 42–53.

3 MENTAL HEALTH SERVICES: WHAT WORKS?

Matthijs Muijen

INTRODUCTION

Despite the fierce and often emotional arguments in favour of or against the closure of mental hospitals over the last few years, in reality the move towards community care started in the 1950s, and has gained momentum ever since. The number of patients occupying beds for the mentally ill has gradually been reduced from about 144 000 in 1954 to 57 000 in 1990, a reduction of 60%. This has been accompanied by a large number of services aiming to reduce the need for hospital care, often based on local initiatives, including many types of residential care for the long term mentally ill, day care and home care. Concern has often been expressed, however, that the amount of reprovision is insufficient (Audit Commission, 1986).

As with the building of the large asylums in the nineteenth century, the changes in care practice seem to have been based on concern about existing practices (Goffman, 1961; Bennett, 1983), rather than on a precise understanding of the potential consequences of change. Some evaluation took place in the 1950s and early 1960s, at about the same time as psychotropic drugs were introduced. Outpatient clinics and domiciliary services were initiated instead of admitting everybody in need of treatment to hospitals (Carse et al., 1958). The first studies reporting the value of day hospitals were conducted (Smith and Cross, 1957; Craft, 1958), and the comparison of a district including components of community care to a traditional service almost exclusively relying on hospital beds (Brad and Sainsbury, 1968) suggested the potential of such services.

The case against change without evaluation is strongly made in the chapter by Fuller Torrey, describing events in the US. Even more extreme change occurred in Italy, which experienced a revolution based on radical legal reforms in 1978. It appears that these reforms have led to improved care in the affluent north, but neglect in the poor south, where hardly any alternative resources were provided (Jones and Poletti, 1985). Often used as arguments against community care, a fairer interpretation is that poor planning and lack of resources are very unlikely to lead to well balanced services.

Some evaluations have taken place, however, and allow some conclusions on the potential benefits and costs of community care. These evaluations can be divided into three types: organizational studies, i.e. the effectiveness of community care as compared to standard hospital care; intervention studies, investigating the benefits produced by specific types of treatments; and process studies, exploring the implications of a new service for staff and patients. This chapter will address each of these areas.

ALTERNATIVES TO STANDARD HOSPITAL CARE

The objective of psychiatric care can be described as aiming to improve the functioning of people suffering from mental health problems and facilitating an optimal quality of life. This includes several dimensions such as psychopathology, social functioning, employment, housing, finances and user and carer satisfaction.

Hospital care concentrates on psychopathology, based on a medical illness model. Patients are admitted for the severity of their symptoms and are discharged when remission has occurred. Social factors such as lack of support, unemployment or homelessness are considered as contributory factors which can hasten admission or delay discharge, but not as core responsibilities of the psychiatric service. Referral to the social worker is the main response to social problems. The effectiveness of hospital care was consequently assessed in terms of relapse and re-admission. A consistent finding is the relapse rate of about 40% within a year following discharge for patients with psychotic disorders, possibly because hospital treatment does not lead to improved community functioning (Anthony et al., 1972, 1978).

The objective of alternatives to inpatient care such as day and home care are to maximize independence and teach skills which are relevant to community functioning. People are supported and treated in their own environment so that skills required for daily living can be taught where they are required. This means that the emphasis is on social functioning, with the underlying expectation that an improvement of the interaction with the environment will lead to greater quality of life and reduced symptomatology, and protect against relapse. Several evaluations have taken place in day care and home care settings to investigate whether the theory is borne out by practice.

Day care

Day care is a generic term for a service which provides treatment and/or support during working hours. Its objective can either be to prevent hospitalization, to offer a course of treatment for specific conditions or the maintenance of patients with a long-term mental illness.

Day care as an alternative to inpatient care has consistently been found to be at least as good as inpatient care. Studies report little difference in outcome on measures such as psychopathology or social functioning between the two types of care after 12 months follow up (Wilder et al., 1966; Herz et al., 1971; Creed et al., 1990). Both patients (Dick et al., 1985) and their relatives (Michaux et al., 1974) preferred day care to hospital care. This is likely to improve compliance, and thus outcome. Furthermore, day treatment is considerably cheaper than hospital care (Fink et al., 1978; Dick et al., 1985). For many patients day care is not feasible due to behavioural, physical or social problems, and not all patients benefit equally from day care. Severely psychotic patients may gain from an initial period in hospital followed by day care, while the immediate advantages of day care for affective and neurotic disorders are strong (Wilder et al., 1966; Michaux et al., 1974; Dick et al., 1985).

Not all patients could be cared for by day care, however. About 40% of all patients who would usually have been admitted could be cared for in a day hospital without further need of inpatient care (Wilder *et al.*, 1966; Herz *et al.*, 1971; Creed *et al.*, 1990). Such results argue for an expanded role for day treatment in the care of many seriously mentally ill patients.

The long term mentally ill are the largest number of patients attending day centres, funded by the local authorities, and also day hospitals, provided by the health service. Facilities for this group are often poorly coordinated and lacking in provisions such as rehabilitation, leisure activities, and support of relatives (Wing, 1982). Treatment programs tailored for individual patients are required, but difficult to implement because of poor staffing levels. Many day care facilities demand either too much initiative or offer too little stimulation, resulting in demoralization. The likely consequence is a high drop-out rate and a risk of neglect. Some day centres allowed patients to use the centre as a social meeting place, and the patients' appreciation was expressed by an improvement in attendance.

Day care has not become very popular in the UK, with numbers of patients attending having remained static during the last decade despite the reduction in hospital beds. The reason for this is unclear, but may be due to its half-way position between hospital and home care. The absence of skills' acquisition in the home environment and the lack of support during the night, often the time that people are most at risk, means that day care combines some of the weaknesses of the other forms of care, but few of their strengths. Ironically, a night-hospital might resolve some of the objections, but such a model has never been developed.

Home care

Home care can be defined as the care of patients sensitive to individual needs at their own place of residence in order to maximize independent functioning and minimize handicaps.

Patients are at risk of neglect if home care does not accept responsibility for the integration and comprehensiveness of care. All hospital functions, including asylum, need to be transferred into the community, but in addition community care has also to take on elements that are not traditionally considered to be the responsibility of psychiatric services, such as benefits and housing. This is the objective of case management, which will be described later and in chapter 5.

The essential components of a community care team have been specified by the National Institute for Mental Health in the USA for community support programs (Turner and Ten Hoor, 1978), and are pertinent to community care in general. These are:

1. Identification of the target population and outreach that can offer appropriate services to those willing to participate;
2. Assistance in applying for benefits;
3. Crisis intervention in the least restrictive setting, with hospital beds available as a last resort;
4. Psychosocial rehabilitation;
5. Supportive services of indefinite duration, including employment and housing;
6. Medical and mental health care;
7. Support to relatives, friends and others;
8. Involvement of concerned community members in order to optimize support networks for patients;
9. Patient advocacy;
10. Case management.

Services need to be available 24 hours a day, 7 days a week. The range and intensity of interventions requires input from a multidisciplinary team, with a high staff–patient ratio. These guidelines are useful as standards to qualify the excellence of services, even though few community services are able to comply with all points (Bachrach, 1981).

Evaluation of home care

Several randomized studies evaluated the efficacy of home care for seriously mentally ill patients who were due to be hospitalized and followed these patients up for a year or more (Pasamanick *et al.*, 1967; Langsley *et al.*, 1969; Polak *et al.*, 1976; Test and Stein, 1980; Fenton *et al.*, 1982; Pai and Kapur, 1982; Hoult and Reynolds, 1983; Marks *et al.*, 1988; Muijen, 1991). Some of these studies have been reviewed by Braun *et al.* (1981) and Kiesler (1982).

The most comprehensive studies were conducted in Madison, Wisconsin (Stein and Test, 1980), Sydney (Hoult and Reynolds, 1983) and London (Muijen, 1991; Muijen *et al.*, 1992). The London and Sydney studies replicated the Madison one, so many features are similar. Inclusion criteria were intended admission for serious mental illness in the absence of brain damage or primary addiction. Patients presenting with aggression, no fixed abode or no social support were accepted. Results in all 3 studies were very similar. Hospital use was reduced by 80% compared with community care. After about a year of care, both home care and hospital groups had improved considerably on psychopathology, with slightly greater recovery for home than hospital care patients. Improvement in social functioning was similar for both treatment groups in all studies.

This lack of improvement in social functioning with home care as compared to standard care is disappointing. Leisure time activities were poor for the majority of patients in both treatment groups in Sydney and London. Despite intensive care, many patients remained unable to work or lead satisfactory social lives. Community burden, measured by police contacts and suicide attempts, was not affected by type of care in any of the projects (Test and Stein, 1980; Fenton et al., 1982; Reynolds and Hoult, 1984; Muijen, 1991).

The London and Sydney study found that home care was strongly preferred by both patients and relatives after a year. Similarly, satisfaction with life and self esteem was significantly higher for home care than hospital care patients in Madison. It is interesting that satisfaction with services was the same after 3 months, suggesting that the greater satisfaction with community care after a year was due to lack of continuity care in the hospital group. This is confirmed by the reduction in satisfaction with care of the hospital patients and their relatives between 3 and 12 months, whereas home care patients and relatives reported unchanged level of satisfaction (Muijen, 1991).

An important aim is to determine which patient groups would benefit most from community care. Muijen (1991) and Hoult and Reynolds (1983) found that first admissions responded better to community care, but the differences were non-significant, possibly due to the low numbers in subgroups. Chronic patients showed fewer gains with home care, but even for this group home care substantially reduced inpatient stay and improved clinical symptoms somewhat.

Little further improvement is achieved beyond six months of care in these studies. Care needs to continue beyond six months, however, to maintain gains. When home care was discontinued at 2 years and 14 months respectively, follow-up studies of the Pasamanick (Davis et al., 1972) and Stein and Test (1980) patient samples found that any gains made with community care were gradually eroded.

None of these studies claimed to offer a cure. The main claim of these projects was that they maximized time spent in the community and the quality of life, leading to greater satisfaction of patients and their relatives. Patients continued to suffer from their mental illnesses, however, as illustrated by poor employment records and need for continuing care.

An important aspect of community care is its cost. An incentive for the development of community services are the supposed savings, based on the results of some of the above programs, which have claimed savings between 4% (Weisbrod *et al.*, 1980) and 25% (Hoult and Reynolds, 1983). Such savings are unlikely to be realized if the extent to which support services will have to be developed are taken into account. As so often, one can expect to get what is paid for, and good quality community services will not come cheap.

COMMUNITY CARE FOR PEOPLE WITH LONG TERM MENTAL HEALTH PROBLEMS

The objective to improve the quality of life of the long term mentally ill has led to the shrinking of the large mental hospitals with a large scale transfer of the most dependent residents. Many health authorities, often in partnership with local authorities and the voluntary sector, developed small scale units in the community with varying degrees of independent living and staff support (see chapter 12). Wing and Furlong (1986) propose the stairway analogy: patients can gradually climb upwards to more independent settings until they have reached their optimal level in residential, occupational and recreational functioning.

The reduction of places in mental hospitals has not been matched by alternative provisions everywhere, which may have caused some neglect and suffering (Bassuk and Gerson, 1978; Weller, 1989). Recent evaluations of hospital closures have shown that districts did provide the required reprovisions, and no evidence was found that patients were discharged with nowhere to go. More likely is that patients leave their alternative homes or hostels, are lost to the services and will suffer increasing neglect. This cannot be wholly attributed to poor community services, but is probably a complex consequence of an increased opportunity for residents to decide for themselves, failure of quality control of residential care, poor coordination between services and lack of housing and other facilities in general. Care management and the care program approach were intended to minimize the risk of patients falling through the cracks between the services supposedly working closely together, and the effectiveness of such initiatives are being investigated (Ryan et al., 1991).

Some studies have evaluated the efficacy of model placements for chronic patients. Patients have been transferred to hostels and foster homes, both with satisfying results. Well staffed hostels, designing individual skill-based treatment plans for about 10 patients produced noticeable improvement in functioning in most patients (Garety and Morris, 1984; Goldberg et al., 1985). These projects were not controlled, and the high staffing levels with an increase in attention may have been the effective component, rather than the transfer of care.

Foster care, the placement of a patient in a traditional family setting, has been used for centuries in Gheel, Belgium, presumably with acceptable results. Linn et al. (1977, 1980) applied this model in Miami, and evaluated its effects on patients and families. The community group as a whole showed significant improvements in adjustment and functioning. Individually, 50% of patients had improved, 25% remained unchanged and 25% had deteriorated. Several foster home characteristics predicted the outcome: children in the house and two or fewer other patients correlated with improvement, and more than 10 occupants or more than 2 other patients correlated with deterioration. A high level of activity and frequent supervision by hospital staff or the fostering person were associated with improved outcome in non-schizophrenic, but a deterioration in schizophrenic patients.

Other studies confirm some of these findings. Stressful environments and lack of support are invariably associated with poor community adjustment and relapse, whereas type or condition of accommodation seem less important (Goldstein and Caton, 1983; Davies et al., 1989). Not every type of pressure causes a deterioration of schizophrenic patients. The empty existence of many patients in hostels without purpose or satisfaction is no improvement on hospital life (Lamb, 1972). When patients with chronic schizophrenia on discharge from hospital were randomized to either a high expectation rehabilitation program or low expectation hostels, relapse rates were similar after 2 years, but social functioning and vocational skills were superior in the high expectation group (Lamb and Goertzel, 1972). Whatever the care setting, a careful balance seems necessary to create an environment which is sufficiently stimulating to improve functioning without increasing psychopathology.

EFFECTIVE COMPONENTS OF CARE

Continuity of care

An essential issue is which factors lead to good outcome. On the face of it, the many projects evaluating alternatives to hospital care differ on more characteristics than they have in common. Many took place in different countries at different time periods, looking after different patient groups with varying staff mix and staff patient ratios, using different philosophies. Nevertheless, outcome was consistently slightly better for home care or day care programs as compared to standard hospital care. This may suggest a commonality between studies responsible for their efficacy other than the site of care being outside hospital. A variable present to varying degrees across the experimental projects, but not in many standard hospital treatments, is continuity of care. This is defined by Bachrach (1981) as the orderly, uninterrupted movement of patients among the diverse elements of the service delivery system. Such coordination of care is essential if patients are to receive comprehensive but efficient interventions, based on individual needs. The provision of continuity of care is the core function of case-management.

The home care studies found that community teams using continuity of care did better than standard care, but when continuity of care was withdrawn the differences disappeared (Davis *et al.*, 1974; Stein and Test, 1980). In contrast, projects not offering continuity of care found reduced gains of experimental gains initially (Langsley *et al.*, 1969) and none at follow up (Wilder *et al.*, 1966; Herz *et al.*, 1971).

Several uncontrolled studies confirmed the value of continuity of care after discharge from hospital, especially for schizophrenic patients (Winston *et al.*, 1977), but not all found that aftercare protected against relapse (Purvis and Miskimins, 1970; Mayer *et al.*, 1973). Interpretation of these findings must be very cautious, since their designs were generally poor. Several may have selected patients for continuing care on the grounds of better prognosis, and patients at highest risk of relapse may have selectively refused care.

Continuing care seemed most effective for patients with serious mental illness (Kirk, 1976). Patients receiving no or regular care functioned better than those seen only a few times, although this generalization hides important differences between subgroups. Of 579 patients followed up after discharge, 31% of the patients who had not received aftercare were re-hospitalized as compared to 41% of patients who had been followed up (Kirk, 1976). Within the group receiving aftercare, readmission occurred in 55% of those who had 1 to 10 visits, but in only 20% of patients who had been seen more than 10 times during the 2–3 years of follow-up. Aftercare only seemed to benefit chronic patients. Patients with good pre-morbid functioning suffered a relapse rate of 30%, independent of follow-up. Among chronic patients aftercare reduced the relapse rate from 50% to 30%. Beard *et al.*, (1978), in a controlled study of chronic patients, also found a positive correlation between continuous outreach, regular attendance at a rehabilitation centre and lower relapse rates, with shorter hospital stays when admission was required. Continuing community care for the long-term mentally ill can also improve their social networks (Thornicroft and Breakey, 1991).

Although continuing care is important, no evidence suggests that this has to be provided by the same person or team. Relapse rates after discharge were similar for schizophrenic patients followed up by either their hospital therapist or a new one (Winston *et al.*, 1977). When patients after 5 years of community care were transferred to another team, their functioning remained constant (McRae *et al.*, 1990). It appears that the provision of continuing care is the effective component, although further research on the importance of therapist variables is needed.

Case management

The coordination of all available resources on an individual basis is essential in order to achieve the most efficient care for dependent and vulnerable groups of patients (Intagliata, 1982; Harris and Bachrach, 1988). This coordination of services by an identifiable professional (the case manager or key worker) allows greater accessibility for the patient and better accountability (Intagliata 1982), and is an essential component of the UK community care policy (Griffiths, 1988; Department of Health, 1990). Studies evaluating case management models offered to patients after discharge reported improved functioning, greater satisfaction with life and increased community tenure as compared with standard follow-up care, consisting of out patient appointments (Bond et al., 1988; Goering et al., 1988; Wright et al., 1989). Less important is the organization of case management models; a team approach in which staff share the responsibility seems to lead to good results (Stein and Test, 1980; Hoult and Reynolds, 1983). The team approach may also reduce the risk of patient dependency, and lessen the interpersonal closeness many patients find hard to manage (Bachrach, 1981). Moreover, it may reduce the intensity of the work for staff, diminishing the risk of burn-out.

Some variations of results of studies evaluating case-management are noticeable. Programs concentrating on psychosocial rehabilitation achieved major gains in this area without affecting hospital use (Goering et al., 1988), while a community support program with a greater emphasis on medical care reduced hospital use by 80% as compared to the period before entry, similar to the reduction achieved by most of the controlled home care projects discussed above, with less emphatic results on social functioning (Wright et al., 1989). This suggests that improvements in any outcome area do not generalize, and that programs need to provide comprehensive interventions for vulnerable patient groups for years (Borland, 1989). It may be possible, however, to reduce the amount of support offered after stabilization has been achieved, since patients whose care was transferred after 5 years of care in a case management program with a staff–patient ratio of 1 to 8 to a community mental health centre with a ratio of about 1 to 50 remained relatively well (McRae et al., 1990). The intensity and duration of case management input required for optimally efficient results is another important area of future research.

In conclusion, it appears that continuity of care is a major and probably essential component of community care, which should be combined with case management. The inclusion of these elements in services for the seriously mentally ill seems to be based on strong evidence. A further important issue for research concerns the specific components of care provided by any service to its various subgroups of patients, particularly those with schizophrenia, which use most resources (Davies and Drummond, 1990).

PRACTICAL EXPERIENCES

So far this chapter has presented research data, on which much of the debate about the feasibility of community care has been based. Just as important are staff experiences, since community care will only fulfil its promise if teams can implement the proposed models. It can be anticipated that the shift from hospital to the community is complex, and the experiences of the Daily Living Programme (DLP) at the Maudsley Hospital, the results of which have been given above, are described here.

Preparation

A major initial problem was the lack of experience of home care in the UK. No services existed aiming to care for the severely mentally ill at home in 1987. Therefore, the senior registrar and senior nurse went to Madison to learn from the experiences of the Mendota Mental Health Centre and the Pact programme, both of which were products of the original Madison study (Stein and Test 1980). Impressions of this visit were published elsewhere (Muijen and McNamee 1989).

The team was recruited by the senior nurse and the senior registrar. The response to advertisements was very poor, so an open day was held, attracting some staff. Eventually almost all applicants were appointed. No staff of the Bethlem–Maudsley Hospital had applied, despite frequent talks about the project on wards, and despite the promise from management that jobs would be secure after the possible closure of the project at the end of its 3-years funding. The manager–coordinator started a fortnight before the project began. At that time the house where the project was due to be based contained not a single desk or chair.

Staff training and team building was minimal, and lasted for a week before patient intake started, organized by the senior registrar and the senior nurse. This consisted of introductions, discussions about care principles, some role playing, and meetings with representatives from the hospital and local services including the police. A problem in organizing this training week was that nobody had a clear idea of what to expect, and what skills were essential in practice. No tested formal training in community care existed anywhere. Even the Madison and Sydney studies had not specified the precise skills necessary for the endeavour. A source of friction at this early stage was the therapeutic approach. The problem-orientated approach was shared by the consultant and the senior nurse, but other staff preferred different approaches. At selection it had not been made clear that the approach would be problem-orientated, nor what it implied clinically. The clinical expertise in applying this approach to the seriously mentally ill was absent, and insufficient time was available for training during the introduction period. The problem solving approach was wrongly associated by staff with behavioural modification techniques, and seen as an imposition. The objective of formulation and rating of problem and target statements was poorly understood, and training in this was resented. The unexpectedly fast build-up of caseloads meant that little opportunity was found later to remedy this. In addition, a resistance to training had developed within the staff team because they considered the issue as extraneous to their daily clinical practice, and they believed that the constant practical problems they were confronted with were ignored. Often painful arguments during case presentations resulted, upsetting everybody involved.

The training period was inadequate regarding important areas such as problem solving, case-management, mental state assessment, crisis-intervention, rehabilitation techniques, family support, the benefit system and working in a multidisciplinary team, and no homogeneous approach evolved which was supported by the whole team. Decisions dealing with leadership problems and hierarchy within a multi-disciplinary team were avoided. Training sessions were regularly initiated, but attempts to maintain these proved impossible, due to the shift system rarely allowing the full team to be present and the constant absence of several of the staff because of clinical engagements. Support and supervision was organized internally by the nursing staff, the senior nurse supervising the charge nurses who in turn each supervised two staff nurses. The social worker and the occupational therapist received dual supervision, both from within the team and from their own department. Staff liaised closely with other services both in and outside the hospital, including the Maudsley Emergency Clinic for crisis cover at night, the occupational therapy department for basic skills assessments, and Day Centres for day-time activities.

Staff experiences

Staff applying for positions in progressive services tend to be young, dynamic, idealistic and dissatisfied with traditional services, and this was a fair description for the first generation DLP team. An exceptionally high motivation to support patients showed itself by willingness to work long hours and take on many tasks. Staff were also very keen to prove the superiority of the project, but expectations were very high. Staff expected exciting and rewarding crisis-intervention work, saving grateful people from misguided institutional care and medical interventions. The reality was constant and endless hard work with the severely mentally ill, often achieving least results with the most demanding patients. Hospital admissions and psychotropic medications had to be used more often than anticipated, and many patients rejected advice. Demoralization was noticeable after about a year, affecting some staff quite badly.

A second aspect of community programs that can present problems is the multi-disciplinary nature of the team. If functioning well the various disciplines can complement each other, but frequently tensions arise, as each discipline within a team regards itself as more important than others. This is caused by a poor understanding of the skills that other disciplines can contribute. Inter-disciplinary rivalry generates unwillingness to accept that others possess skills unique to their background. The large proportion of nurses in the DLP team meant that many problems were approached from a nursing perspective. Nurse training emphasizes generic and non-specialized interventions, and the other disciplines (occupational therapists, social workers and to a lesser extent psychiatrists) had to fight to maintain a balance between on one hand exclusively using their specific and specialized skills and being at risk of marginalization within the team, and on the other hand becoming generic key workers, losing their professional identity. The social worker was initially expected to take on many tedious visits to social services, but it was soon accepted that she would be used as a resource instead, taking on her own case-load. In contrast, the occupational therapist had to convince staff of her specific qualities, such as work-assessments. An attempted solution was the holding of regular staff support meetings which started after a few months, later with a psychotherapist from the psychotherapy department as facilitator. The facilitator allowed greater freedom of expression. Disagreements were discussed in often productive ways, addressing a range of issues including the role of some staff. A regular training program with multi-disciplinary input would have fostered better understanding of each discipline's potential to the team.

An important staff role in community care is the key-worker (case-manager) system. Patients and staff need to know who is responsible for the care of specific patients. Clients can easily 'fall between the cracks' unless someone is responsible for assessing their needs comprehensively, and coordinating and monitoring their care. From the client's perspective an identifiable staff member is a resource he or she can rely on to be an advocate and supporter in times of crisis, and this is likely to result in increased satisfaction and compliance. The staff member who takes this central place in the care of the patient is called the key-worker (case manager is increasingly used as a synonym). This closeness between patient and staff was a two-edged sword. Dependency developed with some patients reluctant to see team members other than their key-worker, and some staff reluctant for others to see their patients. This increased the risk of relapse when the key-worker was not available.

Use of key-workers also had implications for staff. While staff enjoyed the responsibility and direct care involvement this allowed, the close relationship could also be counterproductive when no progress was apparent or setbacks occurred. The three suicides and homicide in particular severely traumatized staff who may have felt guilty and worried that relatives and friends of the patient may have held them responsible.

These stressors can lead to burn-out characterized by lack of interest, tiredness and irritation. Case management should involve sharing of tasks among team members while allowing the case manager to remain accountable for implementing the care program. This not only alleviates the burden on the worker, but also improves quality of care and diminishes the risk of burn-out (Bond 1988). Burn-out was probably a major but unrecognized problem in the DLP, explaining some of the later resentment and lethargy showed by some of the staff, and contributing to several leaving. The attrition rate was no higher than that of the hospital, but the reasons for leaving may have differed: burn-out vs career improvements. Prevention of burn-out is an essential part of community care projects.

Clients and relatives

Staff were surprised by the appreciation from patients and relatives of DLP attempts to prevent hospitalization. It had been expected that admission would be demanded as the presenting problems were often severe. After being told that the DLP provided constant support, patients and relatives became positive about care at home. Those relatives who continued to be worried usually had good reasons for this, and mostly agreed with the DLP team's assessment of the patient's need, such as constant supervision because of suicide risk or aggressive behaviour. As soon as discharge was considered, usually within a couple of days, this was prepared together with clients and their supporters. Rarely did relatives object to a patient being discharged after a brief admission. Contact with some families was maintained even where clients no longer wished to see the DLP. Family sessions were mainly held in the home, and aimed to solve problems created for the family by the patient's behaviour. Families often positively contrasted their close and regular contact with the DLP team with the neglect they had experienced in the past.

Patients' satisfaction was reflected in their very low drop-out rate. Only three patients refused further contact with the DLP beyond the first few weeks, and these functioned well by then, having entered with acute neurotic conditions which required no further care. Several patients refused to see the team for a while, but returned on their own initiative when they needed help. Most patients felt that the DLP was working with them on their identified problems, such as finances, housing and work. Medication compliance was poor initially, but improved over time, possibly as a result of education and the development of trust. The DLP engaged well with Afro-Caribbean patients, many of whom were young males with schizophrenia who lived alone. Very few of this group dropped out of care, despite others finding them very hard to engage (Pepper et al., 1981). Advocacy and the continuity of care seemed important.

The hospital and local authorities

Bethlem–Maudsley staff slowly began to accept the value of the DLP, but no changes of hospital policy ensued. Scepticism revived after a furore in the media in the third year, blaming the homicide on community care.

Emergency Clinic staff who were exposed regularly to the DLP often expressed regrets when a patient was randomized to hospital care, commenting that 'this person would have done so well in your program'. Staff of various wards were usually willing to care for patients during short admission periods and to accept DLP decisions to discharge them early. Resentment occurred at times when ward staff disagreed with the contrasting treatment received by DLP patients, which did not always fit in with some wards' practices, e.g. use of psychodynamic or therapeutic community principles, and much longer inpatient stays.

The local authority contacts were important and constructive. Housing offered DLP priority status, and communications were regular and sympathetic. Day-centres accepted some DLP patients despite being nominally full. This positive attitude may have resulted from the DLP's willingness to continue responsibility for patient care rather than transferring it.

Clinical limitations

The DLP could not provide a comprehensive range of interventions in the absence of other facilities such as day hospitals, hostels, drop-in centres and temporary accommodation. The few day centres in South Southwark cared for the long term mentally ill, and could accept DLP patients with acute symptoms. The lack of sufficient facilities in an impoverished inner city area imposed a great burden of care on DLP staff. Not all patients could be maintained in the community permanently. Three years after entry, a young schizophrenic man had to be referred to a secure unit for long-term care because of the risk he posed, partly due to his psychotic thinking.

It says much about the motivation of the staff that the service was relatively successful despite these disadvantages, but it is doubtful whether such devotion to care could continue indefinitely in community teams. The experience of the Mendota Mental Health Centre, which succeeded the original Madison project (Stein and

Test, 1980), suggests that some reduction in enthusiasm over time can be expected after conversion from a model programme to a regular service (Muijen and McNamee, 1989).

CONCLUSION

Community care is feasible, provided the quality is sufficiently high in terms of resources, coordination of services, continuity of care and range of available interventions. It can be questioned whether the traditional hospital system provided a better service to the majority of patients, and much of the criticism against community care seems to demand much higher standards than were ever asked of hospital care.

The major concern of community care, and the main area of criticism, is the poor living conditions of some of the dependent mentally ill transferred from hospitals to unacceptably low-standard replacement facilities, without adequate follow-up services, as portrayed in colour supplements of Sunday newspapers. These are an important warning that complacency is unwarranted. However, as David Abrahamson describes in his important chapter in this book, and as experienced elsewhere, if deinstitutionalization is undertaken with care, the condition of vulnerable patients remains at least stable and often improves, with a consistent gain in patients' satisfaction. Besides, community care is not only about reprovision, but also about optimizing the quality of life of people who in the past would have embarked on a long career as a hospital patient.

The challenge of community care is to develop a model of care which combines the best of the many developed interventions, whilst not losing touch with the range of needs of the mentally ill. It is likely that different models are required, based on local characteristics as well as on their specific task. This is illustrated by the variety of approaches of the several exciting services described elsewhere within this book.

REFERENCES

Anthony, W.A., Buell, G.J., Sharratt, S. and Althoff, M.E. (1972) The efficacy of psychiatric rehabilitation. *Psychological Bulletin*, **78**, 447–456.

Anthony, W.A., Cohen, M.R. and Vitalo, R. (1978) The measurement of rehabilitation outcome. *Schizophrenia Bulletin*, **4**, 365–383.

Audit Commission for Local Authorities in England and Wales. (1986) *Making a reality of community care*. HMSO, London.

Bachrach, L.L. (1981) Continuity of care for chronic mental patients: a conceptual analysis. *American Journal of Psychiatry*, **138**, 1449–1455.

Bachrach, L.L. (1982) Assessment of outcomes in Community Support Systems: results, problems and limitations. *Schizophrenia Bulletin*, **8**, 39–60.

Bassuk, E.L. and Gerson, S. (1978) Deinstitutionalization and mental health services. *Scientific American*, **238**, 46–53.

Beard, J.H., Malamud, T.J. and Rossman, E. (1978) Psychiatric rehabilitation and long term rehospitalization rates: the findings of two research studies. *Schizophrenia Bulletin*, **4**, 622–635.

Bennett, D.H. (1983) The historical development of rehabilitation services. In: *Theory and practice of psychiatric rehabilitation*. (F.N. Watts and D.H. Bennett, eds). Wiley, Chichester.

Bond, G.R., Miller, R.D. and Krumwied, R.D. (1988) Assertive case management in three CMHCs: a controlled study. *Hospital and Community Psychiatry*, **39**, 411–418.

Borland, A., McRae, J. and Lycan, C. (1989) Outcomes of five years of continuous intensive case management. *Hospital and Community Psychiatry*, **40**, 369–376.

Braun, P., Kochansky, G., Shapiro, R., Greenberg, S., Gudeman, J.E., Johnson, S. and Shore, M.F. (1981) Overview: deinstitutionalization of psychiatric patients, a critical review of outcome studies. *American Journal of Psychiatry*, **136**, 736–749.

Carse, J., Panton, N.Y. and Watt, A. (1958) A district mental health service: the Worthing experience. *Lancet*, **I**, 39–41.

Cheung, H.K. (1981) Schizophrenics fully remitted on neuroleptics for 3–5 years–to stop or continue drugs? *British Journal of Psychiatry*, **138**, 490–494.

Craft, M. (1958) An evaluation of treatment of depressive illness in a day hospital. *Lancet*, **ii**, 149–151.

Creed, F., Black, D., Anthony, P., Osborn, M., Thomas, P. and Tomenson, B. (1990) Randomised controlled trial of day patient versus inpatient psychiatric treatment. *British Medical Journal*, **300**, 1033–1037.

Davies, M.A., Bromet, E.J., Schulz, S.C., Dunn, L.O. and Morgen-
stern, M. (1989) Community adjustment of chronic schizophrenic
patients in urban and rural settings. *Hospital and Community
Psychiatry*, 40, 824–830.

Davies, L.M. and Drummond, M.F. (1990) The economic burden
of schizophrenia. *Psychiatric Bulletin*, 14, 522–525.

Davis, A.E., Dinitz, S. and Pasamanick, B. (1972) The prevention
of hospitalisation in schizophrenia: Five years after an experimental program. *American Journal of Orthopsychiatry*, 42,
375–388.

Davis, J.M. (1975) Overview: Maintenance therapy in Psychiatry:
I. Schizophrenia. *American Journal of Psychiatry*, 132, 1237–
1245.

Dayson, D. and Gooch, C. (1990) Clinical and social outcomes of
the long-term mentally-ill after one-year in the community:
results from the first three cohorts. In: *Better out than in?* Report
from the 5th annual conference of the Team for the Assessment
of Psychiatric Services, July 1990.

Department of Health (1990) The care programme approach for
people with a mental illness. *HC(90)24/LASSL(90)11*.

Dick, P., Cameron, L., Cohen, D., Barlow, M. and Ince, A. (1985)
Day and full time psychiatric treatment—a controlled comparison. *British Journal of Psychiatry*, 147, 246–249.

Fenton, F.R., Tessier, L., Struening, E.L., Smith, F.A. and Benoit,
C. (1982) *Home and hospital psychiatric treatment*. Croom
Helm, London.

Fink, E.B., Longabaugh, R. and Stout, R. (1978) The paradoxical
under-utilization of partial hospitalization. *American Journal of
Psychiatry*, 135, 713–716.

Fuller Torrey, E. (1986) Continuous treatment teams in the care of
the chronic mentally ill. *Hospital and Community Psychiatry*, 37,
1243–1247.

Garety, P. and Morris, I. (1984) A new unit for long-stay psychiatric
patients: organisation, attitudes and quality of care. *Psychological
Medicine*, 14, 183–192.

Goering, P., Wasylenki, D., Lancee, W. and Freeman, S.J.J. (1984)
From hospital to community. Six month and two-year outcomes
for 505 patients. *The Journal of Nervous and Mental Disease*, 172,
667–672.

Goering, P.N., Wasylenki, D.A., Farkas, M., Lancee, W.J. and

Ballantyne, R. (1988) What difference does case management make? *Hospital and Community Psychiatry*, **39**, 272–276.

Goffman, E. (1961) *Asylums*. Pelican, Harmondsworth.

Goldberg, D.P., Bridges, K., Cooper, W., Hyde, C., Sterling, C. and Wyatt, R. (1985) Douglas House: a new type of hostel ward for chronic psychotic patients. *British Journal of Psychiatry*, **147**, 383–389.

Goldstein, J.M. and Caton, C.L.M. (1983) The effects of the community environment on chronic psychiatric patients. *Psychological Medicine*, **13**, 193–199.

Goldstein, M.J., Rodnick, E.H., Evans, J.R., May, P.R.A. and Steinberg, M.R. (1978) Drug and family therapy in the aftercare treatment of actue schizophrenia. *Archives of General Psychiatry*, **35**, 169–177.

Grad, J. and Sainsbury, P. (1968) The effects that patients have on their families in a community care and a control psychiatric service—a two year follow-up. *British Journal of Psychiatry*, **114**, 265–278.

Griffiths, R. (1988) *Community care, agenda for action*. H.M.S.O., London.

Harris, M. and Bachrach, L.L. (1988) *Clinical case management. New Directions for Mental Health Services*, **40**. Jossey-Bass, San Francisco.

Harris, M. and Bergman, H.C. (1988) Clinical case management for the chronically mentally ill: a conceptual analysis. In: *Clinical Case Management*. M. Harris and L. Bachrach eds.)

Herz, M.I., Endicott, J., Spitzer, R.L. and Mesnikoff, A. (1971) Day versus Inpatient Hospitalization: a controlled study. *American Journal of Psychiatry*, **127**, 1371–1381.

Hoult, J. and Reynolds, I. (1983) *Psychiatric Hospital versus Community treatment: a controlled study*. Department of Health, New South Wales.

Intagliata, J. (1982) Improving the quality of community care for the chronically mentally disabled: the role of case management. *Schizophrenia Bulletin*, **8**, 655–674.

Jones, K. and Poletti, A. (1985) Understanding the Italian experience. *British Journal of Psychiatry*, **146**, 336–341.

Kiesler, C.A. (1982) Mental hospitals and alternative care. *American Psychologist*, **37**, 349–360.

Kirk, S.A. (1976) Effectiveness of community services for discharged mental hospital patients. *American Journal of Orthopsychiatry*, **46**, 646–659.

Lamb, H.R. and Goertzel, V. (1972) High expectations of long-term ex-state hospital patients. *American Journal of Psychiatry*, **129**, 471–475.

Langsley, D.G., Flomenhaft, K. and Machotka, P. (1969) Follow-up evaluation of family crisis therapy. *American Journal of Orthopsychiatry*, **39**, 753–759.

Linn, M.W., Caffey, E.R., Klett, C.J. and Hogarty, G. (1977) Hospital vs community (foster) care for psychiatric patients. *Archives of General Psychiatry*, **34**, 78–83.

Linn, M.W., Caffey, E.M., Klett, C.J., Hogarty, G.E. and Lamb, H.R. (1979) Day treatment and psychotropic drugs in the aftercare of schizophrenic patients. *Archives of General Psychiatry*, **36**, 1055–1066.

Linn, M.W., Klett, C.J. and Caffey, E.M. (1980) Foster home characteristics and psychiatric patient outcome. *Archives of General Psychiatry*, **37**, 129–132.

Marks, I., Connolly, J. and Muijen, M. (1988) The Maudsley Daily Living Program. *Psychiatric Bulletin of The Royal College of Psychiatrists*, **12**, 22–23.

Mayer, J., Hotz, M. and Rosenblatt, A. (1973) The readmission patterns of patients referred to aftercare clinics. *Journal of the Bronx State Hospital*, **1**, 4.

McRae, J., Higgins, M., Lycan, C. and Sherman, W. (1990) What happens to patients after five years of intensive case management stops? *Hospital and Community Psychiatry*, **41**, 175–179.

Michaux, M.H. Chelst, M.R., Foster, S.A., Pruim, R.J. and Dasinger, E.M. (1974) Post release adjustment of day and full-time psychiatric patients. *Archives of General Psychiatry*, **29**, 647–651.

Muijen, M. (1991) The first year of the Daily Living Program: A controlled study. PhD: Institute of Psychiatry, University of London.

Muijen, M., Marks, I., Connolly, J. and Audini, B. (1992) The 3 months' outcome of the Daily Living Program: A randomised controlled study evaluating home care versus hospital care. *British Medical Journal*, **304**, 749–754.

Pai, S. and Kapur, R.L. (1982) Impact of treatment intervention on the relationship between dimensions of clinical psychopathology, social dysfunction and burden on the family of psychiatric patients. *British Journal of Psychiatry*, **12**, 651–658.

Pasamanick, B., Scarpitty, F.R. and Dinitz, S. (1967) *Schizophrenics in the community*. Appleton-Century-Crofts, New York.

Pepper, B., Kirschner, M. and Rylewics, H. (1981) The young adult chronic patient: overview of a population. *Hospital and Community Psychiatry*, **32**, 463–469.

Polak, P.R. and Kirby, M.W. (1976) A model to replace psychiatric hospitals. *Journal of Nervous and Mental Disease*, **162**, 13–22.

Purvis, S.A. and Miskimins, R.W. (1970) Effects of community follow-up on post-hospital adjustment of psychiatric patients. *Community Mental Health Journal*, **6**, 374–382.

Reynolds, I. and Hoult, J.E. (1984) The relatives of the mentally ill, a comparative trial of community oriented and hospital oriented psychiatric care. *Journal of Nervous and Mental Disease*, **172**, 480–489.

Ryan, P., Ford, R. and Clifford, P. (1991) *Case Management & Community Care*.

Smith, S. and Cross, E.G.W. (1957) Review of 1000 patients treated at a psychiatric day hospital. *International Journal of Social Psychiatry*, **2**, 292–298.

Stein, L.J. and Test, M.A. (1980) Alternative to mental hospital treatment. 1, Conceptual model, treatment program and clinical evaluation. *Archives of General Psychiatry*, **37**, 392–397.

Test, M.A. and Stein, L.I. (1980) Alternative to mental hospital treatment. 3, Social cost. *Archives of General Psychiatry*, **37**, 409–412.

Thornicroft, G. and Breakey, W.R. (1991) The Costar program: I. Improving social networks of the long term mentally ill. *British Journal of Psychiatry*. In press.

Turner, J.C. and Ten Hoor, W.J. (1978) The NIMH support program: Pilot approach to a needed social reform. *Schizophrenia Bulletin*, **4**, 319–349.

Wasylenki, D., Goering, P., Lancee, W., Fischer, L. and Freeman, S.J.J. (1985) Psychiatric aftercare in a metropolitan setting. *Canadian Journal of Psychiatry*, **30**, 329–336.

Weisbrod, B.A., Test, M.A. and Stein, L.I. (1980) Alternative to mental hospital treatment. 2, Economic benefit-cost analysis. *Archives of General Psychiatry*, **37**, 400–405.

Weller, M.P.I. (1989) Mental illness—who cares? *Nature*, **339**, 249–252.

Wilder, J.F., Levin, G. and Zwerling, I. (1966) A two year follow-up evaluation of acute psychotic patients treated in a day hospital. *American Journal of Psychiatry*, **122**, 1095–1101.

Wing, J.K. (Ed.) (1982) Long-term community care: experience in a London borough. *Psychological Medicine Monograph* (Supplement).

Wing, J. and Furlong, R. (1986) A haven for the severely disabled within the context of a comprehensive psychiatric community service. *British Journal of Psychiatry*, **149**, 449–457.

Winston, A., Parides, H., Papernik, D.S. and Breslin, L. (1977) Aftercare of psychiatric patients and its relation to rehospitalization. *Hospital and Community Psychiatry*, **28**, 118–121.

Wright, R.G., Heiman, J.R., Shupe, J. and Olvera, G. (1989) Defining and measuring stabilization of patients during 4 years of intensive community support. *American Journal of Psychiatry*, **146**, 1293–1298.

Zwerling, I. (1976) The impact of the community mental health movement on psychiatric practice and training. *Hospital and Community Psychiatry*, **27**, 258–262.

4 PRIMARY CARE AND COMMUNITY PSYCHIATRIC SERVICES: CHANGING PATTERNS AND RESPONSIBILITIES

G. Strathdee

INTRODUCTION

This chapter focuses on four areas in the relationship between primary care and community psychiatric services. Firstly, the extent and nature of psychiatric morbidity encountered in the primary care setting is reviewed and recent indications of changing patterns discussed. Secondly, the traditional role of general practitioners in the management of patients with psychological disorders is examined and the extension of this role in the presence of community psychiatric services delineated. Thirdly, the nature of the relationship between the specialist and generalist services is explored and recent research identifying the needs of general practitioners presented. Fourthly, models of community psychiatric services which focus on collaboration and integration with primary care are described. Throughout, particular emphasis is given to the arrangements for those with severe, long-term mental health problems.

THE EXTENT OF PSYCHIATRIC MORBIDITY IN PRIMARY CARE

In Great Britain the extent of psychiatric morbidity presenting to primary care was first established by Shepherd et al. (1966). In a large-scale study of London general practices they found that of 15 000 patients at risk in any 12 month period, 14% consulted at least once for a condition diagnosed as entirely or largely psychiatric in nature. Goldberg and Blackwell (1970) found that this represented the 'conspicuous' psychiatric morbidity detected by the general practitioner, and that a further 10–12% went 'hidden' or unrecognized by the doctors. The majority were assessed to have either neurotic or personality problems. Regier et al. (1985) in the US found, similarly, that approximately 30% of primary care patients had a diagnosis of mental disorder. Approximately 9% of the defined population in both studies suffered chronic disability, having symptoms continuously present for at least one year, or requiring prophylactic treatment. These figures demonstrate that general practitioners play a major role in the care of those with both acute and chronic psychological disorders.

GENERAL PRACTITIONERS AND THE CARE OF CHRONIC PATIENTS

Murray Parkes et al. (1962), following up a cohort of schizophrenic patients discharged from London mental hospitals, found that almost three-quarters had seen their GP in the year after discharge with more than half consulting over five times. Just less than 60% of the sample had attended hospital outpatient clinics in the same time and of these, over half had been seen less than five times. Evidence of this continuing significant contribution of primary care in the management of the severely chronically ill has come more recently from a number of disparate sources.

Pantellis et al. (1988) in the South Camden Schizophrenia Study found that only three-fifths of the known schizophrenics in the area were in contact with the psychiatric services. Lee and Murray (1988) studying the long-term outcome of a group of depressed patients found that over half had lost contact with the hospital services. Johnstone et al. (1984), following a cohort of discharged schizophrenics similar to that of the Murray Parkes group, found that 24% were seeing only their GP in a five year follow-up period.

THE EXPANSION OF THE PRIMARY CARE WORKLOAD

The implementation of community care is likely to affect the workload of GPs by virtue of the alterations in clinical practice and organizational structures. In their review of deinstitutionalization Thornicroft and Bebbington (1989) delineate the possible effects of transferring the functions of the psychiatric hospital to the community. Of particular significance for primary care are: the decrease in bed numbers resulting in the locus of treatment being transferred to homes; the decrease in respite facilities with subsequent increase in burden of care for relatives; the removal of institution staff to meet the needs for physical assessment and treatment.

In addition, length of stay in hard pressed district units (50% of patients stay less than one month) has led to patients remaining with carers or relatives, who look to their family doctors for support and intervention. The increasing number of mentally ill among the homeless, especially in the inner cities, stretch the GP services. The growth of group homes, hostels and other forms of sheltered accommodation inevitably lead to increased demand for both physical and psychiatric care from the local GPs. While patients reside in the community, whether or not they have contact with the secondary services, GPs form the point of first contact in emergencies.

In a major survey of 500 GPs in the South West Thames Region, Kendrick *et al.* (1991) found that while 90% of the doctors were happy to undertake the physical care of patients with long-term mental health illnesses, most were reluctant to accept full responsibility for the psychiatric care. Three-quarters wanted the psychiatric services to maintain primary responsibility and four-fifths believed that the community psychiatric nurse should be the key worker. However, almost all were willing to undertake shared care with the secondary services.

THE ROLE OF PRIMARY CARE IN THE CHANGING PATTERNS OF PSYCHIATRIC CARE

While many psychiatrists have been concerned about the move to the community in the absence of realistic levels of funding and resources (Weller, 1985, see also Chapters 1 and 2), others argue that unlike most countries struggling to develop community care, Great Britain already has a unique resource. Tyrer (1986) asserts that the primary care infrastructure constitutes the most appropriate focus for community care. This view concords with the WHO declaration (1973) 'that the primary care physicians should form the cornerstone of community psychiatry' as they 'are best placed to provide long-term follow-up and be available for successive episodes of illness'. This is endorsed by the Royal College of General Practitioners (1984) which considers that GPs are particularly well placed to practise prevention at both the primary and secondary levels. Horder (1988) contends that the opportunities for 'interested and well-trained GPs to work in this part of medicine differ little from those of psychiatrists—opportunities to detect disturbances, to define problems and to respond with basic psychotherapy, medication or social interventions'. The debate can be informed by an examination of the specific functions that GPs are expected to perform in dealing with the severely mentally ill in the community. These functions will be delineated below together with the extent to which GPs have the necessary skills, training, time and interest required to undertake them.

IDENTIFICATION AND ASSESSMENT OF PHYSICAL AND PSYCHIATRIC MORBIDITY

The British GP is often best placed to first identify and assess psychiatric morbidity. In Great Britain, 98% of the population is registered with a GP and of these 60–70% consult at least once each year. Only 10% fail to consult in any three year period (Sharp and Morrell, 1989). However, there is a nine-fold variation in the doctor's ability to detect psychiatric dysfunction (Shepherd et al., 1966; Davenport et al., 1987). Marks et al. (1979) found that detection improved with the ability to conduct a simple mental state in an empathic manner and the recognition of the association of psychiatric morbidity with social dysfunction. Goldberg et al. (1980) and more recently A.P. Boardman (1987) have demonstrated that videofeedback training can improve the accuracy of assessments.

The treatment of physical illness is the natural forte of the GP and of particular value in the treatment of the long-term mentally ill who are particularly vulnerable to physical morbidity. In a study of 145 long-term users of hospital and social services day psychiatric facilities, Brugha et al. (1989) found that 41% suffered medical problems potentially requiring care. General practitioners will need to familiarize themselves with the spectrum of physical morbidity most likely to occur in such patients and the difficulties of under-taking comprehensive assessments (Thornicroft *et al.*, 1991).

THE MANAGEMENT OF PSYCHIATRIC DISORDER

In the era prior to the development of community care, GPs had relatively few options to employ in dealing with patients suffering from psychiatric disorders. They could either treat the patient themselves with drugs and 'Balint type' psychotherapy or refer to the almost exclusively hospital based services. A number of initia-tives have been directed at extending psychological interventions into primary care. The majority of work has concentrated on the neurotic disorders (Paykel *et al.*, 1982; Catalan *et al.*, 1984; Marks, 1985; Johnstone and Shepley, 1986), with a focus on depression (Blackburn *et al.*, 1981; Teasdale, *et al.*, 1984). Others have concen-trated on training GPs themselves to undertake and apply psycho-logical treatments (France and Robson, 1986). However, there has been no dedicated work to examine the ability of GPs to undertake the psychiatric treatment of the long-term mentally ill, particularly those with psychotic illnesses. Knowledge of the range and thera-peutic efficacy of modern antipsychotics, together with an under-standing of the interaction of medication and psychological therapies, requires particular attention. In the future, the cost to budget holding practices of these frequently consulting patients requiring expensive medication may cause doctors to be reluctant to take them on to their lists and this should be carefully monitored.

FIRST POINT OF CONTACT IN CRISIS

In their follow-up study of schizophrenic patients in the com-munity Murray Parkes *et al.* (1962) concluded that 'while the hospitals and outpatient clinics were responsible for initiating most of the treatment required for maintaining the patients' health, it was the general practitioners who played the major role in dealing with the crises and relapses that occurred in over half the cases'. Eighty per cent of Kendrick's GPs asserted that often patients with long-term mental health problems only came to their attention when a crisis arose (Kendrick *et al.*, 1991). In reviewing the community care experience of the US, Bachrach (1984) has cautioned that the decrease in beds has led to excessive use of emergency services by young psychotic patients who use no other facilities. The system of open access to British primary care services may increase the role of primary care teams in this regard. For their more stable population GPs are well placed to practise prevention as they can use their frequent contacts with patients to recognize changes in behaviour or consultation habits (Widmer and Cadoret, 1979). Over time they can play a key role in working with patients, carers and relatives in establishing premorbid patterns of relapse and enabling timely, tested and individually appropriate levels of medication to be instituted (Birchwood et al., 1989). GPs have themselves identified a need for training in the implementation of the Mental Health Act (Strathdee, 1990) and clarification of their role in relation to social workers.

FAMILY AND CARER EDUCATION AND SUPPORT

The most apposite work for family intervention has come from Falloon (Falloon et al., 1984; Falloon, 1989) who has developed an effective, family-based treatment package for schizophrenia. The patient-orientated management combines optimal neuroleptic drug therapy, rehabilitation, counselling, problem-solving psychotherapy, crisis intervention, and practical assistance with problems such as finances and housing. The approach seeks to enhance the stress reducing capacity of the individual and family through improved understanding of the illness and training in behavioural methods of problem-solving. Falloon et al. (1990) advocate the application of this approach to the primary care setting with referrals processed initially by community psychiatric nurses based in general practices.

REFERRAL AND LIAISON

The family doctor has always had at his disposal the facility to refer patients on to specialist care but has traditionally used this option for only one in twenty of his psychologically ill patients. Goldberg and Huxley (1980) have postulated that the referral decision depends on three interrelated factors—the nature of the patient, the attitude and training of the GP and the nature of the service. Kaeser and Cooper (1971) found that clinical severity accounted for only a proportion of referrals to hospital outpatient clinics, with patient or relative pressure, doctor's therapeutic impotence or failure and social disruption being significant other variables.

With the proliferation of referral destinations since the development of community services, the determinants of the referral decision are less clear but appear to depend more on the availability and organization of services. Low and Pullen (1988), in a Scottish case-register study, found that when a range of services is available GPs tend to refer along a spectrum of severity. Psychotic patients were preferentially referred for emergency care in the form of domiciliary consultation. This finding has been replicated in England where approximately one-third of referrals to domiciliary visits and crisis intervention services are for the treatment of the seriously ill with psychotic illnesses (Boardman *et al.*, 1987a; Sutherby *et al.*, 1991). In contrast, the Scottish group found that only the neurotic end of the spectrum were referred to psychiatrists working in the primary care setting. This appears to be a regional variation, as the more common pattern, found in English studies, is that the severely and chronically ill are well represented in referrals to the service (Browning *et al.*, 1987; Brown *et al.*, 1988; Strathdee *et al.*, 1990).

Although the burden of care for GPs has increased as a result of community care policies, there has also been a corresponding change in the number, range and accessibility of mental health services and professionals available to work with primary care and share the load. The role of the community psychiatric nurse (CPN) is central to this and is discussed in Chapter 6. Most initiatives, however, have focused on patients at the neurotic end of the spectrum and less on the chronically ill (Paykel, 1990).

RESPONSIBILITY FOR COMMUNITY HOMES AND HOSTELS

With the decrease in psychiatric beds in hospital settings many residents are placed in sheltered accommodation in the community. Horder (1990) studied the establishment of three hostel and group home facilities for patients discharged from Friern Hospital. Her aim was to establish the burden of extra responsibility placed on the local GPs and to ascertain the nature of the medical care needed. She found that the residents had a relatively high sickness rate and had higher rates of consultation than the population at large (an average of seven to eight, compared to the population norms of four). Despite this, the unanimous opinion of the GPs involved was that the work had not been unduly arduous or difficult, and that off-duty work was minimal. Three-quarters of the doctors had no regrets about taking on the patients and several were spontaneous in commenting on its interest and value. She concluded that the amount of work devolved to GPs in community facilities depends on such factors as age and health of residents, staffing levels, training, experience and morale in the homes, the standard of local community services and the involvement and interest of the GPs and psychiatrists.

THE RELATIONSHIP BETWEEN PSYCHIATRIC SERVICES AND PRIMARY CARE

The burden on general practitioners in providing community care is naturally influenced by the provision and organization of psychiatric services. The First Contact in Mental Health Care Working Group of the World Health Organization (1983) deliberated whether the model which mental health services should employ in the interface with primary care should be one of *integration* or *collaboration*. In the former, work is always undertaken through and with the primary workers with supervision and direction provided. In the latter, the specialists act as the first-contact workers dealing directly with the families in the community. Before a definitive model can be identified it is interesting to examine the extent to which the traditional relationship between the primary and secondary services is successful in meeting the expectations and needs of GPs. For example, until the advent of community care, consultation services were provided in the main by hospital outpatient clinics. Evaluation of the service (Kaeser and Cooper, 1971; Johnson, 1973a, 1973b; Skuse, 1975; Clare, 1983) has demonstrated referrer dissatisfaction with many aspects including long waiting lists, delay in communications, and disappointment with treatment strategies. Communication difficulties have been one of the major areas of discord between GPs and hospital based doctors (Strathdee, 1990;

Pullen and Yellowlees, 1985). Hansen (1987) found primary care dissatisfaction with a hospital based system of care. The main reasons included too little contact with mental health professionals for consultation on difficult cases, too few possibilities for direct referral to specialist services and too few patients discharged back to primary care after discharge from in-patient status.

As indicated above, the primary care team plays a major part in the crisis management of patients with mental health disorders. Emergency services have in the main been provided by domiciliary visits, casualty departments in general hospitals, or in a very few areas, dedicated emergency clinics. There has been little substantive evaluation of either outcome or satisfaction among GPs with these services. Sutherby et al. (1991) found that while domiciliary consultations present one of the few opportunities for senior psychiatrists and practitioners to work together, in recent years the practice of joint visits has almost disappeared. As this service caters particularly for the severely ill many useful training and liaison opportunities are thus being lost.

The key issue is whether any of the new community services such as crisis intervention teams, community mental health centres with their teams, primary care liaison clinics, the attachment of CPNs and other professionals to the primary care setting have resulted in any improvement in the parameters of outcome identified above. The history of most medical services is that they arise without the benefit of evaluation and often continue despite evidence that they are not optimal in either format or outcome. Regrettably most of the new community provisions have been developed without any prior assessment of primary care needs for the mutual benefit of patients.

IDENTIFIED PSYCHIATRIC SERVICE NEEDS FOR PRIMARY CARE

Horder (1988) identified the needs of individual practitioners as requiring help with interview technique, and the recognition of early symptoms, signs and life events most likely to contribute to illness. He asserts that personal contact between psychiatrist and GPs is of fundamental importance and should be considered in terms of clinical work, education and organization.

In an attempt to examine organizational structures from a 'bottom-up' approach, all GPs in the district of Camberwell (Strathdee, 1990) were consulted to obtain their views on the development of a community psychiatric service. The approach was to identify the components of the existing emergency, consultation and other services which they found most apposite in meeting their needs and those of their patients, with the aim of building on these in future service development. Within the emergency facilities the provision of immediate access to a specialist opinion, personal contact with a senior psychiatrist, and the assessment of patients in their own homes were regarded as of major importance and the doctors advocated the provision of more outreach facilities such as a crisis intervention team. Ferguson (1990), in an audit of GPs in Bassetlaw, also found a preoccupation with obtaining rapid response to crisis and Stansfeld (1991) was advised that this should be on a 24 hour basis.

The Camberwell doctors believed that outpatient facilities should be improved by: having shorter waiting lists, decreased time between referral and appointment, the introduction of information packs explaining the treatments available (e.g. cognitive therapy) and what constituted appropriate cases for referral, with named personnel to contact. Particularly for chronic patients the doctors stressed the need for good communications including a statement of the objectives and rationale of treatments and an estimation of their length and possible side-effects and complications. Open access to community psychiatric nurses and psychologists was regarded as very useful by the doctors who were less convinced of the need for professionals such as psychiatrists and psychologists to hold regular session in the surgeries.

Although 'sectorization' was not specifically mentioned, it was considered good organizational practice to have a named consultant and team responsible for demarcated geographical patches. For patients admitted to hospital they requested automatic and prompt notification of admissions, and follow-up at least in the short term by a member of the psychiatric team after discharge. In summary, the GPs wanted a service which facilitated continuity of care, improved communication and coordination.

MODELS OF COLLABORATION BETWEEN PSYCHIATRY AND PRIMARY CARE

A number of models of community psychiatric services have been developed which focus on the primary care base and provide, in varying degrees, the attributes listed above. At the most basic level has been the devolution of outpatient clinics from hospital sites and the establishment of consultation clinics in primary care settings; 19% of all consultant general adult psychiatrists in England and Wales (Strathdee and Williams, 1984) and half the Scottish psychiatrists (Pullen and Yellowlees, 1988) work in this way. In a survey of the participants in such services it transpired that the impetus for their inception came from grass roots psychiatrists. Among the rationales given were dissatisfaction with the lack of coordination of care exemplified in the hospital outpatient setting, accompanied by the determination to establish and expand community services and to improve liaison and communication between primary and secondary care (Strathdee, 1988).

The clinics are conducted in a variety of formats (Strathdee and Williams, 1984; Mitchell, 1985). General practitioners have expressed a preference for the 'consultation' style wherein the psychiatrist and referrer jointly make an assessment and the primary care professional undertakes the treatment with supervision. In the 'shifted outpatient model' the specialist sees the patients from the immediate catchment area in the local surgery rather than at the often distant psychiatric hospital. This enables them to provide crisis intervention and perform assessment and short-term treatment. In longer standing arrangements the liaison-attachment model evolves with an integrated approach between the specialist and primary care teams in the management of patients. This model is regarded as being cost-effective in that the psychiatrists can contribute to the care of more patients by providing advice on patients not seen, treating others through supervision and enhancing the skills of the primary care team (Creed and Marks, 1989; Darling and Tyrer, 1990).

An early criticism of the clinics was that specialists in the primary care setting would inevitably, as with the American community mental health centres, drift towards seeing the 'walking well'. However, a number of authors have demonstrated that the proportion of patients with serious and long-term mental illness seen, is at least equal to that encountered in hospital outpatient clinics (Tyrer, 1984; Browning et al., 1987; Brown et al., 1988; Strathdee, 1990). In fact there is evidence to suggest that the clinics provide for the previously unmet need of chronic patients reluctant to attend hospital follow-up clinics, especially women, schizophrenics, those with paranoid illnesses (Brown et al., 1988) and the homeless (Joseph et al., 1990).

A model in which the primary care liaison clinics form an important component is the 'Hive' model described by Tyrer (1985). Tyrer advocates that truly comprehensive care can only be achieved by a system that integrates community psychiatry with the hospital base, which should be cited within reach of all parts of the catchment area. Closely coordinated sub-units of care such as day hospitals, community clinics, or mental health centres should be located in the areas with the greatest psychiatric morbidity. Links can then be made with all the actual and potential psychiatric services, including the primary care teams in the locality. In Nottingham, where the 'hive' model has been developed, Tyrer found that with GP clinics incorporated into the sub-unit structure, there was a 20% fall in admissions to hospital. He perceived additional benefits to be the earlier detection of psychiatric illness and a greater ability to prevent relapse in those patients who traditionally are poor attenders at hospital clinics, such as the young and those who feel stigmatized by the process.

In Norway Hansen (1987) has experimented with a model which involves an even greater degree of integration with primary care, including not only primary health care but also social and other agencies. The community psychiatric service was organized separately from the hospital service and functioned exclusively as a second level service. The psychiatric teams were based in a number of primary care agencies and participated in joint meetings. Referrals from both community and hospital agencies were accepted only if a primary care agency assumed responsibility for the future continuity of care. Both day and night emergencies were dealt with by the primary care teams who had rapid access to the psychiatric services if they felt this to be necessary. Referrals for admission were always undertaken by the primary care coordinator even when the judgement that it was necessary had come from the psychiatric team. The three main aims formulated for the service were that it should replace admissions with consultation and treatment within primary care, provide access to consultation for all primary care workers and agencies, regardless of profession, and execute ambulatory treatment without the patient being disconnected from the primary care provider. An 18% reduction in admissions was achieved over a two year period. Hansen, commenting on the experiment, considered that the role of primary care must be a core concern in any attempt to shift the emphasis of psychiatric treatment from an institution to the community.

STRATEGIES FOR THE FUTURE DEVELOPMENT OF COMMUNITY SERVICES

It is evident that even before the introduction of community psychiatric services GPs played a major role in the management of the mentally ill in the community. The indications are that their workload will increase, particularly in providing care for the severely ill. Patients will only get the best service if an alliance between primary and secondary care is actively pursued with consideration of the organizational, clinical and education entities outlined in Horder's (1988) paradigm.

In planning community services organizational structures are of crucial importance. As Tansella counsels, 'what is important in community care is not only the number and characteristics of various services but the way in which they are arranged and integrated'. Jones (1986) too, cautions that 'unless attention is given to finding administrative solutions to the repeated official exhortations (DHSS, 1975, 1978, 1981; Griffiths, 1988) for collaboration and co-operation with GPs we will fail to provide the mix of services needed'. One approach has been hailed as achieving success in this regard. Workers, both abroad (Lindholm, 1983; Hansson, 1989) and in Great Britain (Tyrer et al., 1989), consider that an essential infrastructure for the establishment of better working practices between specialists and generalists is the delineation of small, geographically defined areas or sectors as the unit of service provision. However, there has been little substantive evaluation of the model and reliable measures of process and outcome, as well as costs and benefits, need to be developed (Tansella, 1989).

The recent involvement of GPs into research in this area has resulted in pragmatic, yet innovative, suggestions to improve practice. Kendrick (1990; Kendrick *et al.*, 1991) proposes the establishment of practice policies for the care of patients with long-term mental health disorders. He advocates the development of registers of the 20 to 30 long-term mentally ill individuals on each practice list. This offers opportunities for coordination of care and the development of systems of case management inherent in the directives of the National Health Service and Community Care Act. The latter requires that social services and health authorities jointly formulate community care plans for this vulnerable group (see also Chapter 5). Horder (1990) has defined practical guidelines for the functioning of community hostels including that they should be within easy access of shops, sports facilities, cinemas, day centres, workshops and pubs. There should be a well formulated plan for medical cover before the admission of residents achieved by detailed discussion with all staff members, especially GPs, if they are to be involved and agreements made about spheres of responsibility, emergency work, prescribing and communication.

The three audit studies cited above (Strathdee, 1990; Kendrick *et al.*, 1991; Stansfeld, 1991) provide information on the structure and organization of services necessary to help GPs in the care of seriously ill patients. For the future, the move to develop contracts between family health service authorities and provider primary care practices may facilitate joint audit and the development of consensus in defining good practices in the provision of care.

The need for GP trainees to obtain appropriate post-graduate experience by working in the community, rather than hospital based settings, has been frequently reiterated (Royal College of General Practitioners, 1980; Lesser, 1983). As with psychiatrists, there is a need to recognize that working in the community can only be achieved by the acquisition of new skills beyond the purely clinical (Sturt and Waters, 1985). Success depends on the development of expertise in management, communication, administration and the recognition and mobilization of resources.

REFERENCES

Bachrach, L.L. (1984) The young adult chronic psychiatric patient in an era of deinstitutionalisation. *American Journal of Public Health*, **74**, 382–384.

Birchwood, M., Smith, J., Macmillan, F., Hogg, B., Prasad, R., Harvey, C. and Bering, S. (1989) Predicting relapse in schizophrenia: the development and implementation of an early signs monitoring system using patients and families as observers, a preliminary investigation. *Psychological Medicine*, 18, 649–656.

Blackburn, I.M., Bishops, S., Glen, A.I.M., Whalley, L.J. and Christie, J.E. (1981) The efficacy of cognitive therapy in depression a treatment combination. *British Journal of Psychiatry*, 139, 181–189.

Boardman, A.P. (1986) The General Health Questionnaire and the detection of emotional disorder by general practitioners: a replicated study. *British Journal of Psychiatry*, 165, 373–381.

Boardman, A.P. (1987) The mental health advice centre in Lewisham. Service usage: Trends from 1978–1984. Research Report No. 3. The National Unit for Psychiatric Research and Development, Lewisham.

Brown, R., Strathdee, G., Christie-Brown, J. and Robinson, P. (1988) A comparison of referrals to primary care and hospital outpatient clinics. *British Journal of Psychiatrists*, 153, 168–173.

Browning, S.M., Ford, M.F., Goddard, C.A. and Brown, A.C. (1987) A psychiatric clinic, in general practice: a description and comparison with an out-patient clinic. *Bulletin of the Royal College of Psychiatrists*, 11 (4): 114–117.

Brugha, T.S., Wing, J.K. and Smith, B.L. (1989) Physical ill-health of the long-term mentally ill in the community. Is there an unmet need? *British Journal of Psychiatry*, 155, 777–782.

Catalan, J., Gath, G., Edmonds, G., Bond, A., Mertin, P. and Ennis, J. (1984) Effects of non-prescribing of anxiolytics in general practice, 1. controlled evaluation of psychiatric and social outcome; 2. factors associated with outcome. *British Journal of Psychiatry*, 144, 593–610.

Clare, A. (1983) Use and abuse of the psychiatric consultation. *Medicine International*, 1, 1579–1581.

Creed, F. and Marks, B. (1989) Liaison psychiatry in general practice: a comparison of the liaison-attachment scheme and the shifted outpatient models. *Journal of the Royal College of General Practitioners*, 39, 514–517.

Darling, C. and Tyrer, P. (1990) Brief encounters in general practice: liaison in general practice psychiatry clinics. *Psychiatric Bulletin*, 14, 592–594.

Davenport, S., Goldberg, D. and Millar, T. (1987) How psychiatric disorders are missed during medical consultations. *Lancet*, ii, 439–440.

Department of Health and Social Security. (1975) *Better Services for the Mentally Ill*, Cmnd 6233. HMSO, London.

Department of Health and Social Security. (1978) Collaboration in community care. Central Health Services Council. HMSO, London.

Department of Health and Social Security. (1981) *Care in Action*. HMSO, London.

Falloon, I.R.H. (1989) Behavioural approaches in schizophrenia. In: *Scientific Approaches on Epidemiological and Social Psychiatry, Essays in Honour of Michael Shepherd* (P. Williams, G. Wilkinson and K. Rawnsley, eds). Routledge, London.

Falloon, I.R.H., Boyd, J.L. and McGill, C.W. (1984) *Family Care of Schizophrenia*. Guilford Press, New York.

Falloon, I.R.H., Shanahan, W., Laporta, M. and Krekorian, H.A.R. (1990) Integrated family, general practice and mental health care in the management of schizophrenia. *Journal of the Royal Society of Medicine*, **83**, 225–228.

Ferguson, B. (1990) Clinical audit—a proposal. *Psychiatric Bulletin*, **14**, 275–277.

France, R. and Robson, M. (1986). *Behaviour Therapy in Primary Care*. Croom Helm, London.

Goldberg, D.P. and Blackwell, B. (1970) Psychiatric illness in general practice: a detailed study using a new method of case identification. *British Medical Journal*, ii, 439–443.

Goldberg, D.P. and Huxley, P. (1980) *Mental Illness in the Community. The Pathway to Psychiatric Care*. Tavistock Publications.

Goldberg, D.P., Steele, J.J., Smith, C. and Spivey, L. (1980) Training family doctors to recognise psychiatric illness with increased accuracy. *Lancet*, ii, 521–523.

Griffiths, R. (1988) *Community Care: An Agenda for Action*. HMSO, London.

Hansen, V. (1987) Psychiatric service within primary care. Mode of organisation and influence on admission rates to a mental hospital. *Acta Psychiatrica Scandinavica*, **76**, 121–128.

Hansson, L. (1989) Utilisation of psychiatric in-patient care. *Acta Psychiatrica Scandinavica*, **79**, 571–578.

Horder, E. (1990) Medical care in three psychiatric hostels. Hampstead and Bloomsbury District Health Authority. Hampstead and South Barnet GP Forum and the Hampstead Department of Community Medicine.

Horder, J. (1988) Working with general practitioners *British Journal of Psychiatry*, **153**, 513–521.

Johnson, D.A. (1973a) An analysis of out-patient services. *British Journal of Psychiatry*, **122**, 301–306.

Johnson, D.A. (1973b) A further study of psychiatric outpatient services in Manchester. *British Journal of Psychiatry*, **123**, 185–191.

Johnstone, A. and Shepley, M. (1986) The outcome of hidden neurotic illness treated in general practice. *Journal of the Royal College of General Practitioners*, **36**, 413–415.

Johnstone, E.C., Owens, D.G.C., Gold, A., Crow, T.J. and MacMillan, J.F. (1984) Schizophrenic patients discharged from hospitals—a follow-up study. *British Journal of Psychiatry*, **145**, 586–590.

Jones, K., Robinson, M. and Golightley, P. (1986) Long-term psychiatric patients in the community. *British Journal of Psychiatry*, **149**, 537–540.

Joseph, P., Bridgewater, J.A., Ramsden, S.S. and El Kabir, D.J. (1990) A psychiatric clinic for the single homeless in a primary care setting in inner London. *Psychiatric Bulletin*, **14**, 270–271.

Kaeser, A.C. and Cooper, B. (1971) The psychiatric out-patient, the general practitioner and the out-patient clinic; an operational study: a review. *Psychological Medicine*, **1**, 312–325.

Kendrick, A. (1990) *The Challenge of the Long-term Mentally Ill*. The Royal College of General Practitioners. Members Reference Book. Sterling Publications, London.

Kendrick, A., Sibbald, B., Burns, T. and Freeling, P. (1991) Role of general practitioners in care of long term mentally ill patients. *British Medical Journal*, **302**, 508–511.

Lee, A.S. and Murray, R.M. (1988) The long-term outcome of Maudsley depressives. *British Journal of Psychiatry*, **153**, 741–751.

Lesser, A. (1983) Is training in psychiatry relevant for general practice? *Journal of the Royal College of General Practitioners*, **39**, 617–618.

Lindholm, H. (1983) Sectorised psychiatry. *Acta Psychiatrica Scandinavica*, **67**, Supplement 304.

Low, C.B. and Pullen, I. (1988) Psychiatric clinics in different settings: a case register study. *British Journal of Psychiatry*, **153**, 243–245.

Marks, I. (1985) Controlled trial of psychiatric nurse therapists in primary care. *British Medical Journal*, **240**, 1181–1184.

Marks, J.N., Goldberg, D.P. and Hillier, V.F. (1979) Determinants of the ability of general practitioners to detect psychiatric illness. *Psychological Medicine*, **9**, 337–353.

Mitchell, A.R.K. (1985) Psychiatrists in primary health care settings. *British Journal of Psychiatry*, **147**, 371–370.

Murray Parkes, C., Brown, G.W. and Monck, E.M. (1962) The general practitioner and the schizophrenic patient. *British Medical Journal*, **1**, 972–976.

Pantellis, C., Taylor, J. and Campbell, P. (1988) The South Camden schizophrenia survey. *Bulletin of the Royal College of Psychiatrists*, **12**, 98–101.

Paykel, E. (1990) Innovations in mental health in the primary care system. In: *Mental Health Service Evaluation* (I. Marks and R. Scott, eds). Cambridge University Press, Cambridge.

Paykel, E., Mangen, S., Griffith, J. and Burns, T. (1982) Community psychiatric nursing for neurotic patients: a controlled trial. *British Journal of Psychiatry*, **140**, 573–581.

Pullen, I.M. and Yellowlees, A. (1985) Is communication improving between general practitioners and psychiatrists? *British Medical Journal*, **290**, 31–33.

Pullen, I.M. and Yellowlees, A. (1988) Scottish psychiatrists in primary health-care settings a silent majority. *British Journal of Psychiatry*, **153**, 663–666.

Regier, D.A., Burke, J.R., Manderschied, R.W. and Burns, B.J. (1985) The chronically mentally ill in primary care. *Psychological Medicine*, **15**, 265–273.

Royal College of General Practitioners (1984) Combined Reports on Prevention. Reports from General Practice, 18–21. London.

Sharp, D. and Morrell, D. (1989) The psychiatry of general practice. In: *Scientific Approaches on Epidemiological and Social Psychiatry. Essays in Honour of Michael Shepherd* (P. Williams, G. Wilkinson and K. Rawnsley, eds). Routledge, London.

Shepherd, M., Cooper, B., Brown, A. and Kalton, G. (1966) *Psychiatric Illness in General Practice*. Oxford University Press.

Skuse, D. (1975) Attitudes to the psychiatric outpatient clinics. *British Medical Journal*, **iii**, 469–471.

Stansfeld, S. (1991) Attitudes to developments in community psychiatry among general practitioners. *Psychiatric Bulletin* (in press).

Strathdee, G. (1988). Psychiatrists in primary care: the general practitioner viewpoint. *Family Medicine*, 5, 111–115.

Strathdee, G. (1990) The delivery of psychiatric care. *Journal of the Royal Society of Medicine*, 83, 222–225.

Strathdee, G. and Williams, P. (1984) A survey of psychiatrists in primary care: the silent growth of a new service. *Journal of the Royal College of General Practitioners*, 34, 615–618.

Strathdee, G., King, M., Araya, A. and Lewis, S. (1990). A standardised assessment of patients referred to primary care and hospital psychiatric clinics. *Psychological Medicine*, 20, 219–224.

Sturt, J. and Waters, H. (1985) Role of the psychiatrist in community-based mental health care. *Lancet* 507–508.

Sutherby, K., Srinath, S. and Strathdee, G. (1992) The Domiciliary Consultation Service: outdated anachronism or essential part of community psychiatric outreach? *Health Trends*, 24, 103–105.

Tansella, M. (1989) Evaluating community psychiatric services. In Williams P., Wilkinson, G. and Rawnsley, K. (eds) *Scientific Approaches on Epidemiological and Social Psychiatry. Essays in Honour of Michael Shepherd.* Routledge, London.

Teasdale, J.D., Fennell, M.J.V., Hibbert, G.A. and Amies, P.L. (1984) Cognitive therapy for major depressive disorder in primary care. *British Journal of Psychiatry*, 144, 400–406.

Thornicroft, G. and Bebbington, P. (1988) Deinstitutionalisation: from hospital closure to service development. *British Journal of Psychiatry*, 155, 739–753.

Thornicroft, G., Boocock, A. and Strathdee, G. (1991) Symptomatic and Social Functional changes in long-term patients after trans-institutionalisation. Unpublished research report.

Tyrer, P. (1984) Psychiatric clinics in general practice: an extension of community care. *British Journal of Psychiatry*, 145, 9–14.

Tyrer, P. (1985) The 'hive' system: a model for a psychiatric service. *British Journal of Psychiatry*, 146, 571–575.

Tyrer, P. (1986) What is the role of the psychiatrist in primary care? *Journal of the Royal College of General Practitioners*, 36, 373–375.

Tyrer, P., Turner, R. and Johnson, A. (1989). Integrated hospital and community psychiatric services and use of inpatient beds. *British Medical Journal*, **299**, 298–300.

Weller, M.P.I. (1985) Friern Hospital: where have all the patients gone? *Lancet*, **i**, 569–570.

Widmer, R.B. and Cadoret, R.J. (1979) Depression in family practice: changes in pattern of family visits and complaints during subsequent developing depressions. *Journal of Family Practice*, **9**, 1017–1021.

World Health Organization (1973) *Psychiatry and Primary Medical Care*. WHO Regional Office of Europe.

World Health Organization (1983) *First Contact Mental Health Care*. WHO Regional Office for Europe, Copenhagen.

5 SOCIAL SERVICES CARE MANAGEMENT

P. Ryan

INTRODUCTION

In April 1993, social services departments became 'lead agencies' for coordinating community care, not only for the mentally ill but also for the elderly and people with learning difficulties. In many ways this represents the culmination of trends in social policy and service delivery that have their roots some thirty years ago.

In 1959, the Minister of Health introduced the Mental Health Act by saying: 'One of the main principles we are hoping to pursue is the reorientation of the mental health services, away from hospital care and towards community care.' In fact, hospital inpatient numbers had begun to fall a few years earlier, in 1954, when they reached 148 000 (Busfield, 1986). Social service departments did not themselves come into existence until 1968, when as a result of the Seebohm Report the previously disparate and specialist social work groupings were amalgamated under one corporate roof. The 1989 White Paper *Caring For People* (DOH, 1989) designated local authorities with the lead responsibilty for '. . . assessing individual need, designing care arrangements and securing their delivery within available resources'. As we enter the 1990s, it is these still relatively new organizations that will become the cornerstone for community care. By the same token, care management will therefore be the dominant framework through which community care for the mentally ill will be delivered. This chapter will attempt to:

1. Give a brief overview of the antecedents in policy and practice which have culminated in the new community care reforms.

2. Describe the main constituent elements of care management.
3. Critically review the opportunities and risks that care management presents.

ANTECEDENTS

A decade and a half on from the 1959 Mental Health Act, a Labour government produced a report on the progress made towards establishing community care for the mentally ill. Four main policy objectives were outlined:

1. Local authority social services departments were to expand their provision of residential, day care and domiciliary support.
2. Specialist services were to be relocated in local settings, either at the district general hospital (DGH) or through the build-up of community facilities that provided a DGH-type facility.
3. The establishment of better links between the different agencies involved in delivering services to mentally ill clients.
4. A significant improvement in the staffing of services for the mentally ill.

The report had to admit that there had been failures as well as successes. Though hospital overcrowding had been reduced and inpatient numbers had fallen (to 94 000 by 1972), not a single hospital had actually been closed and community facilities would need to be built up from 'their present minimal level.' There was a depressing conclusion that: 'there is little hope of the kind of service we would ideally like even within a twenty five year planning cycle'. This is a tacit admission that the oil pricing revolution carried out by the organization of petroleum exporting countries (OPEC), three years earlier had drastically undermined the government's confidence that public funding could in fact produce the kind of service it envisaged. Its assumption that local authority social services should be the main providers of such care was intact; its confidence that these services could be delivered was in shreds.

A critical turning point for future developments in community care commenced with the Conservative party's election victory in 1979. In this area of public policy, as in many others, the Conservatives entered office with a reforming zeal. They inherited a welfare state that was creaking at the seams through the expenditure cuts introduced in the latter days of the Labour government (Hills, 1991). An important part of the 'New Right' (Mishra, 1990) agenda with the Thatcher government sought to implement was a radical critique of the underlying assumptions of the welfare state they inherited on entering office. They began by questioning its basic principles of full employment, a universalist/redistributive system of welfare benefits, and comprehensive health and social services. To simplify their critique, the trouble with this was that costs were rising too steeply and in an unsupportable way, the whole system was wasteful in its use of available resources, and there was insufficient consumer choice.

A new direction for community care was soon in evidence, initially with respect to the elderly. The DHSS (1981) policy document *Growing Older* states: 'the primary sources of support and care for elderly people are informal and voluntary. These spring from the personal ties of kinship, friendship and neighbourhood. They are irreplaceable. It is the role of public authorities to sustain and, where necessary develop—but never to displace—such support and care. Care *in* the community becomes care *by* the community.' The gateposts had been changed. Care was now primarily the responsibility of the community itself; the role of the government, and therefore of the public purse, was to enable such support to occur when necessary. This residualist philosophy (Taylor-Gooby, 1991) was expounded more fully to the Conference of Directors of Social Services at Buxton in September 1984. Norman Fowler (then Secretary of State for Social Services) rejected what he called the monopolistic approach, by which local authorities provided all services. Instead, they should develop an 'enabling role'. This concept of the 'enabling authority' has proved central to the Conservative government's new approach to community care. In an influential report (*Making a Reality of Community Care*, 1986), the Audit Commission spelt out in greater detail what this actually meant: 'current arrangements with separately funded agencies requesting services from each other is unsatisfactory. A more traditional way of arranging services would be for one agency to take lead responsibility (and with it control of the budget and accountability for its appropriate use) and to "buy in" services as necessary from other agencies' (Audit Commission, 1986). The government was sufficiently intrigued by its findings and recommendations to set in motion its own response. The Deputy Chairman of the NHS Management Committee was charged with the responsibility of making a report. Sir Roy Griffiths, a business-man from Sainsbury's of impeccable Thatcherite credentials, duly obliged with a document entitled *Community Care: An Agenda for Action* (Griffiths, 1988) Sir Roy made four main recommendations:

1. The appointment of a Minister of State 'clearly and publicly identified as being responsible for community care'.
2. The transfer of all community care—for mentally ill, mentally handicapped, physically handicapped, and the frail and infirm elderly—to local authorities (in effect to social services departments).
3. The provision of earmarked grants 'amounting to say fifty per cent of the costs of an approved programme' by central government.
4. The local authority should be empowered to buy in services from other services, including hospitals, voluntary homes and the private sector (Jones, 1988). This in effect is an endorsement of the concept of the 'enabling authority' which Griffiths further spells out as follows: '. . . the responsibility of social services authorities is to ensure that . . . services are provided within appropriate budget by the public or private sector according to where they can be provided most economically and efficiently' (Griffiths, 1988).

These sweeping recommendations ran into a political minefield. The Thatcher government was simultaneously engaged in a series of battles to restrict the powers of local authorities whether through rate capping, encouraging schools to opt out, or the establishment of local authority bypass operations like the Enterprise Boards.

Nevertheless, the government's own response to the Griffiths Report (*Caring For People*, DOH, 1989) largely accepted most of its recommendations, with the exception of the request for ring-fenced funding. In particular, it accepted the Griffiths proposition that local authorities should be the lead agency for community care. At the same time, the White Paper pulled together a whole series of issues that reflected the ideological stance of the government that created it.

Six main objectives were proposed:

1. To promote the development of domiciliary, day and respite services to enable people to live in their own homes wherever feasible and sensible.
2. To ensure that service providers make practical support for carers a high priority.
3. To make proper assessment of need and good case management the cornerstone of high quality care.
4. To clarify the responsibilities of agencies and so make it easier to hold them to account for their performance.
5. To promote the development of a flourishing independent sector alongside good quality public services.
6. To secure better value for taxpayers' money by introducing a new funding structure for social care.

At the heart of these proposals is a reconstructed role for social service departments, and by implication, for the social worker: 'The Government has accepted Sir Roy's recommendation that social services should be "enabling" agencies. It will be their responsibility to make maximum possible use of private and voluntary providers, and so increase the available range of options and widen consumer choice.' Cost containment, value for money and the efficient use of available resources are of course emphasized. However, what is particularly striking about these objectives is that they highlight, for want of a better phrase, a process of community deinstitutionalization. People are to be encouraged, and supported, to live in their own homes according to their own expressed preferences. The community infrastructure of formal day and residential care services are to be a secondary port of call. People are not simply to be plugged in to whatever services are locally available. On the contrary, assessment of individual need should come first, and should be the driving force and catalyst of community care. Care management can best be understood as the organizational mechanism designed to carry out these objectives. With the passing of the NHS and Community Care Act (1990), these White Paper proposals are now a legislative requirement.

However, before going into further details concerning what care management is and how it works, it is worth asking a pertinent question: are the enormous organizational upheavals that are involved justified: Is the government correct in its original analysis, namely that community care costs were soaring in an unmanageable way, that service coordination was ineffective and inefficient, and that there was inadequate consumer choice?

Costs

So far as the costs of community care are concerned, the evidence is mixed. As Table 1 illustrates, there has been an overall real increase of 11.5% in expenditure on aggregated hospital and community mental health services comparing 1978/79 levels to 1987/88. However, expenditure on hospital inpatient services has increased 7% in real terms from 1978 to 1987/88, despite a drop in patient numbers from 77 297 in 1979 to 56 200 in 1989. Consequently the efficiency of mental hospital expenditure has decreased dramatically over the decade; inpatient costs have risen by 47% over this period of time, from £15 255 per patient in 1979, to £22 468 in 1989. Even more significantly, the overall distribution of expenditure between hospital and community care has remained more or less constant over the decade. In 1978/79, social services mental health expenditure of £36 million accounted for 2.7% of the total budget of £1341 million. In 1987/88, social services had increased their expenditure to £58 million. However, this still accounted for only 3.8% of the total budget, the remaining £1439 million being spent by health authorities (House of Commons Social Service Committee Report, 1990). The evidence for soaring and unmanageable costs in terms of direct budgetary provision is not compelling. The major and severe problem here is the dispro-portionately high expenditure on health authority mental hospital based care, despite a 28% decline of inpatient numbers. Overall social services expenditure itself only increased at a rate of 2.5% per annum throughout the 1980s, a rate which hardly seems excessive (Evandrou, 1990).

The area that has seen a dramatic increase has been social security board and lodging payments. Until the end of the 1970s, board and lodging payments were an insignificant part of the budget of the Supplementary Benefit system. In 1978/79 the cost was £6 million. Two years later this had doubled and it doubled again over the next two years (Land, 1991). During 1983 the cost rose even faster, increasing by £100 million in that year alone (Audit Commission, 1986). By 1987 the figure had reached £489 million and by May 1990, £1 billion (including nursing home care). Throughout the

Table 1 Health, social services mental illness expenditure 1979–89 (£m) (adjusted for real prices)

	78/79	79/80	80/81	81/82	82/83	83/84	84/85	85/86	86/87	87/88	% charge
Inpatient	1179	1186	1205	1222	1216	1211	1214	1202	1197	1267	7%
Outpatient	64	64	64	75	81	81	84	87	86	74	6%
Day Patient	62	61	70	76	77	85	88	93	95	98	72%
Total	1305	1311	1339	1373	1374	1377	1386	1382	1378	1439	10%
SSD Residential	22	24	25	24	25	26	26	25	25	30	37%
SSD Day Care	14	15	16	16	19	21	22	22	25	27	95%
Total	36	39	41	40	44	47	48	47	50	57	58%
	1341	1350	1380	1413	1418	1424	1434	1429	1428	1496	11.5%

From: Social Services Committee (1990).

1980s, social services departments had been suffering financial penalties in terms of reductions in Department of the Environment grants for developing the community services that the Department of Health was keen to encourage. Not unnaturally, off loading direct residential care costs from their budgets, and onto that of the Department of Social Security, seemed like an attractive option. Consequently the 1980s saw a significant drop in the number of local authority sponsored residents in private and voluntary homes; at the same time the overall numbers of clients using these facilities increased significantly (Evandrou, 1990). The government, however, could be forgiven for considering such rapid increases as a threat to their strategy of cost containment. One of the attractions of care management from the government's perspective is that it offers a solution to this problem—the social security subsidy element of care costs are transferred to social services departments, but within the framework of an annual cash-limited budget. In this way, the Department of Social Security (DSS) is prevented from offering an open chequebook to community care.

Coordination

What of the issue of poor service integration and coordination? Are things really as bad as all that? The often quoted Audit Commission (1986) is in no doubt in this matter.

> Unfortunately, the present community care management arrangements do not promote the essential integrated service and operation planning. In particular:
> 1. The structure of local community-based services is confused, with responsibility and accountability for elements of the services fragmented between tiers of the NHS and within local government.
> 2. As a result, the joint planning arrangements need to be complex and are particularly time consuming to operate to ensure adequate liaison between all the various interests involved.
> 3. The difficulties posed by the confused structure and complex planning arrangements are compounded by the lack of incentives and differences in the organization styles of the different agencies concerned.
>
> Each of these problems might be solvable in isolation; but, together, they have combined to make it extraordinarily difficult to manage the transition to community-based care at the local level.

Client-centred approach

What of the third issue highlighted by the government: consumer choice? Because of the patchiness and relative scarcity of community care resources in many areas, it must be conceded that there is often very little on offer in terms of consumer choice. The more common situation is of a considerable shortfall in basic community provision. Because of this, it is very difficult to argue that individual and distinctive needs are taken into account. More often than not, clients are plugged in to what is locally available, whether or not it is especially relevant to their particular needs and circumstances. This is certainly the conclusion of a recent report, which examined the assessment systems of four social services departments (DOH, 1991):

Assessment arrangements were:

a) service-led rather than needs-based
b) separate for each service, preventing the holistic assessment of needs
c) not clearly separated from service provision
d) not clearly differentiated by type or level
e) based on the assumption that services would be provided by the statutory sector
f) not promoting the active participation of users and carers
g) not monitored against specific quality standards

In conclusion, there does appear to be evidence that board and lodging costs in particular have greatly increased over recent years, that community care services are indeed poorly coordinated, and that for a variety of reasons there is very little consumer choice. There *is* a case for change, a case moreover that has been very widely accepted. In this context, it is easy to understand the interest shown in case management by the 1989 White Paper. Here was an approach to community care that 'provides an effective method of targeting resources and planning services to meet specific needs of individual clients.' (DOH, 1989, 3.3.3) Moreover, it had been successfully developed in the UK with respect to work with the frail elderly (Challis and Davies, 1986; Davies and Challis, 1986). Yet almost immediately, a major complication arose, in the sense that two widely different interpretations of the term were utilized (Challis, 1992). In one part of the White Paper (3.3.2) there is clear recognition that case management had been developed to work intensively with small caseloads of especially vulnerable people: 'Where an individuals care needs are complex or significant levels of resource are involved, the Government sees considerable merit in nominating a "case manager" to take responsibility for ensuring that individuals' needs are regularly reviewed, resources are managed effectively, and that each service user has a single point of contact.'

However, in the very next paragraph, the White Paper takes what essentially amounts to a leap in the dark: 'The Government believes that the wider introduction of the key principles of case management would confer considerable benefit, and will seek to encourage their application more widely' (3.3.3). In other words, the major institutional vehicle for community care, the social services department, is to be based upon the principles of case management. Certainly so far as the UK is concerned, knowledge concerning the validity and effectiveness of case management is based upon its application in teams working intensively with relatively small numbers of highly vulnerable individuals (Davies and Challis, 1986). In this sense, care management represents a major national experiment. Nobody knows yet whether these same principles can be applied across the board in large complex bureaucracies.

THE ELEMENTS OF CARE MANAGEMENT

By the time the 1990 policy guidance was published, the term case management had been dropped from official usage, on the basis that it was demeaning and stigmatic to clients. It was replaced by the term care management, which has tended to refer to the second application mentioned above, namely the design of whole, complex organizational systems rather than small intensive teams. The basic elements of care management are succinctly described in the White Paper itself:

> In future, Social Service Departments will have the following key responsibilities:
>
> * carrying out an appropriate assessment of an individual's need for social care (including residential and nursing home care), in

collaboration as necessary with medical, nursing and other caring
agencies, before deciding what services should be provided;
* designing packages of services tailored to meet the assessed needs
of individuals and their carers;
* securing the delivery of services, not simply by acting as direct
providers, but by developing their purchasing and contracting role
to become 'enabling authorities';
* establishing procedures for receiving comments and complaints
from service users;
* monitoring the quality and cost-effectiveness of services, with
medical and nursing advice as appropriate;
* establishing arrangements for assessing the client's ability to
contribute to the full economic cost to the local authority of
residential services. (DOH, 1989, 3.1.3)

Over the ensuing two years, a series of policy guidance documents
have flowed from the Social Services Inspectorate (DOH/SSI, 1990,
1991a, 1991b). The task of the SSI has been to advise how the
general principles expounded in the White Paper and the NHS and
Community Care Act 1990 can be turned into operational reality.

In order to turn social service departments into 'enabling
authorities', the SSI is requiring them to undertake a purchaser–
provider split:

Care Management is based on a needs-led approach which has two
key aspects:

* a progressive separation of the tasks of assessment from those of
service provision in order to focus on needs, where possible having
the tasks carried out by separate staff;
* a shift of influence from those providing to those purchasing
services. (DOH/SSI, 1990)

The guidance goes on to specify a new purchaser role within social
services, that of the Care Manager: 'Care Managers should in effect
act as brokers for services across the statutory and independent
sectors. They should not therefore be involved in direct service
delivery; nor should they normally carry managerial responsibility
for the services they arrange ... Care Managers should be able to
assume some or all of the responsibility for purchasing the services
necessary for implementing a care plan.' (DOH/SSI, 1990, 3.10)

About a year later, two more volumes of guidance emerged from
the SSI, one a managers' and the other a practitioners' guide to

the new reforms. The Practitioners' guidance (1991) has usefully conceptualized care management into seven sequential core tasks:

Stage 1: Publishing information
Making public the needs for which assistance is offered and the arrangements and resources for meeting those needs.

Stage 2: Determining the level of assessment
Making an initial identification of need and matching the appropriate level of assessment to that need.

Stage 3: Assessing need
Understanding individual needs, relating them to agency policies and priorities, and agreeing the objectives for any intervention.

Stage 4: Care planning
Negotiating the most appropriate ways of achieving the objectives identified by the assessment of need and incorporating them into an individual care plan.

Stage 5: Implementing the care plan
Securing the necessary resources or services.

Stage 6: Monitoring
Supporting and controlling the delivery of the care plan on a continuing basis.

Stage 7: Reviewing
Reassessing needs and the service outcomes with a view to revising the care plan at specified intervals.

Inherent within the first two stages is the important issue of gate-keeping: defining the targeted client group and determining who gets access to what level of resource. The guidance suggests six discrete levels of assessment, ranging from simple to complex and comprehensive. It is likely that resources that are either specialist or expensive or both will only be available once their justification has been proven through carrying out a comprehensive or complex assessment. Local authorities will also have to devise a charging policy, in order to clarify how much clients will have to pay for what kind of service.

CONCLUSIONS

There is no doubt that the care management reforms are a bold and radical break with the past. They represent a 'brave new world' for the future of community care. However, it may be recollected that Aldous Huxley's vision of the future turned out to be a dystopia rather than a utopia. Changes as fundamental as those which are proposed inevitably carry with them some risks. These attendant risks will be discussed under three headings.

1. The role of the care manager

The single most controversial aspect of the care management proposals is the separation of assessment from provision of services. This does of course have the backing of legislation; Section 47 of the NHS and Community Care Act 1990 places an explicit duty on local authorities to carry out an assessment before providing services.

There is an excellent case to be made in favour of the principle of progressive separation, well made by the guidance itself:

> Care management and assessment constitute one integrated process for identifying and addressing the needs of individuals within available resources, recognising that those needs are unique to the individuals concerned. For this reason, care management and assessment emphasise adapting services to needs rather than fitting people into existing services, and dealing with the needs of people as a whole rather than assessing needs separately for different services ... If services are to be made more responsive, it is necessary to identify the disparity between assessed needs and currently available services. This is most effectively achieved where the responsibility for assessing need is separated from that of delivering or managing services (DOH/SSI, 1991, 3/5, Managers' Guide).

The principle of separation does, however, imply a major restructuring of social services departments, and consequently a major restructuring of the role of the social worker. The role of the care manager will be in the forefront of these changes. It is the care manager who will be responsible for assessing individual need, developing a care plan, purchasing the ensuing package of care, and monitoring its delivery. For many social workers, becoming a care manager will require them to wean themselves away from providing the direct work with clients they were previously doing. There is an obvious dilemma here. The separation of assessment enables due weight to be given to a client-centred, needs-led approach. On the other hand, by detaching care managers from direct ongoing provision, there is a risk that they will become excessively distanced from the client. There is also a risk to the client, in that the person who controls resources essential for their survival in the community does not directly know them or their circumstances especially well, and therefore is not someone they can easily turn to when in difficulties. Key workers may well know them better, but through being on the provider side of the split will have no access to controlling resources.

The most recent guidance on this matter (DOH/SSI, 1991) has been flexible. It makes the useful general point that: 'Separation has to be done in such a way as to recognise the interdependence of assessment and service provision. Assessment must remain rooted in an appreciation of the realities of service provision, and services must be sensitive to the changing needs of recipients' (DOH/SSI, 1991, 23). It goes on to acknowledge that it may in fact not be sensible to entirely separate the care manager from one kind of ongoing direct work with the client: '. . . it is not intended that distinguishing assessment from provision should result in a rigid or doctrinaire separation that sacrifices organisational strengths . . . The counselling component of assessment may be carried over into the subsequent monitoring and reviewing phases, but where it shades into a therapeutic intervention in its own right, for example, family therapy, it should be regarded as a service to be provided by a different practitioner' (DOH/SSI, 1991, 1.12/13). The guidance goes on to outline nine different models of care management (DOH/SSI, 1991, 2.40), one of which explicitly recognizes the possibility of continuous ongoing direct work with the client (model 8). The major lesson to be drawn from this most recent guidance is that it encourages flexibility in applying care management to local conditions, and a sensitivity to the particular needs of particular groups of clients.

The role of the care manager is a particularly critical issue for people experiencing long-term mental health difficulties. They are often highly vulnerable people who may experience considerable difficulties in communication. Both in cognitive and behavioural terms, they may be highly disturbed. With this client group, it makes very little sense to distinguish between engagement and assessment, or to separate either out from a limited amount of ongoing direct work such as supportive counselling or working on accommodation issues or welfare benefits. These processes tend to become intertwined, and for very good reasons. Clients are unlikely to express their worries or concerns until they have established a relationship of trust with their care manager. This may take some time. Often, a good way to establish trust is to undertake some degree of direct work as an immediate response to need. It would seem ironic and unnecessary in an approach to care that is needs-led, if meeting a particularly urgent expressed need had to wait until a further assessment was completed, and a package of care assembled and purchased.

Both the White Paper and the subsequent guidance note the importance of the principle of continuity: 'Care Management will have its greatest impact when most of the processes involved are carried out by a single care manager . . .' (DOH/SSI, 1990, 3.7). From the point of view of the client, there are considerable advantages to developing a relationship of trust with a single known care manager, who can thereby act as a 'travel companion' to the client. One of the features of the model of care management developed by Ryan and Ford (1991) is that it has enabled an ongoing, continuous relationship of trust to develop between the care manager and the client. Similarly, one of the common features of the most successful American models of care management is precisely this principle of continuity of care, mediated through a known individual or team (Stein and Test, 1980; Harris and Bergman, 1987; Rapp and Winterstein, 1989).

There are many obvious advantages to the progressive separation of assessment from provision. There are, however, risks and perhaps the most obvious one is to institutionalize discontinuity of care. Consider a worst case scenario. A vulnerable, difficult to engage client is referred for assessment. A care manager adopting an administrative, brokerage approach attempts to coordinate and collate a variety of specialist assessments, none of which are successful since the client is unable to engage with the wide variety of professionals who turn up on his door asking awkward and difficult questions. The whole process would be stymied before it got started. Or consider another scenario. A sensitive, client-centred care manager engages well with the client and carries out an effective assessment. However, because the split is rigidly adhered to in his department, he then has to rapidly withdraw into a purely monitoring role. The client is bewildered by this, and subsequently is unable to transfer his allegiance to the allocated key worker in the care package that is eventually purchased. The guidance itself cautions against 'rigid and doctrinaire' interpretations of the separation of assessment from provision. It is to be hoped that its own advice will be taken.

2. Needs-led assessment

The enormous potential advantage that care management holds out is that for the first time, needs-led assessment will lead to individually tailored care in the community. By separating out the assessment function into a new departmental purchasing structure, individual packages of care will be ensured, or so the argument goes. But is it really as simple as that? Both the 1989 White Paper, and the subsequent guidance gives messages concerning assessment that to some degree are contradictory, perhaps inevitably so. On one hand, assessment is quite unambiguously being used as a resource filter: only needs of a certain degree of severity will as it were be let into the system, and thus trigger resource allocation. On the other hand, much emphasis is laid on the importance of individuals, who moreover are encouraged to take as active a part as possible in this process. Indeed, it is upon the foundation stone of individual need that the imposing new edifice of care management is to be built. There is of course nothing new in this conflict between the institutional and individual definition of need—except that in care management this dilemma is supposed not to exist.

Both the White Paper and the guidance contain many statements that lend themselves to a client-centred interpretation of need. The White Paper states: 'The objective of assessment is to determine the best available way of helping the individual. Assessments should focus positively on what the individual can and cannot do, taking account of his or her personal and social relationships. Assessment should not focus only on the user's suitability for a particular existing service. The aim should be first to review the possibility of enabling the individual to live at home . . .' (DOH, 1989, 3.2.3). The 1990 guidance continues this theme by stating: 'The individual service user and normally, with his or her agreement, any carers should be involved throughout the assessment and care management process. They should feel that the process is aimed at meeting their wishes' (DOH/SSI, 1990, 3.16). The 1991 *Practitioners' Guidance* comments: 'Care management makes the needs and wishes of users and their carers central to the caring process. This needs-led approach aims to tailor services to individual requirements . . . It is easy to slip out of thinking "what does this person need?" into "what have we got that he/she could have?"' (DOH/SSI, 1991b, 1.19). Yet elsewhere in the same document need is defined in very different, resource-driven terms:

> Need is a dynamic concept, the definition of which will vary over time in accordance with:
>
> * changes in national legislation
> * changes in local policy
> * the availability of resources
> * the patterns of local demand
>
> Need is thus a relative concept. In the context of community care, need has to be defined at the local level. That definition sets limits to the discretion of practitioners in accessing resources (DOH/SSI, 1991b, 12/13).

This does not seem to be very far away from a resource, service-driven approach to need that would claim that a need does not exist if a service is not available to supply it. Yet it is precisely such an approach to need that care management is designed to oppose. The same section goes on to define need as: 'the requirements of individuals to enable them to achieve, maintain or restore an acceptable level of social independence or quality of life, *as defined by the particular care agency or authority*' (DOH/SSI, 1991b, 11). Care managers are later reminded that: 'Ultimately, having weighed the views of all parties, the assessing practitioner is responsible for defining the user's needs' (DOH/SSI, 1991b, 3.35).

The guidance is perhaps merely expressing a long-standing ambiguity in how 'welfare institutions' use the concept of need. The point is well expressed by Plant: 'To say that "x needs y" is not just to state a fact but is to imply, ceteris paribus, that he ought to get it' (Plant, 1974, p. 76). Care management is perhaps on the horns of an impossible dilemma. Social services departments are large, complex bureaucracies undergoing constant change, facing a variety of resource constraints, in the midst of a vortex of competing demands and priorities. Individual clients will necessarily be passed through a process of institutional filters designed to determine access to resources. Furthermore, responsibility for resource allocation decisions is explicitly controlled by the agency.

At the same time care managers are required to base the whole process of care delivery on the expressed needs of individual clients. They are to create a process in which individual clients actively participate, and where the resultant package of care is seen to emerge from the needs expressed by the client. Not an easy task!

3. The cost of community care

No one is in any doubt that adequate resources are crucial to the successful implementation of community care. The 1989 White Paper states that 'adequate resources' will be required; the current and previous Secretaries of State have given assurances that the reforms will be adequately resourced.

Three main revenue sources will be involved in funding community care; in practice doubts are justifiable as to whether any will prove sufficient. The first funding source are the board and lodging payments referred to earlier. The 1989 White Paper states: 'The Government will transfer to local authorities the resources which it would otherwise have provided to finance care through social security payments to people in residential and nursing homes.' As a result or pressure from the local authority associations the government established a joint local authority association and Department of Health working party to calculate this amount—the Algebra Group as it is colloquially called. There is little doubt about the algebra. In essence it involves projecting the amount that the DSS would have spent on the increasing numbers of people claiming income support in residential care homes, had the old system remained in place. Claimants in residential and nursing homes on 31 March 1993 will all have preserved rights—they will retain their rights to income support under the old system. The DSS will continue to pay for this group, which will, however, decline over time through death or through being discharged from care. Consequently DSS expenditure on this group will decrease. The care costs, to be transferred to local authorities, consist of the difference between the amount of money deemed to be required to pay for the care of people in residential, domiciliary or nursing home care after April 1993 and that continuing to be spent on existing claimants with preserved rights.

The Algebra Group has concluded its work, but the two sides are in profound disagreement over the amount which should be transferred. DOH officials are talking about £400 million for the first year, whilst local authorities have estimated the required amount as in excess of £1 billion (*Social Work Today*, 5–6–92). As well as the likelihood of a shortfall in transferred care costs, there are a number of elements of community care which will not in any case be covered by this amount. Most crucially, the transfer does not take account of the shortfall between benefits and actual charges for residential and nursing home care.

The second funding area to consider are the infrastructure costs for actually setting up care management as a system of care. As an example, local authorities estimate the number of new assessments required in the first year as 180 000 (*Community Care*, 12–6–92). The DOH has offered £96 million to cover these additional set up costs, which local authorities estimate at being about half the total amount required (*Social Work Today*, 5–6–92).

The third revenue area is the total grant for personal social services, 1993–94. The new system of Standard Spending Assessment (SSA) continues to attract criticism from counties, boroughs and metropolitan authorities (*Social Work Today*, 1–8–91). The Association of Directors of Social Services has pointed out that a 23% increase in the 1991–92 personal social services expenditure allocation actually resulted in over one-third of councils having to make savings, with a further 22% keeping to a standstill budget (*Social Work Today*, 1–8–91). Illustrative of the revenue pressure local authorities are under is that Nottingham Social Services is running with a £6 million cut in the current financial year, and is projecting a further £6.5 million cut in 1993–94. It is difficult to avoid the conclusion therefore that the first full year of implementing the new reforms will see the traditional conflict between demand and resources, but in a particularly virulent form.

In summary, care management carries a great weight of expectations. It has to carry out a series of complex, difficult and perhaps contradictory tasks. It will have to contain the rising costs of community care, and optimize the efficient use of available resources through more effective coordination. These tasks are essentially the function of a brokerage approach to community care.

At the same time, the whole system is required to operate on a needs-led, client-centred basis. Is client-centred brokerage feasible? Only time will tell.

REFERENCES

Audit Commission (1986) *Making a Reality of Community Care.* HMSO, London.
Busfield, J. (1986) *Managing Madness—Changing Ideas and Practice.* Unwin, London.
Challis, D. (1992) The state of the art. In: *Case Management: Issues in Practice* (S. Onyett and P. Cambridge eds.) University of Kent.
Davies, B. and Challis, D. (1986) *Matching Resources to Needs in Community Care.* Gower, Aldershot.
DHSS (1981) Growing Older.
DOH (1981) L.A. Survey.
DOH (1989) *Caring for People: Community Care in the Next Decade and Beyond.* (Cmnd 849). HMSO, London.
DOH/SSI (1990) *Implementing Community Care.* HMSO, London.
DOH/SSI (1991a) *Care Management and Assessment: Managers' Guide.* HMSO, London.
DOH/SSI (1991b) *Care Management and Assessment: Practitioners' Guide.* HMSO, London.
Evandrou, M. (1991) The personal social services. In *The State of Welfare* (J. Hills ed.), Oxford.
Griffiths, R. (1988) *Community Care: An Agenda for Action.* HMSO, London.
Harris, M. and Bergman, A.C. (1987) Case management with the long term mentally ill. *Am J Orthopsychiatry* **52**, 2 April.
Hills, J. (ed.) (1991) *The State of Welfare*, Oxford.
Jones, K. (1988) *Experience in Mental Health: Community Care and Social Policy*, Sage, London.
Land, H. (1991) The confused boundaries of community care. In *The Sociology of the Health Service* (J. Gabe, M. Calnan, and M. Bury, eds.). Routledge, London.
Mishra, R. (1990) *The Welfare State in Capitalist Society*. Harvester, London.

Plant, R. (1974) *Community and Ideology*. Routledge, London.

Rapp, C. and Winterstein, R. (1989) The strengths model of case management. *Journal of Psychosocial Rehabilitation* **13**, 1.

Robertson, G. and Fimister, G. (1992) Adding up and taking away. *Community Care*, 12 June.

Ryan, P.J. and Ford, R. (1991) *Case Management and Community Care*. RDP, London.

Stein, L. and Test, M.A. (1980) Alternative to mental hospital treatment. *Archives of General Psychiatry* **37**, 392–397.

Taylor-Gooby, P. (1991) *Social Change, Social Welfare, and Social Science*. Harvester, London.

6 A CHANGING PROFESSION: THE ROLE OF NURSING IN HOME CARE

G. McNamee

This chapter will explore the origins of the nurse in the community, describe the community nurse's role with specific reference to particular programmes and discuss potential future developments. The term 'community psychiatric nurse' (CPN) will be used to denote nurses working in the community as this is the most frequently applied title given to psychiatric nurses in community settings. Similarly in keeping with current practice, the term 'client' will be used to denote any individual under the care of a CPN.

HISTORICAL ORIGINS

The move from hospital to community based nursing of the mentally ill has been the result of many factors: the breakthrough in treatment of the seriously ill with the advent of chlorpromazine and other neuroleptics, the 1959 Mental Health Act, which placed a strong emphasis on community involvement in psychiatric care services, the 1970 Local Authority Social Services Act, which replaced psychiatric social workers with generic workers, the 1974 NHS reorganization and a general change in attitudes towards non-institutional care of persons with mental health difficulties.

The first account of psychiatric nurses working in the community is that of May and Moore (1963). They described the working of two nurses seconded from Warlingham Park Hospital in 1954 to see ex-clients in the Croydon community.

The two 'out-patient' nurses, as they were called (this number later rising to four), were employed, on a part-time basis, to provide a follow-up service to individuals principally suffering from schizophrenia or depression. Their role was to monitor compliance with medication, assess mental state, monitor difficulties in personal habits and care (and where possible remedy these) and reassure relatives. They also inquired into the failure of clients to attend clinic appointments. A nurse also attended outpatient clinics, evening aftercare groups for long-term clients and evening social groups. Each nurse had a 'ward' of clients, these clients being discussed at a weekly 'ward' round. The nurse's role was clinical, and investigation of the client's or family's environmental or social needs was not expected (this being a key difference from the role of the psychiatric social worker). The inadequacy of part-time work was recognized and within a year the nurses were working full-time in the community.

In 1957 a community nursing service was established from Moorhaven Hospital. The 'Nursing After-Care' service, as it was known, differed from its counterpart in Croydon in that nurses had a continuing role working in the hospital as well as with clients who had been discharged. The CPN's were expected to form a relation-ship with the client, and by utilizing this relationship, become a therapeutic agent in their own right by evidencing care and support for the client and facilitating change (Hunter, 1974). This develop-ment of the nursing role was also undertaken to enhance the status of nursing at this time.

THE DEVELOPING ROLE OF THE CPN

Hunter (1974) outlines the composite functions of CPNs up to the late 1960s. The nurse would assist the client and family in practical matters such as bathing and shaving. He/she would give advice, support and supervision particularly with respect to medication, and monitor side effects and cooperate with general practitioners and psychiatrists in the amelioration of these. The CPN would be the link between client and hospital to facilitate easy access to hospital in the event of relapse. They would provide continuity of care for a designated group of clients: those suffering from schizophrenia, recurrent depression and organic psychosis. They provided a preventative function to clients not requiring treatment in hospital or clinic. The CPN would supervise the outpatient clinic and enquire into non-attendances. They would also assist in the running of social clubs and other group work. Finally, the CPN would assist the client in gaining accommodation and employment.

The loss of specialist social workers working with clients with mental health difficulties, following the Local Authority Social Services Act 1970, caused much concern among those involved in the provision of community services for the mentally ill. Several authors (Leopold, 1973; Royal Medico-Psychological Association, 1969) concluded that another body of workers was required to fill the social and rehabilitative role vacated by social workers. There was general agreement that CPNs were the group most suited to this.

Consequently, the CPN role continued to develop, with nurses offering continuing care, crisis intervention, group work, psychotherapy, care of the elderly mentally ill and behaviour therapy services (Hunter, 1974).

Community psychiatric nursing services continued to develop, piecemeal, throughout the 1960s and 1970s. The 1966 Royal College of Nursing survey showed 42 hospitals employing 225 nurses, albeit the majority part-time. By 1980 only six health authorities had no CPN service in operation, and there were 1667 CPNs employed nationwide. By 1985 this number had passed 2800 (Simmons and Brooker, 1986), and there has been a further doubling since then. A key influence on the growth of CPN services has been the planned closure of the large pyschiatric institutions and their replacement by smaller units attached to local district hospitals, and the development of day hospitals and community care facilities. Parnell (1977) carried out an intensive study of CPN services, and found that while they were well established, they were of variable quality and operated in different ways.

CPNs as seen above were principally hospital based. They worked within hospital treatment teams and operated a 'closed referral' system with all referrals coming from the hospital consultants. They saw their clients at home or in clinics, and carried out care programmes which were heavily biased towards the medical model.

However, the development of CPN attachment to general practice in Oxford in the early 1970s led to substantive changes in the CPN role. The CPN became a much more independent practitioner, with responsibility for the assessing of clients' needs, developing supportive relationships with clients and significant others, and often responsible for the planning and implementing of an appropriate care package. The placement of CPNs in primary settings increased. Thus, the 'open referral' system became common, with CPNs accepting referrals from many sources, including each other, and by the late 1970s this referral process had become well established.

CPNs began to develop more autonomous roles and became increasingly specialized during the 1970s. Growth in crisis intervention and elderly care services was seen. This development mirrored the increasing specialization of the CPN's medical colleagues, and indeed was in some cases the result of forcible argument by psychiatrists. A case in point was the development of training for nurses in behaviour therapy by Professor Isaac Marks at the Maudsley Hospital in 1972 (Simmons and Brooker, 1986). This has led to the English National Board (ENB) course 650—'Short-term Adult Behavioural Psychotherapy' and CPNs specializing in this area accounted for almost 5% of all community specialists in 1985 (CPNA, 1985). The care of the elderly mentally ill accounted for the greatest area of specialization of CPN work, with 64% of all specialist CPNs working in this area in 1985.

THE CPN BASE

The role of the CPN and the client make-up of CPN caseloads was to a large extent dictated by the working base of the CPN. As we have seen, the development of CPNs was rapid and in most cases the result of local preference. Initially CPNs were hospital based and only later were they attached to general practice or community facilities, such as community mental health centres. Skidmore and Friend (1984) found that there were major differences in the source of referrals depending on CPN base. Primary based CPNs received significantly more referrals from non-medical sources than did hospital based workers. Brooker and Simmons (1985) found base of CPN also had an important impact on the type of client referred.

This factor is most important if we reflect on the concerns of Goldberg (1985), among others, that with a shift in the base of the CPN there is a risk of shift in clients cared for: 'as CPNs drift away from the hospital based service there is a risk that care of the chronic psychotic patients will take second place to work with people with minor affective disorders.' Wooff and colleagues (1988) found that CPNs in Salford were less likely to be involved with the care of schizophrenic clients than were their social work colleagues, and where these were involved with schizophrenic clients the CPNs saw their role as one of maintenance rather than promoting change. It was also noted that CPNs who had undergone post basic community training did not differ in their practice from their untrained colleagues.

It is of interest, if indeed not of worry, that the above concern has been reiterated by Muijen (1990) in an unpublished report detailing service and outcomes of a generic CPN team relating mainly to primary care services in South London. The issue of 'which is best' remains unresolved, but it is of no less concern today, given recent criticisms of community care and allegations of neglect of the seriously and chronically ill.

THE CPN AT WORK

We have already looked at the developing role of the CPN, from the first service through to recognition that CPNs are an integral part of any community service for persons with mental health difficulties. Let us now detail the functions of the CPN at this time.

Carr *et al.* (1980) outlined the role of the CPN as having the following components:

1. A consultant giving advice to other professionals.
2. A clinician carrying out various nursing interventions as appropriate to client need.
3. A therapist employing therapeutic procedures as part of the nursing intervention.
4. An assessor of need and evaluator of the effectiveness of the interventions.
5. An educator of others about the client's problems and needs.
6. A manager of communication networks in the community.

Barratt (1989) found CPNs showed differences in their perceived work functions depending on the referral source of the clients. However, there was broad agreement on the main roles that the CPNs reported. Assessment of clients (needs) was the most mentioned function. Other roles included prevention, counselling, medication, physical care, education, advice, specialist therapies, reassurance/support, monitoring and evaluation.

Where CPNs mentioned their role in physical care, they appeared to do so in the context of assistance with activities of daily living; bathing, clothing, cooking, shopping and budgeting, and the like. Barratt found that the self-reported role of the CPNs was (at least in part) dictated by the conceptual model of care they aligned themselves with.

Lally (1989) describes, briefly, the typical working week of the generic CPN. This involves such diverse roles as offering time limited counselling to persons with adjustment disorders, to providing long-term support to those with chronic psychiatric need. She recognizes that while CPNs have in common the process of assessment, planning, implementation and evaluation in their work, the tools employed by the CPN will vary widely according to the skills and theoretical orientation of the nurse.

Pollock (1988) looked at the process of community nursing, in her study of hospital based CPNs in Scotland.

The CPNs gave as their key philosophy the provision of individualized care, and emphasized that this concept was at the heart of their practice. This involved 'getting to know the patients' and their carers, and served as the data gathering or assessment phase of their care. It also served to give recognition to the fact that the CPN is less in control of the situation in a community setting than is the nurse practising in hospital. In addition to developing a relationship with the client, the CPNs expressed the need to evidence their caring for the client. This 'showing they cared' not only gave legitimacy to the CPN's role, but also facilitated their crisis management, initial treatment and preventative (of hospital admissions) roles. Another component in the 'individualized care' practice of the CPNs was that of promoting independence.

However, Pollock found that contrary to their stated belief in offering care tailored to the individual needs of clients and their carers, CPNs also practised according to available resources. Her data suggested that CPNs did not in fact respond to needs as expressed by the clients or carers, but rather they responded to those needs to which the nurse had an available resource as solution.

She also found that contrary to the CPNs' declarations of being independent and autonomous practitioners, they more often than not sought agreement from peers and other professionals, before undertaking any particular course of action.

She concluded that it was local needs, and the local constraints on meeting those needs, which determined the practice of the CPN. She also found that these very constraints, coupled with the CPNs' 'check first, act later' practice led to the provision of a service which was remarkably uniform and consistent.

Simmons reported on work by Paykel and Griffith (1983) in which clients stated a preference for contact with CPNs rather than with psychiatrists on an outpatient basis. It appears that it is the CPNs' wish to 'get to know' and to 'show they care' for the client which heightens this preference by clients for CPN contact. They also commented that nurses appeared to offer more information to clients and carers than did psychiatrists.

CPNs, of course, work not only with their clients and carers. They provide an interface between the client and the myriad organizations and bureaucracies with which the client must come into contact. The CPN advocates on the client's behalf with such departments as housing, social services, benefits as well as health. Liaison with GPs, health visitors, inpatient services among others is integral to the role of the CPN. Some aspects of the CPN's work appear similar to that of the care manager (see also Chapter 5).

It would appear then that in spite of inadequacies in training available to CPNs and the limited resources facing them in their day-to-day working, CPNs generally succeed in meeting some of the requirements of each of the components outlined by Carr (1980) in his determining of CPN practice.

CPNs AND HOME CARE

Let us now look at a specific community care programme to determine the multiple and adapting roles, and the nature of the experience, of the nurse in home care.

The Daily Living Program was established in October 1987, as part of a Department of Health funded research programme to determine the efficacy of comprehensive community based care for the seriously ill as compared to the hospital based care. The study and outcomes have been described elsewhere (Muijen *et al.*, 1992). Rather, some of the experiences of the nurses working in this innovative programme will be described. Some of the description overlaps with Chapter 3, which refers to the same service, but from a psychiatric perspective.

The nurses on the programme (henceforth referred to as CPNs for simplicity), were the largest professional sub-group of the team, accounting for 7 of the 10 clinical personnel on the team. They comprised 1 senior nurse manager, 3 charge II nurses and 3 staff nurses, on regrading (1988–89) (1 Clinical Nurse Manager Grade I, 3 Senior Community Nurses Grade G and 3 Community Nurses Grade F). There was a very poor response to the initial recruitment drive, with only as many nurses applying as there were posts to be filled. However, as posts were vacated over time, there was an increase in applicant numbers.

The previous experience of the nurses varied in depth and range. While some had wide previous experience in community and acute settings, others had only recently qualified and had only slight experience in community settings.

The nurse manager, whilst having good research and specialist clinical experience as a behaviour therapist, had no experience in leading a team. The nurses as a group were relatively inexperienced in community working, and this combined with the managerial inexperience of the nurse manager accounted for some of the difficulties experienced which are described below.

The CPNs in the team, in common with their colleagues from other disciplines, sought to offer to their clients care, in a way which would 'maximise their functioning in their natural environment with minimum dependence on services' (Muijen *et al.*, 1992). The CPN acted, within the team, as case manager/key worker for individual clients, with shared working of cases being encouraged. CPNs, on rotation, served as duty workers for the team, and with the psychiatrist carried out the initial assessments of new clients being referred to the programme. The CPN thereafter was responsible for carrying out, with colleagues, a detailed assessment, and for formulating, with the client, problem and target statements which were to form the basis of a problem-oriented care plan.

Herein lay the first of the difficulties mentioned above. While the

CPNs shared a common wish to provide a quality community based service, there was, for some time, no real agreement on a central philosophy or model of care. Some CPNs rejected the problem-oriented approach as being too mechanistic and denying of the individuality of the client.

This highlighted the poor understanding of the concepts by the CPNs, not surprising given the lack of adequate induction and training at the commencement of the programme. It also illustrated the managerial/leadership inexperience of the nurse manager who had difficulty enabling the CPNs to adapt to this novel (for many of them) approach.

One consequence of this lack of agreed philosophy was a wide variation in the quality of assessment and care plan documentation, and a feeling among some CPNs that the team meetings (at which this documented data was presented for care planning purposes) were irrelevant to the 'real work'.

Nevertheless, over time there developed a systematic approach to care planning, with nurses becoming adept at presenting their clients in a clear and informative manner. The maintaining of ratings of problem severity and target achievement allowed the team to discuss the relative merits of different interventions and to promote those interventions most likely to result in positive outcome for the client.

The CPNs as key workers to specific clients, and as co-workers in the care of other clients, faced a multitude of problem areas of which they had no previous experience, but which required their input. Because of the socio-economic setting of the programme, the problems facing clients and consequently the nurses, required much ongoing discussion and negotiation with many agencies, such as housing departments, local DSS offices, social services, police and court services among others. While this intensive advocacy with and on behalf of clients was to prove initially quite stressful, it became one of the most rewarding elements of the nursing role. Indeed so successful were the nurses in this area, that other service users, to whom the programme had no responsibility, often called the staff office because they 'had heard that you . . . (the nurses) . . . can get me a flat/money/job'. This advocacy role of the CPN expanded to include the needs of significant others in the lives of clients.

Because of the nature of the mental health and related problems faced by programme clients, the team CPNs developed closer and more intensive alliances with clients than had been their earlier experiences. CPNs were involved in all areas of the client's life, and were frequently known to family and friends. This close relationship between nurse and client was double-edged. On the positive note, it ensured continuity of care over extended periods of time, allowing for a consistent approach to the client and a clear and consistent source of information to the team. The negative aspects were the real risk of fostering dependency among clients, and burnout among nurses. This was particularly so when there appeared to be little or no positive change in the clients' circumstances, with individual nurses feeling impotent and devalued. This was at least in part offset by co-working with different clients, by careful monitoring of incremental changes, and in some cases, by rotating of case manager/key worker responsibilities.

One area which highlighted the changed nature of the nurse–client relationship was suicide. There were three deaths by suicide in the programme.

The response of the nurses who had been key workers for the clients was so similar as to indicate that the impact on the nurses of their client's death was largely due to the nurse–client relationship generally rather than the specific individuals in each case. The nurses reported feelings of guilt, loss and anger, far in excess of that previously experienced by them when faced with suicide at other times in their working lives. The experience of the nurses was more akin to that usually reported on the loss of a friend, or significant other. Paradoxically it was another negative experience which helped some nurses in finally recognizing that the suicides were another unfortunate aspect of their work rather than something for which they might in any way have been, in part, responsible.

Some time after the last of the suicides, there was intensive media coverage of the programme, little of it favourable. It was widely thought that this flurry of attention had been sparked off at the prompting of a fellow mental health professional in the parent hospital. There then followed a call for an enquiry into the tragedies, which further heightened the anxieties of the team. The outcome of this inquiry, however, was to fully exonerate the team, and mention was made of the commitment and enthusiasm of the clinical team.

It is worth noting that this perceived attack, and the perception that the programme was somewhat out on a limb, and isolated from (and at times unsupported by) the larger institution, resulted in the development of a team spirit best described as 'an esprit de corps'.

This team spirit went a long way to enhancing the positive features of the team's working, and lessening the impact of some of the problems discussed earlier.

While the nurses in the programme had negative as well as positive experiences, they did, in time, with their colleagues, develop into a closely knit group, confident and competent in their roles. They, as a matter of course, undertook roles, for which their earlier experience and training had not equipped them, and which they learnt, by hard experience, 'on the job'.

The experience of the CPNs emphasizes the need for training which aims at skills acquisition appropriate to community care of the seriously mentally ill. Similarly there was demonstrated a clear need for unambiguous statments of care philosophy, and clear definition of role function and expectation. To prevent feelings of isolation and reduce risk of burn-out, clear support from managers and senior clinicians is required. Ongoing and adequate supervision and personal development will ensure that the individual CPNs are clear about their role and provide a safety net. Clear operational policies which are regularly updated can provide a working tool offering guidance and clarification to the CPN. Good management and sound clinical leadership can ensure the development and maintenance of a strong working culture providing support and security for CPNs who otherwise would be prone to isolation and stress with risk of burn-out.

SUMMARY

We have seen the development of the practice of nursing in non-hospital settings from those early Warlingham Park nurses in 1954. The role of nursing in home care has expanded in ways which could not have been envisaged by earlier practitioners. The CPN is now accepted and respected as a vital member of community based services throughout the UK.

However, problems remain with regard to how community based psychiatric nursing might be best practised. It has been argued that while the development of the multi-function CPN might be appealing to the profession, it is potentially at the expense of the seriously and chronically ill, a view expressed by others. The argument of specialist versus generalist, independent worker versus multidisciplinary worker remains with us. It may well be that it will remain unresolved.

The training of nurses in the skills required in community services is of paramount importance. Plans are underway to develop such training, and these initiatives must be supported if CPNs are to adequately meet the needs of clients.

Existing syllabi of training in community nursing need revision, access to training must be opened up to wider numbers of nurses, and all courses must be properly evaluated.

Nursing in home care has come a long way in a relatively short time. From humble beginnings, community psychiatric nursing is now at the forefront of nursing practice and developments. Further changes in the nursing role are inevitable. It is for nurses, in close working with their multidisciplinary colleagues, to determine how nursing reacts to these changes.

REFERENCES

Barratt, E. (1989) Community psychiatric nurses; their self-perceived roles. *Journal of Advanced Nursing*, **14**, 42–48.

Brooker, C. and Simmons, S. (1985). A study to compare two models of community psychiatric nursing care delivery. *Journal of Advanced Nursing*, **10**, 783–792.

Carr, P.J., Butterworth, C.A. and Hodges, B.E. (1980). *Community Psychiatric Nursing—Caring for the Mentally Ill and Handicapped in the Community*. Churchill Livingstone, Edinburgh.

CPNA. (1985) *CPNA National Survey Update*. CPNA Publications.

Goldberg, D. (1985) *Mental Health Policies in Lancashire*. Conference Presentation.

Hunter, P. (1974) Community psychiatric nursing; a literature review. *International Journal of Nursing Studies*, **11**, 223.

Lally, H. (1989) All in a day's work. *Nursing Times—Community Outlook*, January.

Leopold, H. (1973) Psychiatric community nursing. *Health and Social Service Journal*, **83**, 489–490.

May, A.R. and Moore, S. (1963) The mental nurse in the community. *Lancet* **1**, 213–214.

Muijen, M. (1990) A report on Community Psychiatric Nursing. Unpublished.

Muijen, M., Marks, I., Connolly, J. and Audini, B. (1992). Home based care for patients with severe mental illness. *British Medical Journal*, 304, 749–754.

Parnell, J.W. (1977) *Community Psychiatric Nurses: A Descriptive Study*. Queen's Nursing Institute, London.

Paykel, E.S. and Griffith, J.H. (1983) *Community Psychiatric Nursing for Neurotic Patients*. RCN, London.

Pollock, L. (1988). The work of community psychiatric nursing. *Journal of Advanced Nursing*, 13, 537–545.

Royal College of Nursing (1966). *Investigation into the role of the psychiatric nurse in the community*. Unpublished.

Royal Medico-Psychological Association. (1969) A Second Memorandum on the Report of the Committee on Local Authority and Allied Personal Social Services. Members Report.

Seebohm, F. (Chairman). (1968) *Report of the Committee on Local Authority and Allied Personal Services*. Cmmd 3703. HMSO, London.

Simmons, S. and Brooker, C. (1986) *Community Psychiatric Nursing: A Social Perspective*. Heinemann Nursing, London.

Skidmore, D. and Friend, W. (1984) Should CPNs be in the Primary Health Care Team. *Nursing Times: Community Outlook*, 19 September, 310–312.

Wooff, K. Goldberg, D.P. and Fryers, T. (1988) The practice of community psychiatric nursing and mental health social work in Salford. Some implications for community care. *British Journal of Psychiatry*, 152, 783–792.

7 SETTING UP SERVICES FOR ETHNIC MINORITIES

D. Bhugra

INTRODUCTION

Ethnic minorities are far from homogeneous. The term is used here to point out some similarities as well as underlying differences. For any service to succeed in providing what patients need is only half the story. The important half is whether patients will use the services. It is difficult to define ethnic identity, which may be assumed to be a natural fact, though in practice ideological, political and economic interests will define groups that may not be divisible by genetic or cultural factors (Cohen, 1974). Ethnic minorities will present with a bewildering mix of languages, cultures and methods of help seeking. Not all members of any given ethnic category may have come from the same geographical region. It is also likely that their reason for and experiences of migration may be completely different. Quite often certain stereotypes of immigrants emerge and some myths persist. The myths are listed in Table 1.

Various types of migrants and reasons for migration exist. These

Table 1   Some of the myths about immigrants

1.	Immigrants are a homogeneous group
2.	All immigrants have the same reason for migrating
3.	All immigrants come from similar backgrounds
4.	A majority of immigrants would return to their country of origin
5.	All immigrants experience cultural conflicts
6.	All immigrants will have cross-generational problems

are discussed in detail by Rack (1982). It would be sufficient for our purposes to mention the classification used by Rack (1982): *Gastarbeiters*, exiles and settlers. In the ever shrinking global village, students as well as businessmen may move around regularly and at short intervals. There are a number of jetsetting people who maintain more than one residence across continents and the stresses experienced by such individuals may be qualitatively as well as quantitatively different from other geographically stable migrants. This chapter will concentrate on the needs of geographically stable migrants and offer principles of service provision.

PRINCIPLES

The primary aim of setting up services in the community has to be provision of equitable services for all users within the same community. This means that quite a lot of spadework needs to be done well in advance of getting the projects off the planning papers. Since the community health movement in the UK draws from the American experience this would be a suitable point to examine the origins of such a movement and lessons derived from it. Because of the growing influence of the civil rights movements the community mental health initiative focused on blacks in particular (Neighbors, 1987). Initially this ideology placed a heavy emphasis on prevention as a means of improving minority mental health (Caplan, 1964). Since stressful social conditions were seen as responsible aetiological factors in mental disorders, it was assumed that any social engineering through environmental change would result in mental health improvements. However, this did not work in practice even though Neighbors (1987) argues that such a preventive strategy shared a common theme with the targets of civil rights movements. The relationships among social variables like race, religion, social class, stress, unemployment, poor housing etc., are extremely complex. Ketterer (1981) argues that attempts to measure these concepts and chart their developmental course have proved complicated. Many prevention programmes thus ended up as poorly conceptualized consultation and education services. Complicating the failure of these initiatives (Goldstein, 1987) were the issues of racism and poverty contributing to mental ill-health. These further added to the failure of preventive community psychiatry which was unable to take a proactive primary preventive action (Neighbors, 1987). In order for community mental health services to succeed, these have to be:

1. Clear in their vision of what is being provided and for whom.
2. Consumer orientated as well as consumer led.
3. Flexible, accessible and local.
4. Comprehensive.
5. Racially and culturally appropriate.
6. Able to identify and provide for special needs.

In this chapter we shall focus on racially and culturally appropriate services. Since the services are district based, the needs of the district are of paramount importance. A top-down approach with little consultation with the community is doomed to failure. The development of a comprehensive district psychiatric service should include in addition to inpatient services, local authority community services and a mechanism for joint planning and operation of services. The local primary care and voluntary organization networks, local morbidity, attitudes and competencies of local clinicians and managers and financial resources will dictate the success of any community based endeavour.

Over the last 20 or 30 years, British psychiatry has had to face up to the fact that black immigrants and their descendants are making demands on the professions which are likely to increase with time (Francis *et al.*, 1989). Francis *et al.* argue that a major dissatisfaction concerns day-to-day experiences of black clients in mental institutions. It is therefore important that these attitudes are not carried over to community institutions. Black people's mistrust and suspicion towards psychiatry needs to be addressed before any service can hope to succeed.

PREPARATION FOR SETTING UP SERVICES

Services should be accessible

If community services are inaccessible geographically or are seen to be so they are bound to fail. Geographical distance is only one of the factors. Access in terms of understanding, language and culture is vital. Potential clients may manage to overcome the physical distance but emotional distance is much more difficult to overcome. The services have to be seen to be user-friendly. To this end the first step has to be a thorough assessment of the ethnic distribution of the local population. For the first time in the 1991 census, the ethnic origin of the population will enable us to have more accurate figures. This will be an essential first step in the direction of providing not only the appropriate physical location of buildings but also appropriate staff who are aware of the cultural, religious and linguistic norms. The social structure of any ethnic groups is dynamic and will be affected by a variety of factors. Quite often such a structure will not resemble in its entirety that of the host country nor that of the country of origin (Fuller and Toon, 1988). As noted earlier the members of any ethnic group may not be migrant. There are likely to be cross-generational differences which would need to be addressed in the planning stages. Thus a detailed view of the potential clientele is vital before the structure can get off the ground. This information will also enable the providers to assess the varying emphasis on various treatment modules, e.g. whether more psychotherapists are needed or whether a lithium clinic needs to be established. The community services wherever possible should be delivered in the client's usual environment and this is no different for ethnic minorities.

Services should be consumer orientated

In addition to being accessible the services must be based on the needs of the clients rather than those of providers. The services therefore have to be flexible and available whenever needed and for whatever duration. Thus complementary models of explanations of aetiology, course, treatment and prognosis have to be understood and utilized (Bhugra, 1993a). In addition as Kleinman (1980) notes, 70–90% of all ailments get treated in personal/folk *sectors*. Hence a knowledge of utilization of these sectors will add to the attractiveness of the services being made available. Furthermore, attitudes to mental illness affect community care (Bhugra, 1989) and a knowledge of these is also likely to be extremely important for making the services appropriate and attractive for ethnic minorities. Successful services empower clients by offering treatment strategies which fit in with their expectations and allow them to enhance their existing skills and also help them retain control over their lifestyes.

It is of little use ignoring the concepts of personal explanatory models which may prevent the clients from taking their medication. This is discussed further below. Over 200 *hakims* (indigenous healers) serve the Indian community in Britain (Rack, 1982) and their role has to be somehow integrated into services for that group. Other groups may have other sources which would need to be employed.

Services should be racially and culturally appropriate

This includes culturally appropriate methods of testing, an awareness of the cultural norms and appropriate research strategies (for a review see Flaherty *et al.*, 1988). Concepts of personhood show much cross-cultural variation. More holistic societies (in contrast with Western models) may mute recognition of the individual and the inner self, stressing social roles in defining identity (White, 1982). Beliefs about control and its value in illness and modes of seeking treatment vary. In India the locus of control is often seen as external (Bhugra, 1993b) and the notions of self–not self are extremely weak, which is bound to affect therapist–client interaction (see below).

Cultural bias has been identified in the form and content of tests, their adminstration procedures and the usage to which they are put (MacCarthy, 1987). Thus the providers have to be aware and knowledgeable about culture-fair tests, and the norms appropriate for the specific ethnicity must be adhered to. Apart from culturally appropriate needs assessment, cross-cultural training for providers, and recruitment of indigenous, local workers and bilingual staff must be provided for before the services take off.

In addition to the above general principles, two specific principles for ethnic minorities should be stressed here. The first is that of interpretation and translation in the services. Psychiatry more than any other medical specialty relies on both verbal and non-verbal communications to reach a diagnosis and formulate a plan of management. All relevant information about the services and educational material should be available in the languages spoken by the local community and interpreters and translators should be readily accessible. There is no point having access to an interpreter who may not be available for a fortnight. All staff should be aware of the urgency and the importance of using such a service when need arises. Quite often the interpreters are accepted in a casual fashion, the problems of interpretation causing frustration and dissatisfaction to professional and client alike (Fuller and Toon, 1988).

The interpreter must be comfortable in both languages and clients must feel relaxed in the presence of an interpreter and confident that their problems will be put across effectively. The therapist must also feel able to accept the validity of the interpretation. Thus translation and interpretation by the husband in a sexual dysfunction clinic on behalf of his wife will bias the interview (Bhugra and Cordle, 1986). Fuller and Toon (1988) recommend using trained advocates who may act as go-betweens for the ethnic group that they belong to and the institution. Apart from interpretation, they also educate the client and the staff—the former about the institution's desires, needs and wishes and the latter about the client's culture and requirements. Having advocates around can be stressful to the staff but they can be most helpful in a two-way educational process. Trained interpreters have their own advantages and disadvantages. Bilingual health workers, especially if they come from the same region, can be extremely helpful. However, as Fuller and Toon (1988) caution, they could be seen by the client as allying with the institution.

For practical reasons, untrained adult interpreters are often used. This practice should not be employed unless absolutely essential. If family members take such roles their interests may conflict with those of the client. Thus an ideal person to interpret is someone who is bilingual, has some medical knowledge and knowledge of the health service, is available for every consultation, and is impartial and can be trusted by both the client and the therapist. The interpreter should be empathic and able to identify areas of difficulties on both sides of the fence. The therapist should allow enough time and arrange the room and run the session in such a manner that all three present are able to maintain eye to eye contact. The therapist should speak directly to the patient while acknowledging the role of the interpreter (see Fuller and Toon, 1988). The therapist must allow the client and the intepreter to develop a relationship and watch client–interpreter interaction. The interpreter should be allowed to 'fail to understand' and to correct the therapist if required. The therapist should take care in discussing the client with the interpreter and should use illustrations and pictures in explaining the procedures and treatment if needed.

In psychiatric services, the interpreter must be able to differentiate between data and judgement and convey this to the therapist. In some situations, rehearsals of the interview with the interpreter may need to be carried out and thus clarify potential areas of conflict, support and worry for both the therapist and interpreter. During such interviews full use must be made of verbal, non-verbal and paraverbal skills. The client must see the same therapist each time. This will avoid a feeling of frustration and of starting from scratch each time. Other factors affecting therapist–client interactions are discussed later in this chapter.

Since the clients come from different backgrounds and are trying to speak a foreign language (i.e. English) it is important to make them feel relaxed with the right atmosphere, and clear speech, and to make an attempt to pronounce their names correctly.

The second important and particularly relevant point to remember is the sensitivity to racial aspects of the interaction between the client and the therapist. Black clients are often brought into mental hospitals against their wishes and often seen as requiring coercion and seclusion within hospitals. As Francis *et al.* (1989) point out, 'The marginal status that the blacks occupy is conventionally and we believe wrongly, attributed to a social pathology of culture. Since such pathology is often located at the individual level, and since it is essentially seen as disruptive, the visible oppression of black peope is founded on themes of law and order, one of control and coercion'. Other authors have argued on similar premises (e.g. Burke, 1974; Fernando, 1988). However, institutionalized racism does not occur in a vacuum.

Ethnic minorities may have been exposed to racial taunts, harassment and racial attacks. They may feel isolated and may feel reticent when seeking help from a health professional which in certain communities may be seen as a last port of call. The therapist may feel uncomfortable or ill-equipped to deal with such issues. However, being aware of the problems will enable the therapist to acknowledge the difficulties and thereby make the client aware of the racial sensitivity of the therapist. An awareness of cultural norms, e.g. rites of passage, religious issues and dietary restrictions, is vital for the provision of services. If, for example, the therapist is not aware of the periods of mourning or rituals of mourning in one community the grief of the client may be seen as abnormal or pathological. The use of alternative therapies by the patient may be seen as a sign of ignorance or slight by the medical profession. The religious taboos on meat, alcohol and tobacco in some communities are very strict and an insensitive therapist while taking history may rub the client the wrong way. Most of the ethnic minorities have been in the UK for at least two decades—thus there is no lack of knowledge about their cultural and religious norms.

Quite often people tend to converge towards religion in times of distress and it would be easy to see this as a delusional phenomenon. Thus racial sensitivity needs to be inculcated in the members of the team from the planning states. Fundamental knowledge about the religious rituals and basis of the religion will enable therapists to use it as a strength rather than a delusional system. Education through groups and courses is a useful starting point.

Any service (for ethnic minorities) that fails to take into account the proximity of the facility to the work-place or residence, the opening hours, the provisions of appointment or drop-in system and the availability of interpreting would in effect be withholding a service from such individuals (Burke, 1989).

DURING AND AFTER ESTABLISHMENT OF SERVICES

While services are in the process of being established, managers and clinicians must keep in touch with the community through meetings with community leaders, attending local meetings and disseminating information through GPs, voluntary organizations, churches or places of religious worship and other agencies. This process too has to be a two-way one. The perceived rates of various mental disorders will have helped the planners identify the potential clientele. The epidemiological data and various possible explanations are reviewed by Leff (1986). Hospital admission rates can offer only one aspect of the true needs of the community. Many people will not attend the services for reasons of hostility, suspiciousness or a perceived inability of the services to look after their needs. GPs' surgeries will be able to help identify potentially vulnerable clients and thus can be used in attracting patients to the community services.

The client–therapist interaction is the nub of the health care

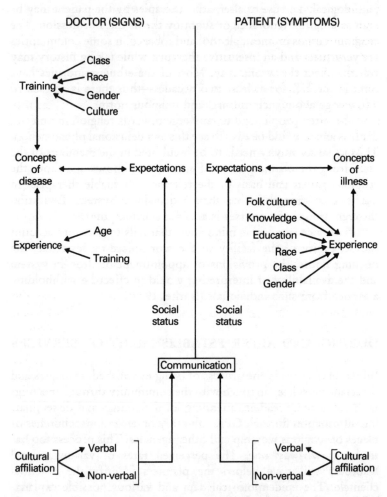

Figure 1 Therapist–client interaction and influencing factors (modified from Leff, 1988).

system. Such an interaction leads to diagnosis, treatment plans and aftercare. The factors in such an interaction can be divided into two categories. These are shown in Figure 1.

In any consultation, clients bring their experiences, attitudes and expectations from previous consultations and the therapist does the same. For the interaction to proceed and succeed these two halves of the equation have to balance. The client attends in order to understand why something is wrong whereas the therapist may be more interested in finding out what is wrong.

By virtue of their previous experiences from the health care system or previous illnesses, clients may succeed or fail in communicating their distress. Various ethnic communities have different ways of communicating their distress. Such distress may be conveyed in a somatic manner. Somatization and its implications are discussed at length elsewhere (see Bhugra, 1993a). As MacCarthy and Craissati (1989) found, Bangladeshi clients were often using their GPs as they would a village elder to help sort out problems rather than simply as a doctor.

The consultation is bound to be affected by the 'cultural distance' between the client and the therapist. Gender of the therapist may be seen as important in some communities. The therapeutic interactions are bound by clear and ambiguous, well stated and not stated rules. The client may thus be very clear on the stated rules and may not understand the ambiguous ones. This may lead to tragic consequences. When the mismatch between the rules becomes apparent, both parties may become frustrated. These rules can be obvious like appointments and not obvious ones like disparity between roles and expectations. Often other members of the family may want to sit in on the client–therapist interactions and may even wish to participate in these. Under these circumstances, if it is the client's wish, their attendance should be arranged. The heavy reliance on intra-familial resources is to some extent brought about by the social isolation of the minorities themselves, which may reinforce the prejudiced, racist outlook that locates the problem within the ethnic minority (Bavington and Majid, 1986).

As noted earlier, within the therapist–client interaction verbal, non-verbal and paraverbal communications can work to both parties' advantage. These are reviewed elsewhere (Bhugra, 1993a; Fuller and Toon, 1988). Suffice it to say that tone of voice, pauses, pace of speech, information giving and gathering, politeness, along with facial expression, gestures, body postures, eye contact, etc., are all important in assessment.

SPECIFIC AREAS OF DIFFICULTY

In assessment, difficulties of language, culture and treatment expectations need to be remembered. In treatment, however, some special problems may arise.

Psychotherapy

Various kinds of psychotherapies available in the National Health Service have their roots in the West and tend to represent a Western ideal which emphasizes a nuclear family model and may ignore or sometimes even contradict the traditional beliefs and ideology of those with different value systems. Western psychotherapy places an unequivocal emphasis on individualism and self-understanding thereby aiming towards a greater maturity of the individual (Bavington and Majid, 1986).

Campling (1989) argues that linguistic difficulties may be one obvious reason for low referral rates of black patients for psychotherapy. Another fear that has been expressed is that by offering psychotherapy, community grass root networks may be undermined. However, there is no reason to believe that the two cannot be worked together.

The essential asymmetry of the psychotherapeutic relationship is open to abuse and misunderstanding, more so if related issues of power are involved. As Campling (1989) cautions, 'we cannot open the door to black patients and hope to exclude the pain and hurt of racism from our therapeutic encounters. It is this we resist, and I believe worries about "cultural sensitivity" are in part a rationalisation.' To counter some of the problems, an intercultural therapy centre was established in north London which can work as a model for similar ventures. The centre was envisaged as having three main functions:

1. Pyschotherapy with adults, adolescents and children.
2. Training.
3. Case consultation with other professions.

The therapy was to be primarily a form of dynamic psychotherapy (Acharyya *et al.*, 1989). The therapy offered is brief, focused, dynamic psychotherapy. Nearly one-third of patients were from south Asia. These authors conclude, 'A major issue is the importance of personal and shared culture in the development of mental distress and the significance of this in the therapeutic process.' Like this project, other projects responding to local needs appear to be functioning well (Francis et al., 1989). Thus there is no reason to believe that clients from ethnic minorities are unable to deal with psychotherapeutic issues—what is lacking quite often is an understanding of the cultural beliefs. In India, for example, modified versions of Western style psychotherapy as well as traditional Ayurvedic models are used (Neki, 1975). As he states, 'these (psychotherapy) systems, of necessity, would make use of the native meta psychologic concepts and idioms for communication with people for whom these concepts and idioms already constitute a part of folklore'. Within the confines of psychotherapy, a number of cross-cultural factors need to be borne in mind. These include issues of dependence and autonomy which vary across cultures; psychological sophistication which may vary within cultures and across cultures; nature of dyadic relationship; personal responsibility and decision-making and nature of guilt; religious and social belief systems (Varma, 1988). The notion of guilt is poor in India whereas that of shame is very strong (Varma, 1985).

The approach may need to be modified depending on the client's needs, cultural beliefs and personality. Briefer, crisis-oriented, supportive, flexible and eclectic therapies, greater use of suggestion and reassurance and less use of dynamic interpretation, and blending the therapy with religious beliefs can often work usefully for Indian clients (Varma, 1988).

In the UK, group therapy has been shown to work successfully using Urdu/Hindi/Punjabi languages (Bavington and Majid, 1986). Therapeutic community models have been used across cultures with some success (Bavington and Majid, 1986). Lau (1986) has demonstrated that it is feasible to develop intervention strategies for working with ethnic minority families. She cautions that the therapist must know the family's cultural and religious background in sufficient detail in order to be able to assess the content of the clinical material. She urges that interventions with extended families must respect the pre-eminence of the family. Once again short-term problem-oriented approaches which do not threaten the family value system are more acceptable for some communities.

Psychoanalysis

Psychoanalysis uses a model of ego development which is the basis on which the analyst explores the analysand's emotional state and behaviour. Where the client and the therapist come from the same socio-cultural background they are more likely to share the aetiological and treatment models of psychological distress and disorder—a process dubbed 'acculturation' by Helman (1990). Here the analysand learns the shared world view and therefore has to acquire an understanding of the concepts, vocabulary and symbols that comprise it. He argues that such a shared view then leads to an exclusion of the family and the community. This is obviously not acceptable where the individual's 'illness' is a family event. The emphasis on the oedipal complex may reflect a position contrary to that seen in joint families where such a complex may be fixed on various elders within the joint family system. Psychoanalyis also reflects a hierarchical relationship which may further be emphasized by underlying race related, power related political formulations. Not enough data is available to encourage one to state categorically that psychoanalysis works among people from ethnic minorities.

Cognitive therapy

This may offer an interesting and potentially useful therapeutic tool. As MacCarthy (1987) observes, techniques such as verifying assumptions and generating alternative solutions and strategies are particularly useful in cross-cultural therapies, since the acceptability of a range of behavioural options within social contexts can be explored as an integral form of therapy. However, many beliefs and values comprising cognitive sets are culturally determined. As noted earlier, in India, the notions of guilt are not the same as in Western depressives. Thus the negative views of the world, the future and the self may differ in quality. This is another area which needs further research.

Behaviour therapies

Behaviour therapies are said to be particularly well-adapted to cross-cultural work largely because these focus on objectively observable phenomena. Some studies have reported excellent results

(Turner, 1982). Bhugra and Cordle (1989) reported that among their Asian patients, behavioural paradigms of treating sexual dysfunction were not being accepted easily. d'Ardenne (1986) reported excellent results with a Bangladeshi sample after she had modified her approach using family elders and handling more educational material.

Attempts to use social skills assessment, assertiveness training, dating behaviour, attitudes to sexuality are all potential areas of discord. Different communities have different attitudes and expectations of social skills. The assertiveness of black patients may be misunderstood or misinterpreted as a potentially violent behaviour. Thus culture-specific measurement instruments and norms are needed. Attempts to modify sexual behaviour in the direction of the therapist's norms may be deeply offensive or theatening, while therapists themselves may risk being offended by culturally-determined sexual stereotypes which contrast with their own beliefs (MacCarthy, 1987). She goes on to caution that careful preliminary negotiation of treatment targets with individual clients, and a willingness to work within a set of expectations which are not the therapist's own, are prerequisites.

Drug therapies

The dosage of drugs required for therapeutic levels may differ among various ethnic minorities. There is some clinical evidence suggesting that Afro-Caribbeans are more likely to be detained under the Mental Health Act (Littlewood and Lipsedge, 1988; McGovern and Cope, 1987; Moodley and Perkins, 1991). Black outpatients are also more likely to receive major tranquillizers and ECT (Littlewood and Cross, 1980). Some studies have reported higher doses of neuroleptics being used among black inpatients (Lloyd and Moodley, 1990). However, the latter study did not match the two groups on the basis of diagnosis. Some authors (Allen et al., 1977; Lewis et al., 1980) have reported that South East Asians and South Asians demonstrate clinical response at lower average levels of neuroleptics when compared to Americans and Europeans. Thus it is obvious that were the same doses given to members of different communities, the levels of response and side effects would differ. Rack (1982) recommends that when new drugs are introduced, their toxicity and efficacy should be assessed for each separate ethnic group and that practitioners should start with low dosages among ethnic minorities and only gradually increase these. Placebo effects of various drugs and their implications are discussed by Helman (1990).

Problems with children and adolescents

The socioeconomic conditions encountered by the ethnic minority population may create obstacles to child development and adolescent adjustment (Black, 1985). Stress among parents and within the family will affect the child's growth and behaviour. Any decisions taken on behalf of the child without any consideration of social issues will remain biased and totally inappropriate. The care procedures predispose to weakening household integrity and the consequences include short-term displacement and categorization as educationally subnormal (Coard, 1971). Burke (1989) concludes that with ghetto-like residence in unsupported social networks there will be a continued build-up of unhappy frustrated, restless West Indian-origin youngsters in Britain. Social deprivation as well as other factors can contribute to problems seen in this age group. Not unlike whites, parents may present with the child as a presenting problem. A holistic approach would therefore clarify the areas of difficulties and enable the therapist to formulate treatment and aftercare.

Ageing

The numbers of elderly among various ethnic minorities are bound to increase. Their needs are different from those experienced by adults. They are more likely to have been in this country longer and may have language difficulties. They may feel left out of the family structure and may find themselves increasingly isolated not only from the host culture but also from their own community. The younger generation may not see them as often or may not show due respect. Other losses may add to their feeling of alienation. They may have stricter dietary rules and may be more religious in their observance of rituals. All these factors may contribute to a different set of problems which need to be addressed rather than being treated only with antidepressants. Bereavement may have its own effects on this population. If rites of passage are not performed as prescribed or ritual mourning period not allowed, it may contribute to 'abnormal grief reactions'.

Other therapies

Occupational therapy (OT) may be seen as irrelevant or worse by members of ethnic minorities. To force them to attend OT classes may further contribute to their feeling of disenchantment. Therapy must be tailored not only to individual needs but also bear in mind the religious, social and cultural beliefs. Bavington and Majid (1986) offer some sensible, practical advice to the unwary. Good clinical practice is to do with listening and understanding what may be expressed as pain and distress. Whichever models and explanations are used, it is important that the therapist works without prejudged, preconceived notions and prejudices.

CONCLUSIONS

To set up user-friendly services which are accessible physically and emotionally is the first step. Implementation of the theory must include recruitment and training of appropriate staff which reflect the constituents of the community. Thus a mix of race, gender, linguistic abilities and professional expertise is essential. Communication with the community through formal and informal links must continue and not stop just because the unit has started functioning. This communication is a two-way process and a feedback loop must be established in order to continue improving the services and meeting the needs of the community.

Sensitivity to racial, cultural and religious aspects is essential if the service is to succeed. An ideal service for ethnic minorities should be aware of the problems it is supposed to be dealing with. It should be flexible, user-friendly, accessible, free of negative stereotypes, should have shedded myths about ethnic minorities, be open to suggestions and prepared to change according to the needs of its clientele.

REFERENCES

Acharyya, S., Moorhouse, S., Kareem, J. and Littlewood, R. (1989) Nafsiyat: a psychotherapy centre for ethnic minorities. *Psychiatric Bulletin*, 13, 358–360.

Allen, J.J., Rack, P.H. and Vaddadi, K.S. (1977) Differences in the effects of clomipramine on English and Asian volunteers: preliminary report on a pilot study. *Postgraduate Medical Journal* 53, suppl 1, 79.

Bavington, J. and Majid, A. (1986) Psychiatric services for ethnic minority groups. In: *Transcultural Psychiatry* (J.L. Cox, ed.). Croom Helm, London, pp. 87–106.

Bhugra, D. (1989) Public attitudes to mental illness. *Acta Psychiatrica Scandinavica*, 80, 1–12.

Bhugra, D. (1993a) Influence of culture on presentation and management of patients. In: *Principles of Social Psychiatry* (D. Bhugra and J.P. Leff, eds). Blackwell. Oxford pp. 67–81.

Bhugra, D. (1993b) Indian teenagers' attitudes to mental illness. *British Journal of Clinical and Social Psychiatry* (in press).

Bhugra, D. and Cordle, C. (1986). Sexual dysfunction in Asian couples. *British Medical Journal*, 192, 111–112.

Bhugra, D. and Cordle, C. (1989) A case control study of sexual dysfunction in Asian and non Asian couples 1981- 5. *Sexual and Marital Therapy* 3, 71–76.

Black, J. (1985) The difficulties of living in Britain. *British Medical Journal*, 290, 615–617.

Burke, A. (1974) Is racism a causitory factor in mental illness. *Inst. Journal of Social Psychiatry*, 30, 1–3.

Burke, A. (1989) Psychiatric practice and ethnic minorities. In: *Ethnic Factors in Health and Disease* (J.K. Cruickshank and D.G. Beevers, eds). Wright, London. pp. 178–189.

Campling, P. (1989) Race, culture and psychotherapy. *Psychiatric Bulletin*, 13, 550–551.

Caplan, G. (1964) *Principles of Preventive Psychiatry*. Basic Books, New York.

Coard, B. (1971). *How the West Indian Child is Made Educationally Sub-normal*. New Beacon Books, London.

Cohen, A. (1974) *Two Dimensional Man*. RK&P, London.

Currer, C. (1975) An attempt to apply the therapeutic community approach to treatment. Cited in Bavington and Majid (1986).

d'Ardenne, P. (1986) Sexual dysfunction in a transcultural setting: assessment, treatment and research. *Sexual and Marital Therapy* 1, 23–24.

Fernando (1988) *Race and Culture and Psychiatry*. Croom Helm, London.

Flaherty, J., Gaviria, F.M., Pathak, D. *et al.* (1988) Developing instruments for cross-cultural psychiatric research. *Journal of Nervous and Mental Disease*, 176(5), 257–265.

Francis, E., David, J., Johnson, M. and Sashidharan, S.P. (1989) Black people and psychiatry in the UK. *Psychiatric Bulletin*, 13, 482–285.

Fuller, J.H.S. and Toon, P.D. (1988) *Medical Practice in a Multi Cultural Society*. Heinemann, Oxford.

Goldstein, M. (1987). Mental health and public health. Cited in H.W. Neighbors: improving the mental health of Black Americans. *Millbank Quarterly*, 65, 348–380.

Helman, C. (1990) *Culture, Health and Illness*. Wright, London.

Ketterer, R. (1981) *Consultation and Education in Mental Health: Problems and Prospects*. Sage, Beverley Hills.

Kleinman, A. (1980) *Patients and Healers in the Context of Culture*. University of California Press, Berkeley, California.

Lau, A. (1986) Family therapy across cultures. *Transcultural Psychiatry* (J.L. Cox, ed.). Croom Helm, London pp. 234–254.

Leff, J.P. (1986) The epidemiology of mental illness across cultures. In: *Transcultural Psychiatry* (J.L. Cox, ed.). Croom Helm, London. pp. 23–36.

Leff, J.P. (1988) Psychiatry around the Globe. Gaskell, London.

Lewis, P., Vaddadi, K.S., Rack, P.W. and Allen, J.J. (1980) Ethnic differences in drugs response. *Postgraduate Medical Journal*, 56, Suppl. 1, 46–49.

Littlewood, R. and Cross, S. (1980) Ethnic minorities and psychiatric services. *Sociology of Health and Illness*, 2, 194–201.

Littlewood, R. and Lipsedge, M. (1988) *Aliens and Alienists*. Unwin Hyman, London.

Lloyd, K. and Moodley, P. (1990) Psychiatry and ethnic groups. *British Journal of Psychiatry*, 156, 907.

MacCarthy, B. (1987) Clinical work with ethnic minorities. In: *New Developments in Clinical Psychology* (F.N. Watts, ed.). John Wiley & Sons, Chichester. pp. 122–139.

MacCarthy, B. and Craissasti, J. (1989) Ethnic differences in response to adversity. A community sample of Bangladeshis and their indigenous neighbours. *Social Psychiatry and Psychiatric Epidemiology*, **24**(4), 196–201.

McGovern, D. and Cope, R. (1987) First admission rates of first and second generation Afro-Caribbean. *Social Psychology*, **22**, 139–149.

Moodley, P. and Perkins, R. (1991) Routes to psychiatric inpatient care in an Inner London borough. *Social Psychiatry and Psychiatric Epidemiology*, **26**, 47–51.

Neighbors, H.W. (1987) Improving the mental health of Black Americans: lessons from community mental health movement. *Millbank Quarterly*, **65** (Suppl. 2), 348–380.

Neki, J.S. (1975) Psychotherapy in India: Past, present and future. *American Journal of Psychotherapy*, **29**, 92–100.

Rack, P. (1982). *Race, Culture and Mental Disorder*. Tavistock, London.

Turner, S.M. (1982) Sexual disorders. In: *Behaviour Modification in Black Populations* (S.M. Turner and R. Jones, eds). Plenum, New York.

Varma, V.K. (1985) Psychosocial and cultural variables relevant to psychotherapy in the developing countries. In: *Psychiatry: The State of the Art* (P. Picot, P. Berner, R. Wolf and K. Thau, eds), Vol. 4. Plenum Press.

Varma, V.K. (1988) Culture, personality and psychotherapy. *International Journal of Social Psychiatry*, **34**(2), 142–149.

White, G.M. (1982) The ethnographic society of cultural knowledge of mental disorder. In: *Cultural Conceptions of Mental Health and Therapy Disorders* (A.J. Marsella and G.M. White, eds). D. Reidel, Dordrecht.

8 A MANAGER'S VIEW: THE NEW TASKS

C. Kirk

The responsibilities of any management are to define:

–the organization by reference to its boundaries,
–its tasks by reference to exclusions,
–its structure by reference to the responsibilities of managers.

Within that framework everyone employed by the organization has to be motivated, to develop skills the better to achieve the organization's goals and to obtain job satisfaction.

All this activity has to be contained within financial targets, because organizations which fail the test cease to exist.

These responsibilities of managers are the same whatever the enterprise. They apply equally to institutional and community care of mentally ill people.

The debate about institutional and community care has more to do with dialectics than reality. Whilst the institutions have dominated public service provision, much treatment has been provided by primary health and social services and most care has been provided by natural carers. The only management assessment of the situation in the United Kingdom, that of Sir Roy Griffiths (Griffiths, 1988), makes this abundantly clear.

Since the mental institutions were recognized as an anachronism by Enoch Powell's 'ten year plan' the proportion of the public service contributed by the institutions has dwindled. In addition the type of contribution has changed, as vacated wards have increasingly been brought into use as places of last resort for seriously demented elderly people.

Management of health services generally is undergoing profound change. Since management has developed a recognizable academic base, it has become respectable in health services. Professional staff are now keen to participate in health service management.

There are marked differences between institutional and community care management. The characteristics of successful institutions include inevitable routines and failsafe mechanisms that are not easily replicated in disparate and dispersed community services. Community services have relied much more on the native wit and common decency of largely independent self-motivating individuals, than on management structures. As greater emphasis is placed on community care an increase in management capacity in public health and social services is timely.

DATA COLLECTION AND PROCESSING

Unlike most other enterprises, public health services have relied too heavily on professional knowledge and judgement rather than sound data. The enormous diversity of tasks undertaken by public health services, which make them a unique enterprise, renders adequate data collection a gargantuan task. This applies equally to patient, staff and financial statistics. Belated massive introduction of information technology into public health services will generate data banks and provide current information on which soundly based decisions can be taken.

Finally, it is often asserted that management cannot be satisfactorily applied in health services, particularly mental health services, because of the impossibility of measuring productivity in terms of quantifying and qualifying outcomes. In fact this problem is common to all service industries and is capable of far more precise resolution than is usually acknowledged.

The conceptual framework, recognized processes and means of data collection now exist to enable much better management of public health and social services than previously, as applicable to mental health services, as to any others. It is possible to establish common goals and common understanding of how to direct available resources effectively.

THE CLIENTS

Any definition of a mental health service has to define the client group. The geographic boundary is easily established, be it a well recognized county boundary or a circuit of streets in a conurbation. The difficult bit in mental health service teams is setting the boundary by reference to the clientele. It is in fact the fundamental management task in the mental health service.

The American experience of denying institutional care to people with seriously disabling long-term mental illnesses, whilst at the same time opening mental health centres to provide counselling and psychotherapy to help reasonably capable people in good health with their problems, needs to be avoided. Desirable as these latter services are, they should be and usually are resourced in different ways.

To an extent this shift in service delivery reflects the preferences of some professional staff. There are clear attractions in successfully satisfying the needs of an appreciative clientele rather than making little progress in trying to help often uncooperative people with profoundly greater needs.

Not uncommonly people exhibiting very violent, aggressive and destructive behaviour are rejected as clients, although obviously in need of help. It is unreasonable of a public mental health service to set its boundaries in a way which excludes such people, whilst taking into treatment well adjusted persons curious about their psychological development.

Because the professionals employed by mental health services are capable of and like carrying out certain procedures and working with certain types of people, this does not mean that those procedures and those clients should be included within the boundary of a mental health service. Clincal psychologists are no doubt excellent at stress management, helping people to cope with normal physiological and psychological reactions. However, psychopathology is central to the treating and caring contribution of a public mental health service and should be given highest priority. To fit within a manageable public mental health service, counselling has to be narrowed down to those areas, such as post trauma counselling, where its absence leaves a high level of risk of psychopathology ensuing. Counselling within staff groups and appropriate circumstances for that are considered later.

There is, therefore, an enormous risk that, as every individual needs to enjoy mental wellbeing, the client boundary can include the entire population, in one way or another. Other than in terms of mental health promotion, this is clearly impractical.

The basic ground rule must be that a mental health service will accept the treatment and care of those most in need of its services. Most importantly, it will not reject clients on the grounds of their needs being too great, in terms of either dependency or difficulty, be the difficulty non-cooperation, aggression or gross antisocial behaviour. This is society's expectation of the service.

A mental health service should not and cannot restrict itself to this client group. It should not because of the many other interventions it can make if adequately resourced. It cannot because it would be impossible for staff to sustain a service with only this clientele. Whereas complete professional self-indulgence cannot be condoned, the motivation and reward of staff working in very difficult services has to feature highly in the equation.

Given the resources, this is readily achievable, still by reference to the client group boundary. Amongst the most damaging of diseases are schizophrenia and dementia. The benefit to prognosis of early diagnois and treatment in the case of schizophrenia and of care programming in the case of dementia is reasonably well-established. In the case of schizophrenia, there is some evidence that the damaging long-term effects of the disease may be reduced by proper intervention during the first 12 months. In the case of both illnesses the ability of natural carers to contribute positively to minimize aggravation, disabilty and dependence is enormously enhanced by early intervention. Psychoses and depressions generally can be more readily contained during the early stages of onset.

Early intervention requires very close cooperation between mental health services and primary care. In particular general practitioners need precision and clarity in statements of diagnostic signs and symptoms to be identified. Here the client boundary is being placed to include people in the very earliest stages of illnesses, which if not tackled early may add to the group of people with long-term mental illnesses of a seriously disabling nature.

The same considerations can be applied in the case of substance abuse, primarily drugs, whether prescribed or illicit, and alcohol. These abuses are also routes into long-term mental ill-health, which mental health services cooperating with primary care can help to avoid, and the client boundary should include them.

The client boundary can then be stated as adults (a) en route to long-term mental health problems if early intervention is not provided, (b) in crisis, and (c) suffering long-term mental ill-health resulting in disability and dependency.

Armed with the geography and the definition of the clients it is possible by epidemiological survey methods to gain some understanding of the number of people with long-term mental health problems, the target population. Over a period of time the number of people removed from that population and added to it can be calculated similarly. Good data collected on an individual patient basis identifies the number of interventions required in a year.

In addition to geography and client group the other organizational boundary to consider is that between the different treating and caring agencies. In spite of all the debate on this subject, public mental health services are funded to meet the treatment needs of people suffering mental ill-health. They are not provided for social welfare. Of necessity treatment, care and aftercare are very often being provided simultaneously, and often aftercare is essential in the preservation of mental health.

There should be no dispute as to which party contributes what. The basic principle is that the health service employs health professionals to treat and provide such care as is required in support of treatment. Social services employ social workers to ensure the welfare elements of the programme. Where the line is drawn within the context of these general principles has to be agreed between the two partners. Once agreement has been reached it should be carefully codified, leaving no area for subsequent dispute, and be available for reference to health and social service staff.

SERVICE DESIGN

Defining the structure of an organization by reference to the responsibilities of its managers assumes an existing service. Ideally all health services for a population should be provided, within their geographic territory. The only exceptions are highly specialized treatments the requirements for which are so infrequent as to require a larger catchment area to support service provision. The determinant then becomes the size of various catchment areas.

The appropriate hierarchy of provision is:

- provision of early intervention as part of primary care, including into the client's home,
- referral to specialist outpatient services, either community or district general hospital based,
- provision of day hospital services where duration of treatment per day exceeds an outpatient attendance but the client is able to live at home and enjoy the amenities of home, with support to carers as necessary,
- provision of inpatient services if unavoidable, for those where home circumstances or the absence of a home require it.

Inpatient services following acute admission should be for short duration of stay at the district general hospital unit. Where a much longer period of inpatient treatment is required, then intensive rehabilitation hostel accommodation is to be preferred, where individual clients' needs for long term care can be catered for. Beyond that a small proportion of clients will need continuing support in hostel accommodation because of residual disabilities and dependency. All these settings, however homely in design and intention, will still be contrived and second best to a home of one's own.

A major group using these residential care settings are homeless people (see also Chapters 9 and 10). Early intervention, crisis care support into the home and rehabilitation are very difficult to provide to homeless people. Unfortunately, severe psychotic behaviour can quickly alienate sufferers from their home environment. Conversely, homelessness is traumatically destabilizing and can be a route into long-term mental illness. Resettlement of homeless people needs extensive forward planning in cooperation with the special needs housing unit.

Before expanding on the above service design, it is important to recognize that this is the contribution of the specialist mental health service. The interventions of that service are secondary to primary care, which provides vast amounts of treatment and care to the whole of the presenting population. Primary care acts as the filter to secondary care, handing over the medical management of clients, who are recognized as needing specialist treatment and care.

This is where cooperation between the secondary specialist and primary services becomes so important, to ensure that the appropriate clients are filtered through at the most beneficial time from the point of view of outcome of treatment.

Sectional specialist interests often overlook the enormous diversity of problems clients constantly present to primary care. It has been assessed that up to 80% of all presenting problems are of a psychological rather than organic nature. An holistic approach would question the meaning of that statistic. However, it does highlight the problem facing primary care in trying to identify clients who may be suffering the early onset of such conditions as schizophrenia and dementia.

Thus, mental health services provide specialist treatment and care to clients, and support to their carers, and cooperate with primary care, which has a more generalist approach. Primary care, working with specialist services, targets on early identification of people showing signs and symptoms of potentially long-term damaging illnesses as described in Chapter 4. These clients are referred for early intervention by the specialist service. People in crisis, whether new to the service or with exacerbations of already identified conditions, require immediate help from both primary health and social services and from specialist mental health care. Admission to inpatient services is restricted to those clients where admission is unavoidable and duration of stay is kept as short as possible. That is achieved by pre-admission domiciliary visiting and programming resettlement from the time of admission.

There are no hard and fast rules about normative levels of provision that can be applied to total population size. However, there is some evidence that an acute inpatient provision of 3 beds per 10 000 total population weighted to take account of deviation from normative levels of people with schizophrenia in the population is adequate. There is further evidence that some 10% of acute admission beds should be provided within a secure enclave of the admission unit for temporary detention of acutely ill people. With an average incidence of schizophrenia, 20 beds per 60 000 plus total population, of which two are provided in a secure enclave, seems a sensible number.

For all the reasons given in the Bonham-Carter Report (1969) it is regarded as most desirable to make these provisions as part of the district general hospital. Thus, with a 240 000 population there would be four 20-bedded acute admission wards with eight of the beds provided within a secure enclave for temporary stays only.

Where longer periods of residential treatment are required, clients are transferred to hostel type accommodation in centres of social amenity away from the district general hospital site. Where, following treatment, continuing care and support is required as part of a longer progress towards independence, a range of residential facilities is required. This will start off with 24 hour staffed accommodation, through staff assisted sheltered accommodation to independent living with occasional visiting as detailed in Chapters 11–13. The whole emphasis throughout is on clients living in their own homes with support according to needs.

All service designs have to be dynamic ones. This is a throughput system. Many of the clients will have limited occasional contacts with the specialist service. Some of the clients will have a lifelong dependency. The whole emphasis is to reduce the latter group to a minimum by early intervention and by reactivating the skills that enable independent living. Throughout, those who currently need support must be provided with the appropriate support and this will always be aimed to care and treat simultaneously, with the emphasis of treatment being on progress to independence. Where there are natural carers, their needs for support and guidance in pursuing the same objectives for the clients are of paramount importance, and specialist team members will concentrate on working to support them, including provision of respite.

LONG-TERM CARE AND MONITORING

The accumulation of clients requring long-term support applies to local district based services in the same way as to institutional ones. It is an error to consider these clients as the long-stay residents of institutions transferred into community care. Some of the clients will have this history, many of them will not. The aim is to avoid adding to the number of these clients by means of early intervention to minimize the long-term crippling effects of untreated mental-illnesses.

The characteristics of the long-term client group are dependence on medication and varying degrees of support, often with exacerbations of acute illness. These clients need to be monitored in the most sensitive way possible.

Many of the long-term client group will avoid involvement with health and social service personnel and in fact often with anyone whom they regard as interfering. The legal imperatives on the health and social services to interfere to avoid clients in crisis harming themselves or others, to the point of removing civil liberties and enforcing treatment, operates against the necessary trusting relationship between client and health and social service personnel. This has to be a primary reason for designing services in such a way that crises are avoided. The incidence of crises and the need to invoke the legal imperatives to deal with them is one measure of the success of mental health services.

There are, then, two monitoring points. There is monitoring to achieve early identification and therefore early intervention at the point of onset of illnesses. Secondly, with the long-term client group, there is a need to monitor to avoid exacerbations of illness reaching crisis point. In terms of social care this second monitoring involves keeping contact with the client and periodically assessing service needs and ensuring they are met.

There is a requirement on specialist services to agree an aftercare package for all vulnerable clients, to be in place at time of discharge from hospital. The specialist services responsibility continues until the specialist considers the client to be no longer vulnerable.

The design of the aftercare package and its implementation requires cooperation between primary and specialist care; both health and social services need to be involved. The social services are responsible for case management and for securing the social care component.

There are strong feelings in some quarters against the registration of people with long-term mental illnesses. Again, this is part of the lack of trust that has arisen from a laissez faire service design, which only catches up with problems at times of crisis and then solves them by imposing legal imperatives. The inadequacy and inappropriateness of this service design is obvious. Here we have an organizational rather than a resource issue (which is not to deny that there may be inadequate resources as well).

Registering long-term clients, follow-up assessments and modification of care plans to meet changing needs is essential.

Health and social services have to maintain contact with long-term clients, and establish a reasonable modus vivendi to enable help and support to be given in a timely way and according to need. There are a number of computer programs specially written to achieve registration with all the spreadsheets necessary for assessment and monitoring of services provided. Their use gives the client legal rights of access to the data held on computer under data protection regulations.

Of course many people leave residential treatment services without formal discharge, often without any indication whatsoever that that is their intention. Enough advance consideration should have been given to the aftercare team to enable it to put together a care programme after the patient has gone. With properly integrated in-house and community services, based on related specialist teams looking after a section of the catchment population, in most cases this ought to be possible.

PHYSICAL RESOURCES

Opportunities to design an entire new service from scratch are rarely available. There almost certainly will never be an occasion when all the buildings and teams available to a service are new ones.

The recent history of the design of purpose built accommodation for specialist mental health services suggests that that is just as well. It is generally agreed that homely accommodation is required. The most readily available homely accommodation is an ordinary dwelling house. Economy of scale in the case of staffed residential accommodation requires either very large houses, built for the affluent few before the First World War, or adjoining houses, which usually have to be bought new.

These considerations do not apply to acute admission accommodation at the district general hospital, where nursing units of around 20 beds, as referred to earlier, are required. These should be built on the small hotel model without any of the trappings usually associated with clinical services.

Large dwelling houses make good day hospital accommodation, good clinic accommodation as well as suitable accommodation for staffed hospitals. The most important requirement is for space both indoors and outdoors.

The components of a specialist mental health service for each locality of 50 000 to 60 000 plus people are:

- Consultation, assessment and counselling space of capacity for client and carers. These can be provided in the client's home, in the health centre, in the mental health resource centre, in the district general hospital outpatient department, maybe in the accident and emergency department. There does need to be some dedicated consultation accommodation available to the relevant professions. This is often provided in the mental health resource centre but there are circumstances when each of the other possibilities mentioned will be preferable.
- Day hospital treatment. Two types of place are needed. About 25 places are needed in an intensive treatment day hospital to help people through acute episodes of illness. About 15 day hospital places are needed to support members of the long-term client group through exacerbations of illness, with modifications to medication and for psychotherapeutic and behaviour modification intervention.
- About 20 acute admission beds, 2 of which will be part of a secure enclave. These beds will be part of the psychiatric department of the district general hospital. The wards of each of the localities within the hospital's catchment area will be grouped together into a loose, mutually supportive, confederation. The relationship emphasis will not be in-house but between the in-house and community services of the locality.
- Intensive rehabilitation unit. The main interventions will be behaviour modification and psychotherapy. Again economies of scale require that this residential care unit has around 20 beds, with the average number of people characterized as suffering schizophrenia in the population. It is reckoned some 5 or 6 beds of this type per locality will be needed.
- A spectrum of staffed hostel accommodation varying from 24 hour staffing, to intermittent daytime staffing, to warden assisted housing, to independent living with occasional staff visiting needs to be provided. This accommodation is needed to house people with long-term mental illnesses. The number of places required is peculiar to the locality. There will be varying numbers of people in this client group who will live with their natural carers with appropriate support. There will be others for whom successful adult fostering places will have been found. There are

many variables and the number of places can only be determined locally. This should be a joint exercise between the housing department, the housing associations, the social services department and the health services. There are many boundary issues involved, which should be ironed out as an early part of the collaborative process essential to good service provision.

Reference has not been made here to crisis houses, day centres or day work centres which are part of the aftercare provision provided by social services. Many of these services can be provided, with advantage to the client and often no disadvantge to the staff, during evenings and weekends. The specialist health services have a contribution to make into these settings in the same way as the primary health and social services have into the specialist service provisions. Parallel services may be provided by voluntary organizations and again cooperative working should be an ever open and available option to build the most comprehensive range of services possible.

STAFFING

Mental health services train and employ staff whose specialized knowledge and skills are designed to equip them for the purpose. All training begins from a holistic base with specialization into the treatment and care of people with mental health problems. In recent years great emphasis has been placed on the maintenance and development of normal interpersonal relationship skills, discarding the professional barriers presumably inadvertently part of previous education and training. Understanding of the potentially thera-peutic or damaging nature of all contacts with clients is part of training. The emphasis is on contact with clients and helping and supporting them.

In most other enterprises division of labour is understood and appreciated. Different staff groups have different contributions to make to the achievement of the collective goals of the enterprise. For a long time this point was lost sight of in mental health services in pursuit of some form of egalitarianism. If the contributions of the different staff groups are equal the organization should clearly employ only those who can be trained most quickly and are correspondingly least costly to employ.

Obviously all staff groups should recognize the contribution each has to make and conduct themselves in an open, honest and approachable way. It is curious that people working in mental health services have sometimes been unable to relate ordinarily to the people they were suposed to help. Although these failings are often characteristics of bad institutions they are by no means exclusive to the institutions. It is a task of management, through training and example, to eradicate the residual vestiges of dehumanizing attitudes, behaviours and practices in the mental health services.

Psychiatrists, psychotherapists, clinical psychologists, psychiatric nurses, community psychiatric nurses, speech therapists, occupational therapists, drama therapists and art therapists make up the clinical staff of a specialist mental health service. They work with colleagues in primary health and social services and have available to them the specialist expertise of approved social workers, who have been trained in legislation relating to the detention, treatment and care of people, who temporarily are considered to be at risk of harming themselves or others. Other specialist contributions are made by civil rights officers administering legislation, welfare rights officers administering patients' affairs, medical secretaries, information staff, ward and clinic clerks, caterers, cleaners, porters, drivers and maintenance staff.

A major management task is to help each staff member develop full potential and the job satisfaction that goes with that. These are fundamental parts of the reward system. Training is an important part of the reward system.

Education and training is largely the responsibility of the schools and colleges. However, all the on-the-job parts of training are supervised by qualified staff working in the service. The presence of young people in training should be an incentive towards the achievement of the highest standards of excellence as an example for them.

All health service workers should be trained in essential basic practical skills. Appropriate training should be included as part of induction. Other than for staff new to the health service refresher training only should be required.

Training skills for staff should not be regarded as dislodging existing skills. Relieving skilled staff of non-skilled work makes sense if it releases more time to perform skilled tasks. It makes no sense at all if skilled staff members have to stand by whilst someone else carries out a mundane task. This is particularly relevant in the case of keying data into computers. The person who understands the data is best able to key it in accurately. It is in fact quicker to do that than either write it down or dictate it for some-one else to copy from.

TEAM WORKING

'A team is not just chaos made into virtue. Team work requires actually more internal organisation, more co-operation and greater definitions of individual assignments than work organised in individual jobs' (Drucker, 1969).

Teams are conceived by managers as a means of concentrating the necessary skills to carry out a defined task efficiently and effectively. Teams work best when the manager with responsibility for carrying out the task selects those individuals with the skills being looked for and subsequently leads the team. Successful management teams are of this kind and the same applies to successful clinical teams.

The problem with many clinical teams is that there are no ground rules and no sanctions, which usually arises from there being no leader. It is possible for a group of professionals, dedicated to carrying out a task and all in agreement as to what the task is, to work extremely well. However, the tensions within the mental health services and the opportunities for opting for a different task and confusing the roles of the team members is too great to leave these essential matters to chance.

Teams with acknowledged leaders, and with clear task and role definitions, will achieve effectively. Efficiency is dependent on a recognition that anyone in the team can carry out generic tasks. The point here is that amongst the skills of any individual are those specific to the profession as against common ones. No-one expects a chauffeur driven car to be available for a doctor or social worker; they are all expected to be able to drive cars these days. It is important then to be aware of what are core skills for a profession and what are generic skills, which anyone can contribute when not being required to contribute core skills. Reference has been made previously to keying data into computers, which will become as natural as driving cars but which some professionals are still resisting.

In all work, task orientation produces the most satisfactory outcomes. This is particularly important in the case of teams, where there are so many potential diversions. The necessity to remain on task at all times must be paramount. There are advantages to team building exercises, where the team pursues a different task than the one for which employed. Similarly review and preview of work is of importance. The problem arises when these activities, which had been marginal ones, encroach on the main task and in some cases swamp it.

There is also a tendency to want to employ facilitators to help teams with problems. This can be helpful or self-indulgent, detracting from the real task. Facilitators can contribute fresh perceptions to problems and help teams analyse their difficulties, so bringing the best out in team members. There are extreme cases where teams look to have a permanent facilitator, which is in general a sign of poor functioning. Teams need assistance through transitions and traumas. Some team leaders will prefer to keep on task during very difficult periods, which is more likely to increase stress. The best team leaders are those who keep the team on task within a set routine which has been found to be efficient and effective but are quick to recognize impending transactions or periods of trauma and ensure that time is taken out to allow the team to work through the difficulties experienced.

Mental health services are provided by a whole range of inter-relating clinical teams, which interface with social workers, voluntary workers and above all friends and relatives acting as natural carers. The potential for confusion, misinformation and general chaos is enormous.

The advantage of the institution is that it has learned over decades a series of set procedures and attitudes that appear to produce order out of chaos. The fact that ordered structure stifles ordinary human response and is intimidating to those not yet institutionalized can be overlooked by those, who value its security above the chaos of normal life.

COMMUNICATIONS

Messages received, understood, will be acted on immediately. This must be the standard aimed for in communications within and between clinical teams. It must be made easy to communicate. Each team should carry out review and preview, briefly but effectively, at an assembly each day. Community teams being mobile are less easy, even with electronic gadgetry, to contact than static ones on wards and in day hospitals. The mobile team should routinely contact the static ones each day to receive any messages about impending patient transfers, recent admission from their patch etc.

The discipline of structured record keeping should also be accepted by everyone. Problem-oriented records dictate tasks and avoid largely useless verbiage, to which, in any case, clients are likely to object and with good reason. As records are increasingly held on computer, they will inevitably be reduced to factual information. Hopefully the response 'I know you have nowhere to live but your problems go much deeper than that' will become a thing of the past.

CONCLUSION: SERVICE DELIVERY

Having identified problem areas and suggested some lines of service development, I will conclude by summarizing a blueprint for an evolving service.

Mental health services, like all service industries, must aim for client satisfaction for a wide range of different people with different needs, who make different levels of demand on the services at different times. There are no parallels in complexity in commerce or industry. Nevertheless, success relies on the same clear thinking about the nature of the task, concentrating effort on carrying it out, and recording and communicating what has been done.

There can be no more intimate task than helping an individual work towards regaining a sense of mental wellbeing, often against an initial response of total non-cooperation. Careful judgements are involved in determining the appropriate opportunity, setting and means of help. This may be with or away from group support, at or away from home, intermittently or during the day or over 24 hour periods. These decisions will often identify the clinical team to be involved, be it domiciliary, outpatient, day patient or inpatient. Many clients will move from one setting to another during a period of treatment.

Clearly if teams themselves are not well structured and task orientated, and the communications between teams are vague, then the potential for client benefit is limited and the possibility of doing more harm than good exists.

Organization of services to the population of a locality of about 60 000 people is usually recommended. This is the upper limit for an average number of people with long-term mental illnesses in the population to be served by a team. The locality manager's responsibility will be to ensure that the needs of those with long-term mental illnesses and those with the potential of becoming so if not treated promptly are met. To achieve this requires:

- registration of those with long-term mental illnesses, identifying their needs, who their case manager is, how their needs are being met;
- simple, straightforward, concise statements of the signs and symptoms of the onset of schizophrenia and dementia, available to primary care and to ensure the earliest possible identification of clients;
- speedy response by specialist community clinical teams where clearly intervention is required and immediate response to crisis situations;
- treatment settings, other than the clients' homes, namely interview rooms, day settings, residential treatment settings; these will vary according to style and nomenclature but should be homely and practical rather than clinical;
- essentially separate clinical teams working in each of the different locations but with flexibility so that team members can gain experience in different settings and follow-through between settings by health service key workers and subsequently by social worker case mangers;
- ready and accurate communication between teams in preparation for and at the time of transfer of clients between teams.

Throughout the clients and their carers must be able to influence the help given, by the offer of alternatives and their exercise of choice. In any conflict of interest the client's choice should always prevail, if practical. The objective of mental health services is to restore the independence on which mental wellbeing is founded.

REFERENCES

Bonham-Carter (1969) *The Functions of the District General Hospital.* The Bonham-Carter Report, HMSO.

Drucker, P.F. (1969) *The Practice of Management.* Heineman, London.

Griffiths, R. (1988) *Community Care: an Agenda for Action.* HMSO.

9 A PRAGMATIC APPROACH TO THE HEALTH CARE OF THE SINGLE HOMELESS: ITS IMPLICATIONS IN TERMS OF HUMAN RESOURCES

D.J. El-Kabir and S.S. Ramsden

Homelessness has always been a feature of urban life, not only in the UK but in most of the Western world. It is felt that in this country the numbers are growing though reliable, comparative figures are few (Canter *et al.*, 1988). Homelessness in recent years may in part be attributed to sociological factors: the current economic situation, and present day social security regulations as well as perhaps the closure of long-stay mental hospitals without adequate provision of aftercare in the community (Lamb, 1984). The disaffection of the young with the social and moral norms and values of their parents and the breakdown of marriages and family life all contribute to this phenomenon. The end-result is a diverse group on the margins of society whose problems and lifestyle lead to frequent and often severe ill-health, combined with difficulties in receiving appropriate health care.

It is the purpose of this chapter to address the diverse nature of the homeless and the difficulties in providing the medical care needed by them. The authors describe the projects that they have developed to meet the challenges presented by sick homeless patients and attempt to analyse what principles underlie the success of such projects and their implications for the medical profession and medical education.

The ill-health suffered by the homeless has been appreciated since the nineteenth century, as has the fear that they may also harbour potentially serious infective disease; typhus in the last century, perhaps tuberculosis in more recent times (Laidlaw, 1956; Ramsden et al., 1988; Shanks, 1982). In the 1950s and 1960s some of the first attempts were made to study the sociodemographic and health characteristics of the hostel dwelling homeless and the remarkable clinics in some of the centres described. A picture emerged of predominantly white males, often of celtic origin and frequently from deprived backgrounds. Illness was common and often almost the norm. In a study of a clinic for the homeless in Edinburgh about half of their patients suffered chronic disease, with epilepsy, tuberculosis and psychiatric problems being particularly noticeable (Scott et al., 1966). The high prevalence of psychiatric morbidity has been shown in a number of studies among the hostel dwelling populations and more recently among those sleeping out (Lodge-Patch, 1971; Priest, 1971; Weller et al., 1989). The picture of illness commonly seen in general practice is predominantly of neurotic problems, especially in middle-aged women (Tyrer, 1984). The pattern among the homeless is, on the other hand, of a very high prevalence of psychosis, personality disorder and alcohol abuse.

The homeless tend to receive primary health care in a different way from the general population. Traditionally most people are registered with a single general practice and consult the same doctor over many years. Access to hospitals is usually through the general practitioner, though in emergencies this may be through casualty departments. The homeless are usually not registered with a general practitioner and their mobility adds to the problems of continuity of care. There are, however, other factors. The homeless tend to behave reactively, not seeking a doctor unless they are too ill to cope with their circumstances. There may also be a reluctance to see doctors who may be perceived as authoritarian and part of the 'establishment'. In our study of the homeless sleeping rough in central London, the vast majority of those without a GP gave their reason for not registering as not being ill (Ramsden et al., 1989). In addition receptionists and appointment systems may be perceived to be further obstacles and waiting rooms feel hostile, when the individual is unwashed, poorly dressed and possibly infested. Inner city GPs may have full lists and some may refuse to see patients who they think are likely to be 'difficult'. For these reasons casualty departments are, for many, the usual primary source of health care. This is an inappropriate use of the departments and less than ideal for the homeless person, as casualty departments are not equipped to deal with the complexities of primary care (Davidson et al., 1983). The homeless are a diverse group of individuals. Some stay in hostels for many years, abstain from drinking and behave in a socially acceptable manner. Such patients are generally adequately served by GPs in their own surgeries or clinics held in hostels. Others can be more difficult to manage. Transience is one problem. Those suffering from personality disorder, alcoholism and substance abuse may be quite unruly, disruptive and sometimes threatening. Still others, mistrustful of contact with others, shy away from all contact with conventional care and their relationship with a doctor may take many consultations before trust is established. This applies particularly to mentally ill patients, especially schizophrenics, who tend to be fragile and reclusive. Clearly, to develop effective and available care for all of these patients a range of services must be made available. General practice as it is organized at present can cope very well with some homeless, particularly as the doctor begins to recognize some of the stresses the patient may be under. However, it is not well designed for many who suffer both physical and mental illness with major psychosocial problems and unpredictable behaviour.

It was in this environment in the 1970s, particularly with the growing appreciation of the plight of young people who gravitated towards a homeless existence in the major cities, with all of the attendant risks such as drugs, exploitation, crime and prostitution, that Great Chapel Street Medical Centre was established.

GREAT CHAPEL STREET MEDICAL CENTRE

In response to these problems, highlighted by various agencies, in 1977 the Department of Health and Social Security (DHSS) set up Great Chapel Street Medical Centre in Soho (El-Kabir, 1982). The Centre was staffed by a full-time administrator, a nursing sister and one of the authors was appointed the physician in charge to provide two sessions a week. It was open every weekday afternoon. There was to be no appointment system, all patients being seen except those who were drunk or grossly abusive. The numbers attending rapidly rose as knowledge of the Centre spread. However, the illnesses and difficulties experienced by the patients soon revealed problems in providing comprehensive and effective health care. In addition to physical ill-health, psychological disability and social problems compounded the picture that many homeless suffer. The operation of the Centre and the way the staff worked had to evolve rapidly. The GP increased his sessions to five per week. The administrator's role in particular underwent change evolving from that of receptionist and administrator to a pivotal figure. He had to interview patients on arriving at the Centre and assess their needs and dilemmas. Medical histories and current medication had to be checked on the spot by contacting previous GPs and hospitals. Patients were then directed to the doctor or nurse as appropriate. Referrals and liaison with support services such as housing, social or probation officers could also be initiated immediately. One other area of need which quickly became apparent was the extent and severity of psychiatric and emotional disturbance. Our experience showed the referring patients on for appointments to hospital clinics was generally unsuccessful. Patients often found appointments hard to keep and the clinics forbidding places where they felt uncomfortable. As a result appointments were often not kept. We were fortunate in being able to arrange drop-in psychiatry (and chiropody) clinics on a regular basis at the Centre. The present psychiatrist, who is an honorary consultant at the Maudsley Hospital, is also a qualified barrister and has developed close links with the courts, who frequently dealt with the homeless but found assessment and recommendations difficult. We now are able to offer same day assessment of the homeless who may be mentally ill and are before the courts. This frequently resulted in patients being rapidly referred to support services rather than remand and was both humane and highly cost effective.

Judging the success of projects needs to be done on a number of levels. Clearly, rising numbers of new and returning patients is an indication and both of these figures have increased annually. We now commonly see over forty patients a day. Another interesting feature came from a study we have completed on the patients attending the psychiatric clinic. Analysing the reattendance figures we found that those most likely to keep reattending were chronic schizophrenics and that the majority of these had been lost to previous psychiatric follow-up. These patients seem to find the clinic acceptable, probably for a number of reasons. The open-ended follow-up means it can be at times that suit them rather than the doctor. The accepting and open attitude of the psychiatrist and staff seems, in addition, to be well received (Joseph et al., 1990). This is particularly encouraging as the findings of Priest and others in common lodging houses suggest that these patients are less likely to attend clinics, preferring the anonymity provided by their homeless existence (Lodge-Patch, 1971; Priest, 1971). The Centre has developed continuously since its inception. It has responded pragmatically to perceived needs and the abilities of those taking part, rather than being planned rigidly at the outset. This may to some extent explain why the Centre has thrived despite the inevitable tensions and strains generated by arduous work of this nature, which could be expected to lead to an inflexible approach or to outright failure of the project as has been the case with a number of other initiatives. There is a common approach and a common sense of awareness of strengths and difficulties among staff which allows flexibility and responsibility, both with the patients and between the members of the staff.

The psychiatric service at Great Chapel Street

Psychiatrists have been encouraged to work within the community and sessions in general practice surgeries are no longer uncommon. The psychiatric services at Great Chapel Street has certain unusual features which are worth noting. The aim is that the service should be readily accessible, and that the minimum of barriers, administrative or personal, should be put between a need and its resolution. The service should be flexible and adaptable to the variety of mental ill-health in this population, there should be continuity of care for the individual, and continuity of support for changing or evolving needs. We have attempted to address these criteria as follows:

1. As with our other clinics, no appointments are necessary to see the psychiatrist. Any inconvenience caused by the fluctuation in numbers is more than compensated by the advantage of being seen to be readily available.
2. The psychiatrist is literally across the corridor from the general practitioner and the contact between them is fluent and frequent.

3. The emphasis in the consultation is to understand the patient rather than diagnose an illness.
4. Great store is set on continuity of care. It is important that the patient is not met with a succession of unfamiliar faces when in need of establishing some sort of therapeutic stability. This is a weakness of the hospital outpatient system that we have been anxious to avoid. It says much for the service that there have been few changes of medical staff in its history—the physician having been in post for 14 years and the psychiatrist for 8 years.
5. Continuity of care also implies continuity of support. The sick bay (see below) has been a vital 'next step' in the provision of care, and its success in individual cases has been quite remarkable. A number of patients admitted in an acutely psychotic state have, with time, developed unexpected personal and social skills and substantially improved the quality of their lives. We have also been moved by the way in which some of our schizophrenic patients have taken to looking after older patients and helping them with their daily necessities. This has encouraged us to think that therapeutic communities of between six to eight people could be established with the collaboration of housing associations. These would be largely autonomous but could be overseen by members of the sick bay staff. Further support would, as now, be continued to be supplied by the sick bay which would function as an unofficial day centre.
6. The psychiatrist is further helped by close liaison with other community services for the homeless, in particular voluntary and statutory housing, day centres, probation agencies and the courts.
7. A further innovation has been the creation through the Family Health Services of the post of Patient Services Coordinator. The present incumbent is a social worker who has dealt with the homeless for many years. His remit is to understand and research the needs of individual patients, and to act as an outreach worker, visiting the homeless where they sleep and helping to slot them into an appropriate agency. He also facilitates dialogue between various services dealing with the homeless; hence further opening up resources to the needs of the individual.

The present state of services is fragmented, limited and often poorly coordinated. We have had to evolve, of necessity, our own community care. As is usual in health care, the most vulnerable and needy must negotiate the least available care. Beginning with availability of psychiatric care, to addressing the need for supportive housing, help with the DSS and daytime support, including therapeutic day centres and alcohol support services, this integrated model of care has become a natural progression. The work is arduous, in large part because of the difficulty in obtaining and maintaining the variety of resources needed to meet the breadth of patients' needs. We hope that as community care becomes the accepted model, the organization and resources needed to make it work effectively and efficiently will become available.

WYTHAM HALL SICK BAY

It was perceived early on in our experience that the homeless sick, because of their circumstances, had needs which could not be met by conventional resources. There was no adequate provision of bed rest for those who, although ill, were not sick enough by normal criteria to warrant hospital admission. Indeed even those staying in many of London's hostels are required to leave during the daytime whether ill or not. Others in hospital may need care in the community after their discharge, but this is not readily available and rarely amounts to more than a bedsitter and an outpatient appointment. The failure of such arrangements is hardly surprising. The creation of a community hospital in Paddington proved to be no answer to this problem. The great majority of homeless admitted there found the rigidity of the routines unpalatable and discharged themselves shortly after admission. It is understandable, given their difficulties in coming to terms with routines or with authority, or with people who, however well meaning, were perceived as authoritarian or condescending. It was in this atmosphere that the idea of creating a sick bay arose.

In the early 1980s a number of Dr El-Kabir's former medical students from Oxford were undertaking clinical studies at the London teaching hospitals. They had worked with the homeless at Great Chapel Street Medical Centre during vacations. The idea evolved that if a property with bedsitting rooms could be found, they could live and study there and at the same time look after a small number of sick homeless. It took about three years of searching and convincing funding bodies before suitable premises were found. In 1984 a large terraced house in Maida Vale became available, with initial funding from the King's Fund and Bloomsbury Health Authority. The ground floor was converted to provide three bedrooms, with six beds, kitchen, bathrooms and a common room. Since then, conservatories and an extra four beds have been added. The majority of patients are referred from Great Chapel Street Clinic and another clinic for the homeless. In addition, hospitals refer patients directly from the wards, when their acute problem has resolved and aftercare with social support needs to be stressed. From the beginning Wytham Hall broke new ground, both in terms of extending the quality of care that can be offered to the homeless and, equally fascinating and important, in extending the often parochial education that medical students experience in the UK.

The sick bay allows us to look after patients with a wide variety of illnesses in a more complete and effective way than had previously been possible, even with the resource of Great Chapel Street Medical Centre. The scope of illnesses that we can deal with has increased to include major mental illness such as schizophrenia, tuberculosis, cardiovascular disease and alcohol withdrawal.

The operation and attitudes underlying the workings of the sick bay are of pivotal importance in achieving its effectiveness. The atmosphere is of seriousness and care administered with a lightness of touch. Regimentation is kept to a minimum: patients can come and go as they please between 9 a.m. and 7 p.m. Reasonable behaviour and an absolute ban on alcohol are the main rules. Each patient has a bed, locker and reading light and there is both a common room for company and television and a conservatory for quiet. When admitted, patients are introduced to the sick bay by the manager. A medical student clerks the patient on the day of arrival and the patient is then reviewed with a doctor. At this initital assessment a clinical plan is formed taking into account he wishes and problems of the patient. Indeed the distinction between addressing the illness and the patient's more global needs is minimal. As doctors and medical students are on-site, the care of the patient is relaxed but attentive to the responses to treatment and the new environment. We were initially surprised at the transformation in many patients within a short time of admission. This is probably due to the attitudes and atmosphere of the sick bay, which is exemplified by calling the patients 'Mr' rather than by the condescending Fred or Bill, an unearned familiarity which limits rather than encourages any rapport with a patient. Introversion and suspicion, a common feature of many of the homeless, frequently disappear, being replaced by self-respect and optimism. Awareness of this change is paramount as plans for housing, follow-up and even compliance with treatment depend very much on individual's capabilities and attitudes. If the maximum potential of the outcome of the stay is to be realized, it demands that we should be alert and sensitive to these factors.

Ward rounds are held once a week when all patients are formally reviewed and an assessment of progress made. Other resources which are available include local psychiatric day centres and workshops. These are made use of to encourage suitable patients to take up drawing, painting or sculpture. These activities prove invaluable, particularly for patients with psychiatric or psychological problems. At ward rounds future plans for housing and follow-up are explored by the staff, the patient being involved in these discussions when the time is right. Housing applications may take weeks or months and the scarcity of accommodation, be it independent flats or supportive houses, makes this task particularly difficult. The average stay at the sick bay is three to four weeks but some, usually with psychiatric or severe physical disability may stay up to 9 months. The guideline for the length of stay is simply that it should be as long as is needed to improve the patient's illness. Since opening Wytham Hall has cared for over 1100 patients, the commonest conditions being psychiatric, respiratory or skin disease, often complicated by alcohol abuse. Some conditions are serious, such as tuberculosis, cardiac failure or schizophrenia. The self discharge rate is around 20% which is remarkably low for such a group of patients, the usual precipitating factor being a return to alcohol abuse.

In addition to the day-to-day running of the sick bay Wytham Hall is also a meeting place. Guest nights are held regularly. People from a wide variety of backgrounds such as doctors, care workers, administrators and those involved in medical politics are invited to see and discuss our work.

The sick bay is run on a voluntary basis, by the doctors and medical students; only the administrator and caterers are paid. In describing the growth, organization and working of the sick bay, it is necessary to discuss the process by which a pragmatic approach to perceived needs, followed up logically, led to the creation and elaboration of the service.

To have a viable and above all consistent service, the following criteria had to be respected:

1. From the point of view of the patients, the approach had to be informal, understanding without being inquisitive, supportive without being overzealous and competent without being coercive.

2. From the point of view of the staff there had to be an atmosphere where creativity was nurtured and encouraged, so that even routine could be seen in a light where responsibility, self-respect and the understanding of others could mature all the time. Medical students in their preclinical years were encouraged to spend some of their vacations at the sick bay before making up their minds as to whether to reside there. There is always a danger that this concept of 'doing good' may attract people with a need to project their own unresolved conflicts onto helping others, with unrealistic expectations or a romanticized view of the underprivileged. In general such potential members are dissuaded from hasty decisions by experiencing the reality of caring for patients which might disappoint their misplaced expectations.

THE MOBILE SURGERY

In 1987 a group of councillors and social workers asked us whether we thought a mobile surgery that visited the sites where the homeless congregate to sleep might provide a useful service, as charitable funds were available to purchase a vehicle. We became interested in the idea and undertook to design the conversion of a Renault Master van into a mobile consulting room and operate the clinic on a regular basis. The interior has a seating area for consultations, an examining couch and a sink. A supply of medicines is taken in a case and there are dressings available. We initially visited Lincoln's Inn Fields in central London one evening a week, where up to 70 homeless sleep, but soon extended the service to the Bullring close to Waterloo station where around 150 sleep out. There have now been over 2000 consultations on the surgery.

An outreach project such as this is to some extent a reversal of the usual way in which someone sees a doctor. The sick person acknowledges that they need the help and advice of a doctor and seeks help as a patient at a surgery or clinic. However, with the mobile surgery we enter the homeless person's 'territory' and make ourselves available to consultation. It is important to recognize this as some may rightly feel this an invasion of their privacy and thus in operating the surgery we have had to show great sensitivity and patience. It took a number of visits to the sites before trust and rapport was established with the homeless but the numbers consulting soon grew. At present we see around 30 patients a week.

The conditions we find are what one might expect among such a population. Chest and musculoskeletal problems are particularly common, and many having injuries. Infestation is very common, often coexisting with other disease. What is surprising is the severity of some of the illnesses: frank osteomyelitis, psychosis, untreated epilepsy and young pregnant girls receiving no antenatal care. The prevalence of severe mental illness is less clear among those who sleep rough and hostel population data may not be applicable. We have just studied the prevalence of psychosis and alcohol abuse in residents of a cold weather shelter at a time of deep snow. Most came directly from the streets. Psychosis was relatively uncommon at 12%, whereas alcohol abuse was diagnosed in nearly two-thirds (Reed et al., 1992).

The picture rapidly emerged of an isolated group, many of whom did not even use day centres or hostels, and who suffer frequent and sometimes severe ill-health. Despite this only 37% in our study had a GP in London and many of those chose not to consult the GP for their illness. When asked why a patient had not registered the usual answer was that they had not been ill. Less than 10% gave as the reason that GPs were not likely to accept them. The patients felt that if they were sufficiently ill to need medical help then they would go to a casualty department. We also had a strong feeling that there was a reluctance on a somewhat deeper level among many homeless to seeing a doctor. This was summed up by one, who when asked why he and others took so long to see us replied 'because we're afraid of what you might find'. We feel that this fear, on both a physical and psychological level, lies behind much of the unusual behaviour that is experienced with homeless patients, particularly at the start of consultations.

The majority of problems can be dealt with by the surgery but follow-up and further investigations are obviously desirable in some. Indeed without the ability to refer patients on for further management the value of the service would be markedly reduced. Follow-up was directed to existing clinics and particularly at Great Chapel Street Medical Centre for patients seen at the nearby Lincoln's Inn Fields. When we studied this aspect of the clinic, we found that about a third of all patients seen at Lincoln's Inn Fields consulted at our medical centre within a month of their first consultation on the mobile surgery (Ramsden *et al.*, 1988). This observation is encouraging as it suggests that the mobile surgery can act as a link between this particular group of homeless and formal sources of health care.

Some patients have had fractures and been taken to a local casualty department in the van. Others have been admitted directly to Wytham Hall Sick Bay for more intensive assessment and treatment. We are aware that some who use the surgery do not want to go to any formal clinics and we accept this. Yet others will not consult on the surgery, despite the ease of access. Without such a scheme our work would miss a large section of the single homeless, who would not otherwise use the facilities. The mobile surgery is not a panacea for the homeless who sleep out, but, aided by flexible back-up, it can make an important difference to the health and lives of those not served by other resources.

IMPLICATIONS

We have described some unusual ways of dealing with a current medico-social problem. One reason setting up these special services for the homeless has been the need to adapt pragmatically to their needs. Perhaps another factor is to be found in the implications of the dynamics of the medical consultation. The patient comes to the doctor because he needs help with a particular problem in his life. He comes with certain needs, certain fears, certain preconceptions of which the doctor needs to be aware. The doctor may equally view the homeless patient with a degree of unease which the unfamiliar or potentially frustrating would engender in the unprepared.

If we can analyse this situation we would have to turn to the variables which bear upon it. The patient frequently finds the routines of life coercive and intolerable; these may be reflected in the authority of the doctor and in the institutions in which he works, the surgery, the hospital outpatient department or the ward. In addition the patient may well be aware, consciously or otherwise, of the fragility of his condition and afraid of its consequences. The doctor has similar dilemmas. He is usually unprepared to meet unconventional situations and the 'medical model' has traditionally been the means by which he interprets the patient's needs rather than seeing those needs in what the ancient Greeks called 'a sense of ecstasy', i.e. a dispassionate appraisal of what is being said by the patient and what is being perceived by the doctor. Nowhere in his education has he been encouraged to ask seminal questions about himself as a decision-maker, of his resources, personal as well as therapeutic, as a provider of care. Many doctors may be nice, sympathetic, and good listeners. Few have been encouraged to think deeply about the social and economic issues, and to see them in a historical perspective or have an attitude to suffering, ageing and death which has been thought out and refined through experience or necessity.

The homeless are often referred to as outsiders, yet we can all be said to be outsiders of one sort or another. We all have feelings that non-one can share, and no-one can share another's death. We consider ourselves insiders because we collude, en masse, like Ibsen's Trolls, into believing that all is well with life and death, with our interpersonal relationships, with our work, with the way we integrate within the social system of our day. To understand and feel for the homeless is thus to further one's ability to feel compassion towards oneself.

The built-in authoritarianism of the medical profession has long been commented upon satirically (for example, by Molière in *Le Malade Imaginaire* and Bernard Shaw in *The Doctor's Dilemma*) or philosophically and sociologically (Foucault, 1973; Illich, 1976; Kennedy, 1981). It is built on the premise that the doctor is ultimately the arbiter of what constitutes another person's illness and therefore as what he chooses to see as within his competence— a sort of restrictive practice of ill-health, which would be absurd if it were to be adopted by say, a plumber or a carpenter; and this in these days where the neuro-endocrine mechanisms, demonstrating the effects on the organism of external and internal stress, have been clearly established (Harris, 1955). This is an illustration of how the profession adapts to the problems it is unprepared to face by 'doubling' (Lifton, 1986), where, for example, a knowledge of the mechanisms of production of endorphins is kept separate from its implications on the phenomena of ill-health. Some have felt that medicine had become 'too scientific' and have stressed the human aspects of practice (Peabody, 1927; Engel, 1971), or a 'holistic' approach where the needs of the 'mind', 'body' and 'spirit' have to be addressed. We are far from advocating that medicine should be less scientific. On the contrary, we feel that it is, in some ways, not scientific enough in its acknowledgement of variables and of observer bias. We equally feel that the sometimes nebulous assumptions of 'holistic medicine' might lead to the substitution of one theology for another. We need a definition of ill-health which would be more apposite to the realities of what patients experience when they are unwell. We propose for the purposes of this discussion to define ill-health as a change in the internal condition of a person which is regarded, subjectively or objectively, to be noxious to him or others.

In the past, the priest, as well as the doctor, could have been the person to whom the problem could be addressed, but it would seem that the doctor will increasingly have to face the demands of the unwell in our society. If we accept this concept, we must agree that the medical course is singularly ill-designed to fulfil the needs of either students or their future patients. It is ironical that one's initiation to the medical course should take the form of dissecting a dead body, and experimenting with the frog gastrocnemius preparation. This is symbolic of the lack of balance in the attitude of didactic teaching, not subjected to an overview of the needs of the student, and heedless of the deadening effect upon curiosity of an inflexible and authoritarian attitude to what is to be taught in the medical curriculum. It is encouraging to note that the profession as a whole is becoming conscious of these deficiencies (Kilpatrick, 1989) and some of the obstacles to reform (Shaw, 1989). Attempts are being made to humanize the medical course (American Board of Internal Medicine, 1985), especially and more radically Harvard (Tosteson, 1990). Wytham Hall was created largely as a result of tutorial situations at Oxford where the attitudes of undergraduates were explored and tested in the manner of a Socractic dialogue. Its success can be seen as evidence of this view of the relationship between the role of the student and the teacher and is echoed in the relationship between the patient and the doctor.

The ideal of community care is a noble one, in which society acknowledges its awareness of the fragility of the human condition and the vulnerability of some of its members. It often, alas, becomes a rather vague concept, where imprecision of thought hides infirmity of purpose. That this need not be so is demonstrated in some measure in the Newcastle experiment (Community Care, 1990), where a shared sense of purpose by voluntary and statutory bodies has elaborated a model of care on a regional basis. We have attempted to state what, to our mind, is needed and can be done to make it a more secure and universal concept in the future.

REFERENCES

American Board of Internal Medicine (1985) *A Guide to Awareness and Evaluation of Humanistic Qualities in the Internist*.

Canter, D., Moore, J., Stockley, D., Littler, T. and Drake, M. (1988). Preliminary Report on Experimental Pilot Count of People who are Homeless in West Central London. Report 1. Department of Psychology, University of Surrey.

Community Care. (1990) *Partnership in Action*. Business Sciences (UK), London.

Davidson, A., Hildrey, A. and Floyer, M. (1983) Use and misuse of an Accident and Emergency department in the East End of London. *Journal of the Royal Society of Medicine*, 76, 37–40.

El-Kabir, D. (1982) Great Chapel Street Medical Centre. *British Medical Journal*, 284, 480–481.

Engel, G.L. (1971) Care and feeding of the medical student. *Journal of the American Medical Association*, 215, no. 7, 1135–1141.

Foucault, M. (1973) *The Birth of the Clinic*. Tavistock Publications, London.

Harris, G. (1955). *The Neural Control of the Pituitary Gland*. Edward Arnold, London.

Illich, I. (1976) *Limits to Medicine*. Maryon Boyers, London.

Joseph, P., Bridgewater, J., Ramsden, S. and El-Kabir, D. (1990) A psychiatric clinic for the single homeless in a primary care setting in inner London. *Psychiatric Bulletin*, 14, 270–271.

Kennedy, I. (1981) *The Unmasking of Medicine*. George, Allen and Unwin, London.

Kilpatrick, R. (1989) In: *Annual Report of the General Medical Council*, p. 2.

Laidlaw, S. (1956). *Glasgow Common Lodging Houses and the People Living in Them*. Glasgow Corporation.

Lamb, H. (1984) Deinstitutionalisation and the homeless mentally ill. *Hospital and Community Psychiatry*, **35**, 889–907.

Lifton, R. (1986) *The Nazi Doctors*, Macmillan, London.

Lodge-Patch, I. (1971) Homeless men in London: Demographic findings in a common lodging house sample. *British Journal of Psychiatry*, **118**, 313–317.

Peabody, C. (1927) The care of the patient. *Journal of the American Medical Association*, **88** 877–882.

Priest, R. (1971) The Edinburgh homeless: psychiatric survey. *American Journal of Psychotherapy*, **25**, 191–213.

Ramsden, S., Baur, S. and El-Kabir, D. (1988) Tuberculosis among the central London single homeless. *Journal of the Royal College of Physicians*, **22**, 16–17.

Ramsden, S., Nyiri, P., Bridgewater, J. and El-Kabir, D. (1989) A mobile surgery for single homeless people in London. *British Medical Journal*, **289**, 372–374.

Reed, A., Ramsden, S., Marshall, J. *et al.* (1992) Psychiatric morbidity and substance abuse among residents of a cold weather shelter. *British Medical Journal*, **304**, 1028–1029.

Scott, R., Gaskell, P. and Morrell, D. (1966) Patients who reside in common lodging houses. *British Medical Journal*, **ii**, 1561–1564.

Shanks, N. (1982). Improving the identification rate of pulmonary tuberculosis among inmates of common lodging houses. *Journal of Epidemiology and Community Health*, **36**, 130–132.

Shaw, D. (1989) In: *Annual Report of the General Medical Council* pp. 16–17.

Tosteson, D. (1990) New pathways in general medical education. *New England Medical Journal*, **4**, 234–238.

Tyrer, P. (1984) Psychiatric clinics in general practice. An extension of community care. *British Journal of Psychiatry*, **145**, 9–14.

Weller, M., Tobiansky, R., Hollander, D. and Ibrahimi, S. (1989) Psychosis and destitution at Christmas. *Lancet* 1509–1551.

10 WORKING WELL WITH PEOPLE WITH LONG-TERM MENTAL HEALTH PROBLEMS: THE PROCESS OF PSYCHIATRIC REHABILITATION

I. Morris

INTRODUCTION

Despite the considerable progress made in psychiatric rehabilitation in recent years, a significant proportion of patients experience an episode of severe mental illness that does not have a favourable outcome (Johnstone *et al.*, 1990; Watt *et al.*, 1983). This group is characterized by poorly controlled symptomatology and social handicap which, to varying degrees, prevents the realization of their previous personal potential. However, much can be done to help people with severe and persistent mental illness to achieve and maintain as good a level of social adjustment as possible. This prevents the downward drift towards passivity, social segregation and loss of independence. Psychiatric rehabilitation addresses these problems and is concerned with preventing the adverse psychological and social consequences of disability. Sometimes the term psychiatric rehabilitation is not fully understood and we will begin by considering this further.

There has been a tendency in the past to equate psychiatric

rehabilitation with the resettlement of institutionalized patients from the large psychiatric hospitals to the community. However, for the purposes of this chapter psychiatric rehabilitation will be considered to have a broader scope. Shepherd (1991) defines this wider perspective as, '. . . the notion that what is important in determining a person's social adaptation is the dynamic interaction between his or her social disabilities and their social environment. Psychiatric rehabilitation addresses this dynamic adaptation and attempts to maximise functioning, while at the same time acknowledging the possibility of relatively fixed disabilities and the necessity of providing supportive environments.' Psychiatric rehabilitation is therefore an approach to working with people with long-term mental illness that considers this complex interaction of disability with social and psychological circumstances.

PSYCHIATRIC REHABILITATION, RESETTLEMENT AND COMMUNITY CARE

Most psychiatric rehabilitation programmes were initially developed in the large psychiatric hospitals (Ekdawi, 1972; Bennett, 1961). They had as their goal the resettlement of long-stay patients in supported accommodation in the community. In this way psychiatric rehabilitation became almost synonymous with resettlement (Bennett and Morris, 1983). However, most people with long-term mental illness do not now reside in hospital. They live in the community with their families, on their own, or in supported accommodation. The process of psychiatric rehabilitation therefore needs to be less associated with resettlement, and more concerned with a general approach to the care of people with long-term mental illness irrespective of where they reside.

The association of psychiatric rehabilitation with resettlement also implied, to some extent, that it is a time limited approach. When long-stay patients left hospital to live in the community the goals of rehabilitation had been achieved. However, if rehabilitation is an approach that is of value to people with long-term mental illness, irrespective of whether they are in hospital or in the community, then it is not a time limited endeavour but a lifelong commitment to the psychiatrically handicapped individual. Viewed in this way, rehabilitation is not an approach leading to one end such as discharge from hospital or engagement in day care, but is an ongoing process of regular assessment of needs, of social adjustment and of support systems.

The need to broaden the scope of psychiatric rehabilitation is all the more important as increasingly services for people with severe and persistent mental illness are developed in the community. Living in the community is not a panacea and, without a positive approach to their care, this can be a disabling, rather than an enabling, experience for people with long-term mental health problems. Indeed, it could be argued that applying the principles of psychiatric rehabilitation is even more important in the community than in the mental hospital. On the long-stay wards of the mental hospital the notion of asylum meant that patients were, to a considerable extent, insulated from the demands of everyday life. In the community those with long-term mental illness are more likely to be exposed to the fluctuating demands, pleasures and uncertainties of an unsheltered existence. Life events, changing social circumstances, and the demands of more independent living might contribute to a more precarious psychological adjustment and an increased likelihood of relapse (Brown and Birley, 1968). People with long-term mental illness living in the community might therefore deteriorate, remain stable or improve over time, and needs for treatment, rehabilitation and social support will be constantly changing. A service founded on the principles of psychiatric rehabilitation will involve regular assessment and the formulation of a community care plan. This will ensure that adequate measures are taken to help people with long-term mental illness adapt to more variable social demands than might be experienced in hospital.

Psychiatric rehabilitation, then, is not necessarily about step by step improvement, but must also take into account decrements in functioning, fluctuation in mental state and changes in a social network that will affect the individual's capacity to meet the challenges of community life.

A further consequence of rehabilitation being synonymous with resettlement is that rehabilitation programmes have been selective, focusing their efforts on the least disabled patients thought to have greatest potential for independent life in the community. This practice has resulted in rehabilitation being deemed inappropriate for some of those most severely disabled by mental illness. Surveying the population of one large psychiatric hospital, Bewley *et al.*

(1981) wrote: 'No rehabilitation was needed or possible for 40% of the patients.' These patients were thought to be too disabled to benefit. Yet this group, perhaps more than any other, need a positive therapeutic approach, with carefully structured expectations, to prevent undue deterioration and depersonalization. There is no evidence to suggest that they do not benefit. Hall *et al.* (1977), in a careful evaluation of a token economy approach, noted that it was the most handicapped patients who benefited the most, though they continued to need a high level of support. When rehabilitation is less closely associated with resettlement it is an approach to care that guides the setting of modest but positive goals for even the most handicapped individual. Wykes (1982) described the value of this style of care for 'new' long-stay residents in a hospital based long-term hostel. In this setting it was assumed that most of the residents would *not* be able to live more independently outside hospital. However, every effort was made to help them reach as good a level of independence as possible by the implementation of the principles of good psychiatric rehabilitation. The hospital-hostel residents were found to improve in their functioning compared with a control group receiving more custodial care.

REHABILITATION, TREATMENT AND HOSPITALIZATION

In reconsidering our definition of psychiatric rehabilitation it is also worth considering the distinction between treatment and rehabilitation. The medical model of psychiatric care brought with it an emphasis on acute treatment and cure. This resulted in a tendency to concentrate resources in units providing acute care. Such a conceptual framework is not helpful when psychiatric problems take a chronic course in which therapeutic success is limited and the ultimate goal of complete recovery is unobtainable. Professional staff can then find it difficult to come to terms with their limitations and their consequent demoralization becomes detrimental to those in their care. This process has been described on acute wards where the frequency of contact and interaction decreases the longer a patient is on a ward (Altschul, 1972). The abandonment of long-term patients to poorly resourced back wards, or to inadequate care in the community, perhaps also reflects the difficulties all disciplines have in accepting their therapeutic failure. To some extent these problems might be attributed to the dominance of the 'treatment' model that has little to offer when treatment has proved wholly or partially unsuccessful. Staff will only work well with people who have long-term mental health problems when they have a different model of care that takes account of treatment limitations. The process of psychiatric rehabilitation begins when there is a recognition of the limitations of treatment, an acceptance of some degree of residual disability, and an understanding that the psychiatric problems are likely to take a long-term course. This is not to argue that maintenance or prophylactic treatment does not play an important part in long-term care. However, it is not enough to ensure a reasonable quality of care that takes a comprehensive account of the difficulties that are experienced by those with long-term mental illness and their families.

The difference between treatment and rehabilitation is to some extent blurred, however, and the difference in emphasis is summarized in Table 1.

The rewards that accompany effective treatment are less easily

Table 1 Distinctions between treatment and rehabilitation

Acute treatment	Rehabilitation
Assumes minimal or no residual disability and social handicap	Assumes some degree of residual disability and social handicap
Frequently, though not always, time limited	Not time limited. Recognition of need for long-term support
Main focus is psychological change, stabilization of mental state reduction of symptomatology	Focus on functioning and promotion of social adaptation in the context of residual or poorly controlled symptomatology
Assumes that the patient will be well enough to return to usual domestic and vocational roles	Assumes that there is likely to be difficulty maintaining previous social roles. Sheltered or supportive environments might be necessary
Progress is more likely to be fairly quick and the work of staff will be demand led	Progress is more likely to be slow with gradual steps being taken to minimize stress and prevent over-stimulation

obtainable when working with those whose problems are long-term or fluctuating. However, rewards can be forthcoming if staff, in partnership with their clients, set realistic and constructive goals to improve quality of life, adopt a positive attitude and monitor the effects of their work carefully. This has been recognized for some time. Brown (1973), writing of the neglect of long-stay hospital patients comments, 'One of the persistent failures of the medical profession in the care of the handicapped has been to ignore the need for setting, in conjunction with other professional groups, a sufficiently graded series of goals which both other professional groups and themselves could use to find the work useful and rewarding. For this it is unnecessary to cure the patient. Once it is recognized how little can be done a worker can be rewarded by quite slow progress.' To be fair it must be added that the fault lies not just with the medical profession, but with all professional groups who tend to find working with the acutely ill more rewarding than devoting their time to those with chronic conditions and associated social disability.

THE ROLE OF THE HOSPITAL IN PSYCHIATRIC REHABILITATION

Given the limitations of the treatment model and the importance of a long-term perspective, it is useful at this stage to consider the role of the hospital in psychiatric rehabilitation. Frequently, reduction of rates of rehospitalization, rates of discharge and length of community tenure have been used as measures of the success of rehabilitation programmes. However, the avoidance of hospitalization, or the minimal use of hospitalization, cannot be judged a success if this results in people with long-term mental health problems not being admitted when they might benefit from inpatient care. Equally unsatisfactory is when clients are out of hospital but living in a state of self-neglect, disturbance or distress. This situation is not uncommon and was referred to in the Report of the Select Committee of the House of Commons (1985) that commented, 'Great difficulties are being experienced in procuring emergency psychiatric care, putting strain on the individuals concerned and their families, (p. cxix, par. 53). Although all should be done to prevent relapse, and minimize the disruption to patients' lives which hospitalization can cause, this should not be judged as a failure of community care. Locally based hospital services are not an *alternative* to community care but one element in the network of services available. The success of hospital services should therefore be judged by the extent to which they are used appropriately to meet the accurately assessed needs of people with long-term mental illness. More sophisticated evaluative measures are needed to assess the value of rehabilitation programmes than the crude indices of readmission rates, and use of psychiatric beds in a local service. Some of these issues are discussed in Chapter 3.

To summarize, rehabilitation is not just about leaving hospital or minimizing the use of hospital care; it is not just about gradual improvement or potential for progress. Rehabilitation is essentially a therapeutic approach that implies finding possibilities for positive work despite severe and long-standing difficulties. It is optimistic in that it assumes that much can be done to alleviate difficulties and enhance and maintain independent functioning. However, it is also realistic in appreciating the problems which clients and their families can experience and in recognizing limits to the degree of success that can be attained. It is, as Creer and Wing (1974) suggest in their account of the experience of living with schizophrenia, only when it is accepted that problems are likely to be long-term, that appropriate and positive adjustments can be made by patients and their families. Over-optimism is not helpful. Models of mental illness that attribute all deficits in functioning to the effects of institutional life, the over-zealous application of the medical model or social stigmatization and segregation are likely to deny the reality of the experience of severe mental illness. This over-simplified perspective can result in the assumption that disabilities will 'melt away' in a normal environment in the community. While, indeed, there is much that can be done to improve problems and minimize ensuing social handicap, unfortunately primary disability is unlikely to disappear. A danger of such an over-optimistic approach is that staff can easily become disillusioned when they are unable to realize high expectations and then fail to take more modest, positive steps that would be beneficial.

Those with social disability resulting from severe mental illness will only be able to make use of opportunities presented by community care if they are enabled to do so by a well thought out programme of rehabilitation. Bennett (1978) has defined psychiatric rehabilitation as '... the process of helping the psychiatrically disabled person to function at as optimum a level as possible in a social setting which is as normal as possible.' The emphasis here is on developing the potential of each individual and thinking carefully about the environmental context. Wing and Morris (1981) suggest that in the process of rehabilitation, 'A thorough assessment of the nature of disablement will form the basis for setting goals of rehabilitation for each patient and for the formulation of a plan of action to achieve the goals. Rehabilitation therefore necessitates a long-term commitment to the individual patient.' The emphasis here is on clarity of purpose and action over extended periods of time. Both definitions place the theory and practice of rehabilitation in a central position in our general approach to the positive care of people with severe and persistent mental health problems.

Finally it must be stressed that rehabilitation is essentially a partnership. Learning from each other, staff and clients will work out together the best ways to improve quality of life and ameliorate the impact of residual symptomatology. In this way the autonomy of people with mental health problems will not be undermined and the process of psychiatric rehabilitation will help to strengthen and maintain their place in wider society.

WHAT NEEDS MUST BE MET?

In the first part of this chapter we have considered the *process* of psychiatric rehabilitation. Now we will turn to the content. What are the needs that must be met if people with long-term mental illness are to achieve the best possible social adjustment and lead respected and rewarding lives in the community? One way to think about this is to consider 'ordinary' needs and 'special' needs.

People with long-term mental illness have ordinary needs like the rest of us. They seek financial security, a place to live, rewarding personal relationships and some purpose in life (Lehman, 1983). However, these modest aspirations can be difficult to achieve in the context of motivational problems, a pull towards dependency, and residual symptoms that impair thinking and concentration. Rehabilitation is about enabling people with long-term mental illness to meet these ordinary needs themselves or with support.

It is also important to think about the special needs that arise as a result of severe and persistent mental illness. These will include the prescription and monitoring of prophylactic medication, the provision of supportive or compensatory environments, family work, and finding ways to develop skills. A comprehensive rehabilitation plan will ensure that both ordinary and special needs are being met.

To explore this further we will now look at some examples of the way in which the principles of rehabilitation can be put into practice to meet the ordinary and the special needs of people with long-term mental illness.

MEETING ORDINARY NEEDS

An ordinary need that we all share is for some sort of structure or framework around which we organize our lives. Often this framework is determined by the demands of paid employment, family responsibilities and domestic routines. However, people with severe mental health problems frequently lose this structure because of unemployment or because of difficulties sustaining social roles. One aim of a rehabilitation programme can be to plan a routine that will be satisfying but will not jeopardize fragile psychological adjustment. Sometimes staff working with this client group are suspicious of the need to create some sort of structure. This is because of their awareness of rigid institutional regimes and an understandable wish to avoid reproducing such practices in the community. However, a clear distinction must be made between *institutional regimes* that apply to all patients irrespective of their individual needs and *personal routines* that reflect individual preferences. The notion that an absence of any routine or structure will benefit people with long-term mental problems is mistaken. They will not be helped by a disorganized existence without structure or boundaries. It is important, however, to ensure that routines are planned in partnership with clients according to their wishes. The following example illustrates this process of helping an inpatient with very severe problems plan a better start to her day.

One common difficulty encountered by people with long-term mental illness (and many of the rest of us), is getting up in the morning. Some might argue that this is not a problem if it reflects the client's choice, but it can be a source of demoralization to people with long-term mental illness. It can also prevent them participating in rewarding activities and can lead to a distorted lifestyle if they sleep all day and are up all night. Other problems such as pacing about at night can be a source of distress to families, or other residents in supported accommodation. Unsafe behaviour in the kitchen, when nobody else is around, can also be a source of anxiety. Establishing a more natural daily pattern can help with these difficulties. The following example describes how this problem was tackled in an intensive rehabilitation ward in a large psychiatric hospital.

Miss A had recently moved to the intensive rehabilitation ward. She had spent many years living on an acute psychiatric ward because of the severity of her problems. She was distressed by very active symptomatology which had never been well controlled. She spent much of the time on her previous ward in bed and despite the efforts of staff, it had not been possible to help her participate in activities that might be a source of satisfaction or make use of her personal strengths. On the intensive rehabilitation unit the staff planned to help her develop a more satisfying daily routine. Attempts by the staff to prompt Miss A to get up had not been successful and had resulted in increased verbal abuse. In a team discussion it was pointed out that we all have preferences regarding the way we like to start the day. The key worker agreed to discuss this further with Miss A who said that she liked to be wakened and then lie in bed for a while before getting up to face the day. She also said that she would find things easier if as soon as she got up she could look forward to a cup of tea and cigarette before getting dressed. This routine was documented on her care plan so that all the staff could respect Miss A's wishes. Staff noted on the care plan evaluation how the plan was going. This way the key worker and Miss A could review progress together.

The above example illustrates the way in which individual wishes can be accepted as the starting point for building up an individual routine. However, very seriously disturbed or institutionalized people might find it difficult to enter a dialogue with staff. For them it is necessary to try different routines and establish the best approach by a process of trial and error. This requires careful behavioural monitoring as progress is likely to fluctuate. For a detailed example of work of this kind see Afele and Morris (1983).

A further issue of relevance when thinking about meeting the ordinary needs of people with severe mental health problems is how help can be given in a way that facilitates learning. Occasionally staff might be concerned that they are giving too much help and therefore are reinforcing dependency. Lamb (1980) has identified this problem and suggested that this type of thinking can mean that help to carry out the ordinary activities of daily living is not provided. There is sometimes the belief that if staff do not offer help the client will gradually assume responsibility himself. This is unlikely to be the case when working with people who have major motivational problems, but it is necessary to think carefully about the way help is given. To use an analogy, nobody would dispute that very young children require considerable help from their parents. This help does not create dependency but gradually promotes the child's autonomy. Watchful parents greet tentative steps towards independence and reduce help in stages as the child gains in competence and confidence. Help which promotes learning in this way has the following features: it is given consistently, note is taken of progress towards independence that is actively encouraged, and support is gradually withdrawn in a consistent way. By thinking carefully about the way help is given independence can be promoted as the following example illustrates.

A resident in a hospital-hostel, Peter, had major difficulties with all aspects of self-care. He was very overweight and had difficulty dressing himself. He neglected to change his clothes which was a particular problem as he was occasionally incontinent and did not clean himself properly after using the toilet. As a result of these problems he needed a good deal of individual help to attend to his personal hygiene in the morning. To give help in a way that might help Peter learn a routine his key worker worked out a step-by-step approach with him. This list was kept in his bedroom and each morning a member of staff consistently reminded Peter of the routine. Peter would note each morning any steps he had managed to carry out independently. Help was then systematically withdrawn in these areas. Over a two year period Peter coped with his morning self-care much more independently.

Peter had mild learning difficulties. He was also disturbed by hallucinations and shouted aloud in an incomprehensible way that could be frightening to people who did not know him. Learning was not easy for him and he would have found it difficult to make progress had help been given by eleven different staff in eleven different ways. The care taken to improve consistency in the way help was given created environmental demands with which Peter could cope. The plan described illustrates an approach using consistency, feedback and fading help out in a systematic way.

Meeting ordinary needs also means helping people with long-term mental health problems to maintain valued social roles in wider society as described in Chapter 14. In psychiatric rehabilitation this aim is reflected in attempts to provide opportunities for employment or sheltered work (Watts, 1983). However, having a range of services is necessary but not sufficient to ensure that people handicapped by long-term mental illness are able to make use of these opportunities. Wansbrough and Cooper (1980), in their review of employment for people with mental illness, conclude that there must be close liaison between facilities offering sheltered work and other mental health services if employment rehabilitation is to be successful. This means that special measures must be taken if those with more severe difficulties are going to succeed. The following plan was worked out to help a woman with major problems cope with some sessions of sheltered work.

Miss B lived in a high support hostel. Although her self-care was quite good her behaviour tended to alienate her from other people. Her family, although fond of her, could not cope with her at home. Despite her problems Miss B was keen to get a job. An attempt had been made to involve her in a local sheltered workshop, but this had not worked out because of her disruptive behaviour and poor concentration. This was a great disappointment for Miss B. At a team discussion it was decided that it might be more successful if Miss B attended the workshop for a shorter period of time. This was agreed with the workshop staff. It was also felt that much of Miss B's disruptive behaviour was 'attention seeking'. What this really meant was that Miss B desperately needed personal contact and reassurance which it was impossible for the workshop staff to provide because of their responsibility for over 30 people. At a meeting with the workshop staff the hostel agreed to send a member of staff with Miss B. This member of staff helped in the workshop but every ten minutes sat down beside Miss B to give her reassurance and encouragement. This method worked quite well and the workshop staff and other workers felt able to cope with Miss B. Eventually, gaining confidence, Miss B was able to cope with the whole hour without a member of the hostel staff having to accompany her. Later on she decided that she would like more varied activities and a mixed programme of work and other activities was agreed. The method used in the workshop was also useful in helping Miss B cope with a wider range of other activities.

This example describes an enabling approach to help someone with major mental health problems make use of service opportunities available. It also illustrates flexibility on the part of the hostel staff and the workshop staff and a willingness to work together with Miss B to help her achieve a more constructive role which brought her some satisfaction.

MEETING SPECIAL NEEDS

In addition to meeting ordinary needs some people with long-term mental illness also have special needs arising from poorly controlled symptoms or secondary behavioural disturbance. Measures then need to be taken to ameliorate the negative impact of these problems. Taking prophylactic medication is one example of special measures which have to be taken. It might not be thought that this has much to do with rehabilitation, but a good rehabilitation team will think beyond pharmacological concerns. Such issues as compliance problems, working towards self-medication, and teaching clients more about the medication which they are taking can be addressed. The value of self-monitoring (Birchwood *et al.*, 1989) can also be explored. All of this will help to involve people with long-term mental health problems in decisions about their care and will help resist passivity and consequent loss of self-esteem.

One danger when working with people whose symptoms are poorly controlled and whose behaviour can be disturbed is to assume that medication is likely to be the only effective intervention. This can result in people with severe problems being maintained on high levels of medication with little impact on their problems. One woman on an intensive rehabilitation unit was periodically behaviourally disturbed. She screamed, shouted and occasionally harmed herself or others in the midst of these attacks. Previously they had been managed by PRN medication. This helped to calm her down but resulted in her being sedated much of the time. The rehabilitation team decided to try a different approach. When Miss M started to scream and shout a member of staff took her to a quiet area of the ward. She was asked if she wanted someone to remain with her or if she preferred to be left alone. Sometimes she found it reassuring to have a member of staff with her, at other times she preferred to listen to music which she found calming. She herself decided when she was ready to join the other patients again. These measures helped control the outbursts to some extent. Although they did not work 100% of the time they did seem to stop the episodes escalating and the staff felt confident to deal with them without resorting to additional medication. Miss M was eventually able to start attending a day centre in the community. At this time of change, the outbursts started to be a problem at the day centre. Miss M said that she liked attending, but her place was in jeopardy because of the behavioural disturbance. The sister of the rehabilitation ward went to discuss with day centre staff the methods which had been effective on the ward. Again these were helpful and the day centre staff encouraged Miss M to use a quiet cloakroom once an outburst started. But one can never be too confident of success. On one occasion Miss M did not calm down and pulled the washbasin from the wall! To their credit the day centre staff persevered and eventually Miss M was able to go and live in a high support house in the community.

Meeting special needs also means having a knowledge of the principles of social psychiatry and understanding the impact of the environment on psychosis. While trying to meet ordinary needs by increasing confidence and competence and aiding the development of meaningful social roles, care must be taken to ensure that this does not have an adverse effect on symptomatology. We know, for instance, that too much passivity or time doing nothing can have a deleterious effect on mental state (Wing and Brown, 1970). On the other hand excessive stimulation or expectations which are too high can also result in relapse (Stone and Eldred, 1959). Consequently, central to the process of rehabilitation is helping each individual to achieve the right balance of stimulation and withdrawal. Other research in social psychiatry points to the importance of the emotional environment (Brown et al., 1972; Leff et al., 1982). This work, mostly looking at family life, has identified factors such as degree of intimacy, over-involvement, critical attitude and an increase in life events, as being related to relapse. It could be hypothesized that these findings would be relevant to rehabilitation services. Staff might also be over-involved or critical in their attitudes. Thinking carefully about a rehabilitation plan should include discussions about the quality of relationships along these dimensions. Expectations which are too high or trying to move ahead too quickly could result in an excessive increase in life events. Care must therefore be taken to ensure changes are gradual and slowly paced.

Meeting special needs therefore means understanding the experience of severe mental illness and the social factors which can help or exacerbate the impact of residual symptomatology. This must go hand in hand with finding ways to enable clients to live valued and rewarding lives in partnership with those who care for them in the community.

CONCLUSION

Much of this book is about service planning and development. Issues such as the size of residential facilities, their location, types of staff to be employed and methods of care coordination are much debated. This debate is essentially about locus of care and organization of services. All of this is important, but absent from this debate, much of the time, is discussion about the way in which we work with clients. Why is this? Is it in some ways a flight from understanding the reality of the experience of being with those who are most severely mentally ill? In the old mental hospitals social distance between staff and patients was one of the features of institutional regimes. With low staffing levels and poor resources, contact between staff and patients was reduced to the essential, custodial tasks. The current preoccupation with policies and service structures perhaps serves to distance ourselves from our clients in a more subtle way. Crucial issues to do with day-to-day practices are neglected. How do we work well with people whose lives and hopes have been damaged by mental illness? How do staff work with clients in supported housing, in day care facilities? How do we work on engaging people with major motivational difficulties in services? How do we help people who are severely socially withdrawn to have rewarding contact with others? What methods are available to us to minimize the negative impact of residual symptomatology and behavioural disturbance? How do we enable people who experience a powerful pull towards passivity to be more active in controlling their own lives? There are no easy answers to these questions but the theory and principles of psychiatric rehabilitation provide a sound knowledge base for practice. From this starting point we can begin to think through conceptually and practically the ways in which we can work in partnership with people who have severe and persistent mental health problems to promote an ordinary life in the community and meet their special needs.

REFERENCES

Afele, H. and Morris, I. (1986) Coming back to life. A case study of a severely regressed, long-stay psychiatric patient. *Nursing Times*, 14 May, 34–36.

Altschul, A.T. (1972) *A Study of Interaction Patterns in Acute Psychiatric Wards*. Churchill Livingstone, Edinburgh.

Bennett, D.H. (1961) A resettlement unit in a mental hospital. *Lancet*, 11, 539–541.

Bennett, D.H. (1978) Social forms of psychiatric treatment. In: *Schizophrenia Towards a New Synthesis* (J.K. Wing, ed.). Academic Press, London.

Bennett, D.H. and Morris, I. (1983) Deinstitutionalisation in the United Kingdom. *International Journal of Mental Health*, 11 (4), 5–23.

Bewley, T.H., Bland, M., Mechen, D. and Walch, E. (1981) 'New' chronic patients. *British Medical Journal*, 283, 1161–1164.

Birchwood, M., Smith, J. and MacMillan, F. (1989) Predicting relapse in schizophrenia the development and implementation of an early signs monitoring system using patients and families as observers. *Psychological Medicine*, 19, 649–656.

Brown, G.W. (1973) The mental hospital as an institution. *Social Science and Medicine*, 7, 407–424.

Brown, G.W. and Birley, J.L.T. (1968) Crises and life changes and the onset of schizophrenia. *Journal of Health and Social Behaviour*, 9, 203–214.

Brown, G.W., Birley, J.L.T. and Wing, J.K. (1972) Influence of family life on the course of schizophrenic disorders. *British Journal of Psychiatry*, 121, 241–2258.

Creer, C. and Wing, J.K. (1974) *Schizophrenia at Home*. National Schizophrenia Fellowship, Surbiton.

Ekdawi, M.Y. (1972) The Netherne Resettlement Unit: results of ten years. *British Journal of Psychiatry*, **121**, 417–424.

Hall, J.N., Baker, R.D. and Hutchinson, K. (1977) A controlled evaluation of token economy procedures with chronic schizophrenic patients. *Behaviour Research and Therapy*, **15**, 201–283.

House of Commons, Second Report from the Social Services Select Committee (1985) *Community Care with Special Reference to Adult Mentally Ill and Mentally Handicapped People*. HMSO, London.

Johnstone, E.C., MacMillan, J.F., Frith, C.D., Benn, D.K. and Crow, T.J. (1990) Further investigation of the predictors of outcome following first schizophrenic episodes. *British Journal of Psychiatry*, **157**, 182–189.

Lamb, H.R. (1980) Structure: the neglected ingredient of community treatment. *Archives of General Psychiatry*, **37**, 1224–1228.

Leff, J., Kuipers, L., Berkowitz, R., Eberlein-Vries, R. and Sturgeon, D. (1982) A controlled trial of social intervention in the families of schizophrenic patients. *British Journal of Psychiatry*, **141**, 121–134.

Lehman, A.F. (1983) The well-being of chronic mental patients. *Archives of General Psychiatry*, **40**, 369–373.

Shepherd, G. (1991) Psychiatric rehabilitation for the 1990s. Foreword. In: *Theory and Practice of Psychiatric Rehabilitation* (F.N. Watts and D.H. Bennett eds), 2nd edn. John Wiley & Sons, Chichester.

Stone, A.A. and Eldred, S.H. (1959) Delusion formation during the activation of chronic schizophrenic patients. *Archives of General Psychiatry*, **1**, 177–179.

Wansbrough, N. and Cooper, C. (1980) *Open Employment after Mental Illness*. London: Tavistock Publications.

Watt, D.C., Katz, K. and Shepherd, M. (1983) The natural history of schizophrenia. A five year prospective follow-up study of a representative sample of schizophrenics by means of standardised clinical and social adjustment. *Psychological Medicine*, **13**, 603–670.

Watts, F.N. (1983) Employment. In: *Theory and Practice of Psychiatric Rehabilitation* (F.N. Watts and D.H. Bennett eds). John Wiley & Sons, Chichester.

Wing, J.K. and Brown, G. (1970) *Institutionalism and Schizophrenia*. Cambridge University Press, Cambridge.

Wing, J.K. and Morris, B. (1981) *Handbook of Psychiatric Rehabilitation Practice*. Oxford University Press, London.

Wykes, T. (1982) A hostel ward for 'new' long-stay patients: an evaluative study of 'a ward in a house'. In: *Long-term Community Care: Experience in a London Borough* (J.K. Wing, ed.). Psychological Medicine monograph Supplement 2. Cambridge University Press, Cambridge.

11 AN INTENSIVE REHABILITATION UNIT: NINE YEARS EXPERIENCE

M.P.I. Weller

Sometimes I think it ain't none of us pure crazy and ain't none of us pure sane until the balance of us talks him that-a-way. It ain't so much what a fellow does, but it's the way the majority of folks is looking at him when he does it. (William Faulkner, As I Lay Dying)

INTRODUCTION

Experience on an Intensive Rehabilitation Unit, initiated by the author and Isobel Morris, over some nine years, in preparation for Friern Hospital closure, has demonstrated that meticulous attention to daily living programmes can produce substantial improvements in social performance over a period of eighteen months to three years. Successful community placements have been achieved with very ill residents. The Unit has provided an important component in the closure of Friern Hospital, providing a valuable interface with supportive hospital accommodation.

The unit aims to create realistic expectations of self-care, and domestic and occupational activity with prompting, feedback and reinforcement by praise and approval, within a comprehensive rehabilitation programme preparing residents for discharge. We maintain close contact with jointly funded ventures during the transition period and with the community support team. Emphasis is placed on taking small, constructive steps and gradually increasing expectations in relation to progress with a highly selected group of severely disabled residents.

The individually tailored behavioural programmes require patience and persistence with constant monitoring and revision.

SOME GENERAL CONSIDERATIONS

Gregariousness knits together the social fabric (Whyte, 1955; Becker, 1975; Reisman *et al.*, 1985) but an enduring tendency to a preoccupation with inner experiences and social isolation is prominent in many schizophrenic patients, who comprise the great majority of remaining long-term patients. As a result, perhaps the most obvious characteristic of our chronic patients is their minimal social contacts.

The more severely disturbed patients tend to come from a background of low social cohesiveness (Schwartz and Mintz, 1963), their friendships are generally weak and their affiliations often superficial. Such patients have withdrawn into an interior, isolated world of hallucinations and delusions. This may be erroneously interpreted as a result of prolonged institutional living, but the same finding occurs in a variety of settings, including a nuclear family environment (Weller *et al.*, 1989, 1990). We perceive our role as seeking to overcome or minimize these characteristics and to foster social interaction and independent living, as far as possible in a community setting.

We try to build on strengths to help the more disabled make the best of their abilities, improve their self-confidence and play the most normal role of which they are capable in society. To assist in these aims we maintain close liaison with community provisions, residents, relatives and friends.

The Unit must be seen as an important link in a chain of rehabilitation steps. We work particularly closely with a local authority managed, jointly funded, hostel, which has provided the main route of discharge from the Unit. Until the creation of this nurse managed facility as part of the Friern Hospital closure programme, discharge facilities were often inadequate to progress to the next phase of social rehabilitation and a more normal environment.

HOSPITAL MILIEU

The importance of environment is implicit in all forms of psychiatric treatment settings.

As hospital beds have been progressively reduced there has been a selective bias with a sifting of treatment resistive cases into prolonged care. Our present emphasis on hospital closures and discharge intensifies this selective tendency. Nevertheless, with refined, individualized measures to evaluate long-term treatment, such as measures of self-destructiveness and violence, and level of treatment compliance, an improvement can be achieved (Allen *et al.*, 1986) and we are anxious to discover the factors favouring to improvement and to develop these.

We have learnt to stress 'long-term' goals; extending improvement by slow degrees. We have come to believe that optimism is best sustained and patients/clients most helped if we first identify and then concentrate on very small gains in independence and social performance. We seek to travel a middle road between an unrealistic quick cure and the abandonment of therapeutic and rehabilitative endeavour in a belief in inevitable chronicity.

PROFILE OF THE WARD

A well resourced, mixed sex, 12 bed, Intensive Rehabilitation Unit was created at Friern Hospital in 1984, soon after the intended closure was announced. Effectively, we enjoyed a near doubling of nursing resources, with a staff : patient ratio of 2 : 1. There are two sessions of a clinical psychologist and six sessions of a psychology assistant and, for much of the time of operation of the ward, a full-time occupational therapist, with appropriate equipment. There is one consultant and a specially designated junior doctor, both with additional responsibilities. Each resident has his or her own room with personal washing facilities, writing space and chair, as well as bedroom furniture, and the atmosphere of the ward is homely. In addition, the residents have access to a variety of occupational departments within the hospital.

We have a budget for rehabilitation purposes, which the staff can use with considerable discretion, and a ward based activity programme. The ward budget is available to help residents develop their own shopping and budgeting skills. Activities and expeditions outside of the hospital are organized routinely, enticing patients into a more outward looking attitude that emphasizes our resettlement objective.

The young patients who are recruited into the Intensive Rehabilitation Unit setting are referred by other consultant colleagues. In large measure, they have persistently failed to progress in other environments and/or have created particular difficulties of containment. The Unit differed from the many other similar projects since all the patients are under compulsory sections of the Mental Health Act 1983 and provides a contained environment within a locked ward. The door is opened on request during free time such as lunch time, late afternoon, evening and during the weekends. We have a seclusion room which is used when patients are disturbed and a risk to other patients and staff. In addition, as an alternative, we have a segregation area, without furniture or door, in which patients can spend time separated from others (time out).

Whilst the importance of the ward milieu is well appreciated, it is difficult to modify, being very much dependent on goodwill, commitment and aptitudes amongst the staff. Wing et al. (1964) showed how patients' achievements are very much affected by the expectations and interest of the staff. The powerful placebo results in many medication trials vividly demonstrate the benefit of the milieu and therapeutic optimism. Schizophrenic patients are particularly sensitive and vulnerable to significant life events and to the emotional climate. Conscious of these factors, in the early stages the staff had meetings under the auspices of a trained psychoanalyst and these meetings continue although the initiator has retired. Mutual tolerance and acceptance is fostered and the ward culture has been happy and optimistic, despite recurring difficulties in sustaining resources, a change in direction away from multidistrict work and an intended relocation.

Despite the constraints engendered by the Unit being located in a dying psychiatric hospital, efforts are made to create opportunities for independence. Residents are engaged as fully as possible in daily

Figure 1   Daily behavioural objectives. ABC = antecedent behaviour and consequences.

DATE	19/10	20/10	21/10	22/10	23/10	24/10	25/10
	MON	TUE	WED	THUR	FRI	SAT	SUN
A) MORNING ROUTINE	3						
1) Getting up	3	2	3	A	3		
2) Personal/oral hygiene	3	2	3		3		
3) General appearance	3	2	2	W	3		
4) Makes bed	3	2	2	M	3		
				A			
B) WEEKLY SELF-CARE							
1) Bath/hairwash	1/1			2/2			
2) Change clothes							
3) Change bed							
4) Room cleaning							
5) Ward chores							
6) Wash/iron clothes							
C) WARD-BASED SESSIONS							
1) Exercise/relaxation	2	*Walk* 2		A	2		
2) Morning group	3	2		W			
3) PM relaxation group				M			
4) News/puzzle group				A			
5) Community group thur	1				1		
6) Social group (mon)	3						
7) Group meal							
8) Individual cooking							
9) *Social skills group*			2				
D) OTHER ACTIVITY							
1) Industrial therapy							
2) Outing							
3) Pottery/snooker							
4) Art therapy				*Absent*			
5) Gym			1				
6)							
7)							

SCALES A–D: 1=no prompting. 2=1–2 prompts. 3=3+ prompts. 4=refusal

COMMENTS (details of outings, ABC entries etc.)

....
....
....
....
....
....
....

domestic tasks. As a prelude to eventual discharge, and to foster domestic skills, we have a well equipped kitchen to help patients/ clients develop their cooking skills and ward based laundry facilities are provided. All residents are encouraged to wash and iron their own clothes, regularly to cook simple meals, bake, make tea and wash up their own crockery (Figure 1).

Individual care plans are devised to combat self-neglect, improve independence and reduce the time that patients habitually are 'doing nothing' (Wing and Brown, 1970) by promoting focused activities. These are often joint activities and thus help the patients to socialize, but whether they are joint or isolated activities, they encourage patients/clients to experience a degree of success through which they enjoy enhanced self-esteem.

In general, the serious illnesses we treat have had an early onset, and the patients have missed out on higher education, work and peer relationships enjoyed by their healthy contemporaries. Such experiences are important for coordinating social perceptions, maturation and development of inner resources.

Gentle but persistent efforts are first made to induce patients/ clients into unit based activities, later to activities elsewhere in the hospital, and eventually to outside day care facilities as a prelude to discharge to a supported environment. These patient efforts have gradually generated an ethos which itself facilitates reinvolvement in communal activity.

Since the resident population is relatively long-term and stay on the ward is long, we have an unusually favourable opportunity to foster a communal spirit, enhanced by unit-based activities, including daily group meetings, which, inter alia, improve communication skills. One meeting a week is devoted to reviewing feedback and review of individual programmes.

The core concepts on which the ward operates include structured individual care plans, clearly agreed and consistent expectations regarding day-to-day functioning, and the use of behavioural measures such as incentive schemes, social reinforcement and feedback. Every effort is made to stimulate interaction with staff and with residents and to improve social learning. The tailored programmes seek to emphasize the acquisition of skills and the reduction of bizarre and inappropriate behaviour. Expectations are carefully adjusted and constantly re-evaluated and efforts to generalize the specific training is assisted within the wide variety of activities available in the hospital setting.

We focus on developing 'social episodes' (Goffman, 1969) through joint action between patient/client and therapist, generally a nominated key worker. The unit provides a context and a set of conventions in which these episodes can be developed and integrated into the flow of everyday life. The relative stability of the resident population and the Unit staff helps create a sense of continuity and shared culture which is central in many therapeutic community projects. This relative stability raises patients/clients' hopes for improvement and fosters the development of self-confidence and self-acceptance through developing trust and learning to value relationships (Yallom, 1985).

Lutz (1988), from an anthropological perspective, emphasizes the inherently social nature of emotional experience, 'by far the most important [method] was my daily listening to people as they described present and past events to each other and made emotional sense of them. Every ethnographer knows the awe which accompanies this listening, as another way of seeing the world and being with others is revealed, sentence by sentence, conversation by conversation' (p. 46). She cites DeRivera (1984) with approval: 'It would be incorrect to say that a situation causes an emotion or that an emotion causes a perception of the situation. Rather the person's situation is always interpreted by some emotion' (p. 47). Russell Davis (1972), approaching the issue from a different perspective, and following the writings of Cameron (1943a, 1943b), emphasizes the need for confirmation of one's perceptions, and considers that social isolation, such as may occur in sensitive people during adolescence, is conducive to the evolution of idiosyncratic perceptions and concepts, which he sees as implicated in the aetiology of schizophrenia. These views extend back at least as far as Mead, who developed an inherently social model of consciousness (Miller, 1973), and occupational and industrial therapies are based on a belief in the beneficial effects of attending to real situations in company.

All residents start off with a ward based daily routine and activity programme, which enables us to observe and modify our programmes very closely and brings them into close contact with one another and the staff, encouraging relationships. As residents progress, sessions are arranged in other rehabilitation departments in the hospital and in suitable day centres in the community. We are fortunate in having particularly well-developed industrial and occupational therapeutic departments, authoritatively described as the best in the world, and a great deal of reliance has been placed on these activities off the ward. Light industrial work is contracted out, consisting of sorting, assembly and packaging. Supervision is supplied by occupational therapists. Patients are paid for sessional work and with additional bonuses. Arrangements have been made to carry forward some of these activities in the near vicinity when we move to a new site.

The occupational therapy programme includes remedial gymnastics, social skills training, speech therapy, art and pottery, music therapy, individual cookery and relaxation sessions. Many of these activities initially take place on the unit and then in the various departments as patients/clients improve.

The individual management programme is designed in consultation with the resident, one of the clinical psychologists attached to the ward and ward nursing staff, after a two week assessment period. We try to identify retained skills and strengths and ensure that residents have ample opportunity for development. A central component in realizing this objective is recognizing and appreciating small gains in competence. This is more easily achieved when experience of mental illness has led to an understanding of the interaction between symptomatology and the patient's social and physical environment (see Lenzenweger et al., 1991).

Many years ago, Welford (1958, 1968) described how cognitive decline is apparent in the elderly, who, however, given optimal conditions, in which thought is given to factors like reduction in the need for switching attention, could perform as well, or nearly as well, as young subjects (and who could perform better on some tasks). Similarly we have paid careful attention to devising appropriate unhurried activities in a (calm) environment.

We seek to provide opportunities to develop shared social activities, believing that all activity is potentially or actually joint action. Conversation is an intricate cooperative skill which can be learnt through cooperative activities such as games and ward chores. At first the staff take the initiative in creating a range of activities, rather as described by Vygotsky (1978) when discussing the development of social interaction amongst young children by what he termed the 'zone of proximal development'. Through participation in these planned and structured activities there is a gradual increase in the residents' interaction, involvement and initiative.

Most of the residents avail themselves of social clubs on the hospital premises, which enable them to maintain contacts outside of the ward in a situation where they can buy refreshments, listen to records, watch television or play snooker. There is a table tennis table on the ward and a variety of exercising equipment. This experience facilitates the later use of day centres and drop-in centres.

An objective evaluation of the Unit, with a matched control group, showed that residents on the Unit made significant progress in social functioning (Janez, 1985). In particular, and most importantly for our ultimate objective, patients on the Unit improved in the areas of self-care, participation in domestic tasks, and their social involvement during free time. Despite severe impairment in social functioning, all the patients cooked at least once a week, did their own washing and ironing, helped with laying the tables, washing up, and with ward chores. These activities are, of course, common in rehabilitation programmes. However, it is encouraging that some of the very handicapped patients met these expectations with one-to-one help.

Low motivation and aimless apathy are common problems amongst chronic psychiatric patients which may cause or amplify apparent cognitive dysfunction in schizophrenia (Summerfelt *et al.*, 1991) and an improvement in motivation, consequential on social reinforcement, is potentially helpful in overcoming difficulties which might be underpinned by an organic deficit.

We are convinced that it is possible to overcome some of the motivational problems within the Unit. Our rehabilitation tools are careful attention to individual abilities, prompting, feedback and reinforcement by praise and approval. This is embedded in a comprehensive rehabilitation programme and we attempt to carry through features of continuity of care by providing supportive community services in the eventual patient placements.

The general low motivation of schizophrenic patients, their apparent lack of 'inner compulsion', which Fromm suggests is a necessary ingredient for social cohesion (Fromm, 1944), makes it difficult to find strong reinforcements. On the other hand, work with the elderly, comparing 'prompting' with and without reinforcement, showed that reinforcement made no perceptible difference (Gotestam and Melin, 1990). In our experience approval in a stable environment with consistent staff, and 'prompting' is a

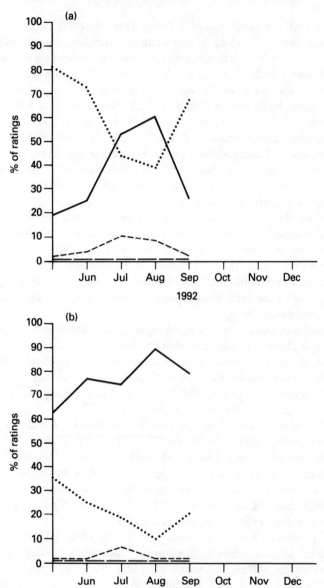

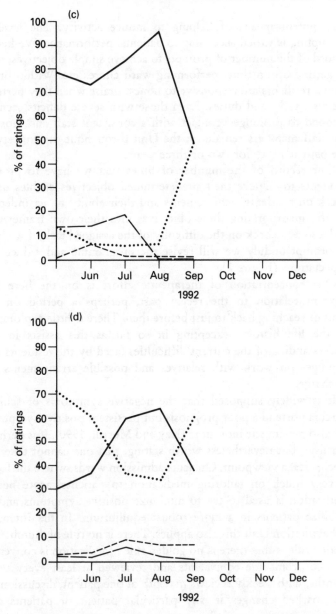

Figure 2 Prompt charts (a) Morning routine. (b) Weekly self-care and cleaning. (c) Other activity. (d) Overall rating. ———, no prompting; ......, 1–2 prompts; ----, 3+ prompts; ————, refusal.

very potent means of helping to induce activity. The level of prompting is varied according to patients' performance. We keep a record of the number of prompts to achieve simple objectives, such as getting up on time, performing ward chores etc. Within broad limits, residents are responsive to honest praise when they perform their set tasks and duties. Even those with severe deficits seem to respond to prolonged contact with a consistent staff and most of the staff members remain on the Unit throughout the entirety of the patient's stay for two or three years.

Our record of the number of times that we have to prompt residents to achieve their predetermined objectives enables us to check on residents' achievements and their ability to act independently, incorporating these objectives into their own framework, and also as a check on the difficulty of the assigned task; if we have to prompt unduly we will revise the programme and reduce our expectations (Figure 2).

Our concentration of therapeutic effort is on the here and now in relation to the recent past, perhaps a period on the Unit or reaching back to just before then. There is little exploration of the life history, excepting in so far as this assists in our understanding of the current difficulties faced by the residents and impinges on work with relatives and possible arrangements for discharge.

It is widely supposed that the negative symptoms of schizophrenia portend a poor prognosis but persistent positive symptoms are also pessimistic indicators (Kay and Murrill, 1990). It is perhaps a truism, but nevertheless worth stating, that one cannot take too mechanical a viewpoint. On acute admission wards, where the focus is very much on tailoring medication to patients' acute needs, medication is used to try to minimize positive symptoms and to stabilize patients in a more robust equilibrium. In the Intensive Rehabilitation Unit this also applies. There is no rule of thumb: 'the golden rule is that there is no golden rule'. Medication is converted to chlorpromazine equivalents and reviewed at least every three months, with weekly reviews in depth of one patient, discussion on any marked changes in any particular patient or patients and overviews of the remainder.

MONITORING AND DOCUMENTATION

Assessment instruments

In the past we have used the MRC Social Performance Scale and an in-house scale devised by a clinical psychologist Tilly Latimer-Sayer, who worked in the Unit, which incorporates the level of prompting. Both instruments have their advantages but we are currently using the Hall and Baker Social Rehabilitation Scale (Figure 3) (Baker and Hall, 1983), scored by the nursing staff, and the Manchester Scale (Krawiecka et al., 1977), a rating instrument for psychopathology applied by the medical staff. Both assessments are at three monthly intervals.

Specific tasks are generally of half an hour duration, to maintain concentration and involvement. Improvements in performance form a baseline for increases in task requirement, such as duration or complexity, or by reducing support. The daily record of all prompts given to residents to achieve their targets, is under constant review. The prompt records are read in conjunction with the Social Rehabilitation Scale and the Manchester Scale enabling us to monitor the patients' difficulties in achieving objectives and to adjust them as appropriate.

Initial asessment

Before residents are accepted into the Intensive Rehabilitation Unit, they have a full assessment of their symptoms and psychosocial functioning. We then invite the patients to attend the Unit over a period of weeks when we make further assessments and also introduce them to the Unit environment. These assessments become our baseline for monitoring progress and adjusting treatment strategies.

All intensive care patients are on compulsory orders, sometimes on Home Office restrictions. This reflects the severity of their psychopathology but it helps us to press patients a little more firmly than would be possible if we were dealing with a voluntary population. No punishment is used on the Unit. Residents are expected to get up, attend to their hygiene, brush their teeth etc., and as they improve to involve themselves in occupational and industrial therapy. We do not require the patients to do anything

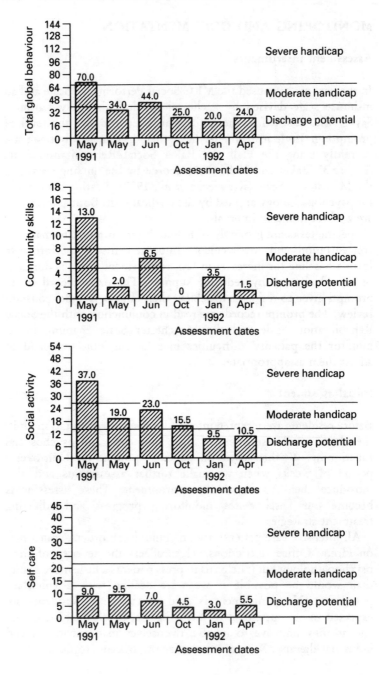

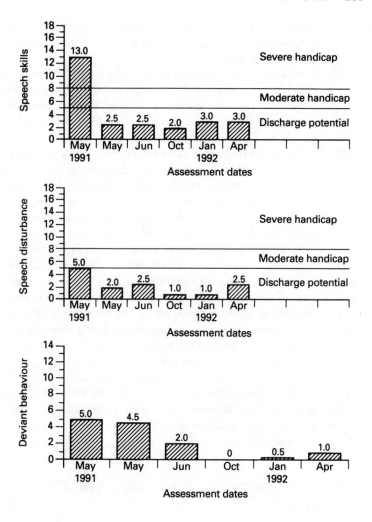

Figure 3 Hall and Baker Social Rehabilitation Scale.

onerous or offensive but to be competent in those areas which would be required for a measure of independent living outside of the hospital environment.

We do not expect patients to achieve all these daily living targets immediately, and, as explained, we are content with very slow progress. Nevertheless, we continue to urge patients to achieve these minimal objectives in our common quest for their discharge (see Figure 1).

We frequently encounter a tacit assumption from community carers that all psychiatric patients are fundamentally the same and are different from normal people only in degree. Psychiatrists recognize a disease concept with a natural history and progression and we seek to distinguish this from variants of normality. However, the so-called 'medical model' also recognizes the importance of the family and the social environment, it is this which engages our closest attention. We emphasize the merits of order, regularity and consistent expectations and in doing so share a common set of concepts with our colleagues outside of hospital.

Our experience above all has led us to advocate a policy of gradual gently increasing expectations, whilst being reconciled to a stuttering progression with many hiccups. We believe that our best work is done when we are especially patient and focused on long-term goals. In the same way that psychotherapy takes a long time but may provide long-term benefit, we aim to provide a secure background and well-thought-out social programme to enable residents to develop and live a richer and more rewarding life outside hospital settings.

DISCHARGE FROM THE UNIT INTO THE COMMUNITY

Transfer generally takes place in a phased manner with increasing leave to a community placement. We keep the bed open for a variable period after phased discharge, depending on circumstances but somewhere around six weeks to three months. When full discharge has been accomplished patients are returned to their donating consultant teams, four in number in west Haringey, and soon to be broadened to encompass another three teams in the east part of the district. We remain engagé in the event of problems or relapse, although readmission is generally routed through the acute admission ward.

It is important for staff morale that progress has been documented and that early expectations are not excessive. Social integration generally remains restricted but improves. It is fair to say that at the end of our rehabilitation programme, our patients/clients often have active symptomatology and profound social disabilities. They continue to need support in social activities, occupational therapy and training for domestic skills and counselling for relatives and supportive psychotherapy. These needs may remain unmet in community settings (Salokangas *et al.*, 1991) and are not readily available in depth in other hospital settings.

Disturbed patients still require a range of suitable facilities to retain skills and enable these to be developed further. It is the most telling indictment of the custodial attitudes of the past that it took so long for them to be challenged. We must not commit the corollary error of expecting too much and providing too little.

DISCHARGE INTO THE COMMUNITY

We have no jurisdiction over ultimate placements and have limited capacity to influence this importance determinant, and the range of supervised accommodation is still limited. Sometimes we can foresee problems. For example, one patient, who was resented by his mother, was, nevertheless, placed in a hostel very close to his mother's home and the arrangement rapidly broke down.

We welcome maintained contact with discharged residents and their carers but this is generally accommodated during a transition period while residents are settling in. The longer-term contact reverts to the donating consultant team in conjunction with the community support team.

Our goals are modest and carefully monitored, which encourages residents and staff at each step. It may seem unnecessary to stress the problems in schizophrenia but when we are discussing the illness with potential caring agencies we emphasize the chronicity of the disorder and the likelihood of this remaining problematic to temper unrealistic expectations. In some of the community placements, we have found that staff have very high expectations of residents' improvement and 'burn out' very quickly. The rate of staff turnover is very high; at first many in our district resigned after six months.

A widely held interpretation of 'normalization' in reality is a laissez-faire philosophy, which abandons residents to the ravages of their illness under the guise of enlightened treatment. Leaving them unsupervised to spend the day in bed and then to expel them from accommodation because they smoke, drink or fail to budget adequately and to pay their rent is to leave them without support when they most need help, on the dubious grounds that they have chosen this situation and exercised an inalienable choice, which has been denied them in hospital.

In the past we have been pessimistic about placements, particularly those which have a list of requirements that imply that residents can be model tenants and have no planned activities. As the service has developed these expectations have increasingly harmonized with ours and our success rate continues to improve.

SUMMARY AND CONCLUSION

In traditional long-stay wards, the mixing of patients with widely differing levels of florid symptoms and handicap diverts attention away from the more deteriorated patient. The Intensive Rehabilitation Unit has achieved some conspicuous successes with many of these residents, who were amongst the most disabled, recalcitrant, difficult and treatment resistant in the entire hospital. They were generally regarded as irredeemably chronic and needing perpetual long-term asylum.

Originally a multi-district ward, we drew from four separate districts and were able, over a typical period of two to two and a half years, to successfully discharge 33 patients/clients to community settings. In many instances, our failures to achieve discharge reflected the inadequacy of community resources and this gap is now being addressed constructively. We are in constant dialogue with a rehabilitation hostel with whom we work particularly closely, and are targeting many of our discharges through this channel. A special hostel for Afro-Car clients has recently come into operation which has three senior nurses on its staff who have had psychiatric hospital experience and which seems very promising.

Tooth and Brook (1961) attributed the decline in resident patients between the years 1954 and 1959 inter alia to the more active rehabilitation of long-stay patients (see Chapter 1). It is clear that new initiatives are required to assist the more disabled residents who have failed to progress in conventional settings. The comparatively small size of the Unit described here reduces impersonality and the high staff : patient ratio is certainly helpful in providing additional support, fostering a more intimate atmosphere and communal attitude. Unfortunately, national norms for nursing resources and concentration on 'efficiency' make the extension of these observations unlikely in general ward settings, where we believe that more rehabilitative effort could be usefully developed prior to discharge.

Rehabilitation is a continuous process. Patients remain fragile and vulnerable and relapse all too readily, sometimes inexplicably. We have tried to foster independence and have been pleased that our experience has had resonances in other areas of practice. Nurses have visited from other wards and the Unit is a designated training ward. We have developed good working relationships with hostel staff and social services. We have learnt that terminology is important in fostering accord. Phrases like maintenance and broadening of daily living skills are more acceptable terms than 'programmes' and, in many ways, a more accurate reflection of our work.

Whatever terms are used, we have done our utmost to nurture self-respect and self-motivation, to broaden horizons and increase capacities. In the final analysis our work has been directed to give our residents a richer and more rewarding life. Many appreciate our efforts, coming to regard us as valued allies in their struggles against the ravages of dreadful illnesses, but our work is best done if patients finally blend into 'normal' society, turn their backs on us and see us no more.

ACKNOWLEDGEMENT

I thank Olga Margolis for her comments on an earlier draft.

REFERENCES

Allen, J.G., Tarnoff, G., Coyne, L., Spohn, H.E., Buskirk, J.R. and Keller, M.W. (1986) An innovative approach to assessing outcome of long-term psychiatric hospitalization. *Hospital Community Psychiatry*, **37**, 376–380.

Baker, R. and Hall J.N. (1983) *Rehabilitation: Rehabilitation Evaluation*. Vine Publishing, Aberdeen.

Barton, R. (1959) *Institutional Neurosis*, 2nd edn., 1966. Wright, Bristol.

Becker, H.S. (1975) *Outsiders: Studies in the Sociology of Deviance*. The Free Press, New York and London.

Cameron, N. (1943a) The paranoid pseudo-community. *American Journal of Sociology*, **49**, 32–38.

Cameron, N. (1943b) The paranoid pseudo-community. *Psychological Review*, **50**, 219–233.

DeRivera, J. (1984) The structure of emotional relationships. In: *Review of Personality and Social Psychology vol. 5. Emotions, Relationships and Health* (P. Shaver, ed.). Sage, Beverley Hills.

Fromm, E. (1944) Individual and social origins of neurosis. *American Sociological Review* IX, 380, reprinted in: *Personality in Nature, Society and Culture* (C. Kluckholm and H. Murray, eds). Alfred Knopf, New York.

Goffman, E. (1969) *The Presentation of Self in Everyday Life*. Penguin, London.

Gotestam, K.G. and Melin, L. (1990) The effect of prompting and reinforcement of activity in elderly demented inpatients. *Scandinavian Journal of Psychology*, **31**, 2–8.

Janez, N.M. (1985) A preliminary evaluation of an intensive rehabilitation unit. MSc thesis. University of Surrey.

Kay, S.R. and Murrill, L.M. (1990) Predicting outcome of schizophrenia: significance of symptom profiles and outcome dimensions. *Comprehensive Psychiatry*, **31**, 91–102.

Krawiecka, M., Goldberg, D. and Vaughn, M. (1977) A standardised psychiatric assessment scale for rating chronic psychotic patients. *Acta Psychiatrica Scandinavica*, **55**, 170–180.

Lenzenweger, M.F., Dworkin, R.H. and Wethington, E. (1991) Examining the underlying structure of schizophrenic phenomenology: evidence for a three-process model. *Schizophrenia Bulletin*, **17**, 515–524.

Lutz, C.A. (1988) *Unnatural Emotions*. University of Chicago Press, Chicago and London.

Miller, D.L. (1973) *George Herbert Mead: Self Language and the World*. University of Texas Press, Texas.

Reisman, G., Glazer, N. and Denney, R. (1985) *The Lonely Crowd. A Study of the American Character*. Doubleday Anchor, New York.
Russell-Davis, D. (1972) *Introduction to Psychopathology*, 3rd edn. Oxford University Press.
Salokangas, R.K., Palo-oja, T., Ojanen, M. and Jalo, K. (1991) Need for community care among psychotic outpatients. *Acta Psychiatrica Scandinavica*, 84(2), 191–196.
Schwartz, D.T. and Mintz, N.L. (1963) Ecology and psychosis among Italians in 27 Boston communities. *Social Problems*, 10, 371–376.
Summerfelt, A.T., Alphs, L.D., Wagman, A.M., Funderburk, F.R., Hierholzer, R.M. and Strauss, M.E. (1991) Reduction of perseverative errors in patients with schizophrenia using monetary feedback. *Journal of Abnormal Psychology*, 100, 613–616.
Tooth, G.C. and Brook, E.M. (1961) Trends in the mental hospital population and their effect on future planning. *Lancet*, i, 710.
Vygotsky (1978) *Thought and Language*. MIT Press, Cambridge, Mass.
Welford, A.T. (1958) *Ageing and Human Skill*. Oxford University Press for the Nuffield Foundation.
Welford, A.T. (1968) *Fundamentals of Skill*. Methuen, London.
Weller, M.P.I., Tobiansky, R.I., Hollander, D. and Ibrahimi, S. (1989) Psychosis and destitution at Christmas 1985–88. *Lancet*, ii, 1384–1385.
Weller, M.P.I., Weller, B.G.A. and Cheyne, A. (1990) Quality of life after discharge from long-stay wards. *Lancet*, ii, 1384–1385.
Whyte, W.F (1955) *Street Corner Society*, 2nd edn. University of Chicago Press.
Wing, J.K. and Brown, G.W. (1970) *Institutionalism and Schizophrenia*. University Press, Cambridge.
Wing, J.K., Bennett, D.H. and Denham, J. (1964) *The Industrial Rehabilitation of Long-stay Schizophrenic Patients*. MRC Memorandum No 42. HMSO, London.
Yallom, I.D. (1985) *The Theory and Practice of Group Psychotherapy*, 3rd edn. Basic Books, New York.

12 HOUSING AND DEINSTITUTIONAL-IZATION: THEORY AND PRACTICE IN THE DEVELOPMENT OF A RESETTLEMENT SERVICE

D. Abrahamson

HISTORY

The notion that houses of different sizes might supplement or even replace large institutions for the long-stay mentally ill is one of those modern seeming ideas in psychiatry that in fact go back well into the last century. The concept originated from the use of two houses which had been built for offices at the Devon County Asylum. They proved to be 'cheerful and home like' and much preferred to the wards by the 'tranquil patients' who later lived in them (Bucknill, 1858). As a result, Bucknill argued for building on the hospital campus 'distinct houses built on a simple plan, retaining as much as possible the ordinary arrangements of English Homes' in which patients and staff would live together. They were to be known as cottages or cottage wards. He suggested that in a model asylum of 300 patients half should be accommodated in this way, in groups of five with married attendants and in larger groups of 'higher class' patients in the houses of medical staff, and the other half in a central hospital.

A cottage specially designed for this purpose by Baron Mundy with 'a comfortable home like aspect' and 'a pretty little garden at the front' attracted considerable attention at the Paris Exhibition (Notes & News, 1867).

Despite worsening overcrowding this approach was not widely taken up, but a number of similar, small cottages in which patients and staff lived together were later developed around the London area by the Mental After Care Association (MACA). They remained the Association's main provision from 1893 until the 1940s when they were replaced by large hostels. The reasons for their eventual closure remain as topical as the concept. These included cost, a degree of social isolation of the residents, and 'the many new and complex regulations connected with the running of Registered homes for the mentally disturbed' (MACA, 1966).

The value of housing was rediscovered in the early 1960s, again initially with hospital houses which happened to be available. This time their success led on to the widespread development of group homes, as the term now became, in the community. The principal aim was to provide for long-term patients who were poorly served by the transitional hostels which had become the main local authority provision (Ryan, 1979). These were intended to be 'halfway houses', with residence usually restricted to 6–12 months, even though suitable accommodation for those with long-term disabilities to move on to was rarely available. They therefore tended to remain beyond the planned time limit, stigmatized—Apte (1968) refers to 'the dependent patient who becomes an unmoveable object'—and without any security of tenure. Some authorities instituted policies that effectively excluded them even at the price of many unfilled places.

Group homes have played an important role in deinstitutionalization, both in practical terms and perhaps as importantly by the positive attitudes to 'chronic' patients they have engendered. They have traditionally been unstaffed houses where residents, supported by visits, live more independently than in the earlier cottages which they shared with staff. As will be described, emphasis has in recent years moved to staffed houses which are in some respects more closely reminiscent of Bucknill's original concept, in a historical circle typical of mental illness services.

DO LONG-STAY PATIENTS WANT TO LEAVE HOSPITAL?

The deinstitutionalization movement gathered increasing momentum from the 1960s onwards, despite surprisingly little information about long-stay patients' own wishes.

The few studies of patients' attitudes prior to the 1980s required them to express their opinions about leaving hospital without being provided with information about where they could go, with whom, and with what level of medical and other support (Freeman et al., 1965; Wing and Brown, 1975).

Later studies at Goodmayes Hospital (Abrahamson and Brenner, 1983; Abrahamson et al., 1989; Cotson et al., 1990) established that in these circumstances the expressed wish to remain in hospital was not explained by the process of 'institutionalism', supposedly representing gradual loss of interest in the outside world with increasing length of stay, that had been postulated (Wing and Brown, 1970). Negative attitudes to leaving were shown to reflect to a major extent patients' lack of information about alternative accommodation and other resources outside hospital and doubts about their own ability to cope which were realistic in this context. The climate of expectations around the time of admission, when for the longer stay the norm would have been to remain indefinitely in hospital, as well as specific events such as loss of home or family during the intervening years, are also likely to have been relevant (Abrahamson, 1987).

THE LOCAL APPROACH

These studies of long-stay patients' attitudes at Goodmayes have considerably influenced local practice. Its main goals have been to develop a range of varied accommodation so as to enable them to exercise choice amongst a variety of options, to provide the information and preparation before discharge and the support afterwards they need to do so as fully as possible, and to promote satisfying social networks.

In these circumstances many of even the very long-stay patients have been prepared realistically, and courageously, to consider leaving and have later made the transition successfully.

Table 1 Evolution of current housing provision

Year	Project	Structure	Places	Staffing	No. of staff
1972, 1973	Group homes	Single houses	7, 4	Peripatetic	
1974, 1975	Group homes	Single houses	4, 4	Peripatetic	
1983	'209'	7 Bedsitters, 11 flats, communal rooms	18	Housing Association	3
1984	Group homes	Single houses	4, 3	Peripatetic	
1987	Cambridge Park	Individual and communal rooms	10	Housing Association	6
1989	Group homes	Single houses	4, 3	Peripatetic	
1989	Group homes	2 sets of paired houses	4 × 3	NHS	9
1990	Group homes	2 single houses	4, 3	NHS	5
1990	Group homes	2 single houses	4, 3	NHS	2
1990	Group homes	2 single houses	4, 3	Housing Association	1
1990	Wakeling Court	15 studio flats, 1 self-contained flat, 3 person house, communal rooms	19	Housing Association	20
1990	Rook Lodge	5 bedsitters, 5 self-contained flats, communal rooms	10	NHS	8
1991	Group home	Single house	5	Voluntary organization	6
1991	Group home	2 adjacent houses	7	NHS	8
1992/3	Group homes	3 single houses	14	NHS	14
1992/3	Magpie Close	Core and cluster	16	Housing Association	16

Evolution of the current provision

Table 1 shows how the pattern of accommodation has evolved in the catchment area of Goodmayes Hospital, since 1972 when the first group home was opened. The catchment area population now totals approximately 400 000, divided almost equally between the London Boroughs of Redbridge and Newham.

Three main phases are evident which broadly represent progression in terms of the levels of disability catered for: an unstaffed group home phase; the '209' flat cluster project; and fully staffed accommodation of both group home and cluster types.

Throughout these phases additional long-stay patients, who attained the necessary level of independence during the preparation to be described later, have been resettled in individual flats obtained from local authority housing departments and a number of housing associations.

All the accommodation provides indefinite security of tenure, which is one of the essential features of a housing approach and is a sine qua non if patients who have spent decades in hospital are freely to choose to leave. This evolving provision has been associated with developments in pre-discharge facilities and community support systems, as well as studies of patients' attitudes and social networks, which will also be described.

GROUP HOMES

The first group home opened in May 1972. Four men and three women had been selected—in fact largely self-selected because of their interest in leaving hospital—and prepared in the occupational therapy department by an equally self-selected group of keen staff.

The house was an obvious success in terms of their ability to cope with practical tasks, the relationships between them, and the homely atmosphere that developed. It was clear that these patients, who together had spent more than 200 years in hospital, retained much more potential than expected. This encouraging experience led on to the development of a series of further unstaffed group homes, as outlined in Table 1.

Experience over the course of twenty years has led to both appreciation of the contribution group homes can make to the care

of long-term patients and to understanding of their limitations. Comments from residents (Keays, 1982) illustrate the balance of individuality and interdependence that is one of their general characteristics, although each house tends to have its own particular atmosphere which evolves slowly and often very subtly.
They included:

> 'More privacy', 'More your own boss', 'More myself', 'I can do more myself', 'More freedom', 'We are all very individual'.

And also:

> 'More support from others living here', 'Learn to help each other', 'All muck in together', 'Understand each other', 'We depend on each other', 'if someone is not well we do their chores', 'If I am ill, the others will look after me'.

The development of this balance is not necessarily a trouble free process, nor is it inevitable. Despite the testing of compatibility inherent in careful preparation, tensions may later develop which cause unacceptable distress to vulnerable individuals living within the close confines of a small house. The complex factors involved include especially differences in assertiveness and dominance. It has proved essential that one resident is not encouraged to become dominant over the others for the sake of more efficient running of the house. Unwillingness to share chores, disparities in conversational ability, and disturbed behaviour are also important negative factors, yet attachments amongst a group of residents may override any of them.

Replacement when vacancies occur is difficult and the more so the more cohesive the group has become. The preparation houses described later have facilitated the gradual introduction of newcomers in consultation with residents. It has also been policy to reduce the number of places in the houses when necessary to provide individual bedrooms. This has been the overwhelming preference amongst both these residents and long-stay patients in general (Abrahamson et al., 1989).

Much further evidence has accrued which illustrates how complex—for both good and bad—group home relationships can be. Tensions are of course inevitable in all close living arrangements but the special vulnerabilities of these clients cannot be ignored, especially as their choice of small group living is inevitably influenced by professionals however much effort is made to avoid pressure (Abrahamson and Brenner, 1982).

Sensitivity on the part of visiting staff is essential for the recognition of problems, as residents may be reluctant to disclose them from a sense of loyalty. It is also important to ensure that strengths are not underestimated. Some groups develop impressively warm and mutually satisfying relationships which every effort should be made to preserve even if, for example, a resident's contribution becomes impaired by age or for other reasons.

It is also possible for residents to live together under the same roof other than as a cohesive group—shared houses rather than group homes (Pritlove, 1985)—and some may prefer to do so despite the loss of companionship. The first Goodmayes house evolved in this direction after three of the initial tightly knit group had moved on to flats. As these moves indicate, the security of tenure provided does not inhibit some residents' eventual wish to try more independent accommodation and may promote it by increasing their confidence.

Support teams

The support arrangements have varied over the years. Two specialist community psychiatric nurses now provide the main input with invaluable help from a social worker. In the last four years the housing association responsible has also developed a small specialist group home team, one of the aims of which is to increase the range of activities available to residents and expand their social networks, partly by forming links between the houses (Mandiberg and Telles, 1990). This team meets regularly with the consultant psychiatrist, community psychiatric nurses (CPNs) and other members of the multidisciplinary Rehabilitation Team, which also holds regular clinical meetings.

Nuclear and extended families

Evidence of the double-edged effect of the interdependence characteristic of group homes together with awareness that the new long-stay patients passing through the preparation houses were increasingly choosing individual flats, in which some tended to become socially isolated, led to fresh thinking in the early 1980s. The aim became the development of accommodation which would provide opportunities for companionship and support without the imposed physical and emotional closeness of group homes. This was conceptualized to some extent as a shift from a nuclear towards an extended family model, which was in keeping with evidence of benefits from the latter for schizophrenic patients (WHO, 1979).

Added to flats and group homes such accommodation would further the overriding aim of offering as wide a range of choices as possible.

THE '209' PROJECT

It was fortunate that at this point a large Victorian house in the East End of London became available to Springboard Housing Association, which already managed the group homes. This not only became an invaluable resource in itself but experience gained from it has much influenced later projects. It proved possible to convert the house into seven bedsitters and three self-contained flats, and to build eight self-contained flats at the end of its large garden: a range of units that allows for individual choices. The main building also includes two lounges and a communal kitchen/dining-room which are open to all residents, including those in the flats. They have the option of lunch on weekdays, prepared by staff with their help, and are otherwise mainly responsible for their own meals. Emphasis at '209', as the project has come to be known, is on privacy and independence combined with opportunities for companionship without pressure to be closer in physical or emotional terms than preferred.

The milieu is firmly housing rather than formally therapeutic, although a good deal of informal emotional support as well as practical help is provided by the project leader and two other staff who are on site during the daytime, Monday to Friday. Residents and staff hold a meeting each week which has mainly the character of a tenants' meeting. The midday meal, afternoon tea which has gradually developed as an informal get together, and the celebration of birthdays and holidays help to promote the sense of community which is evident.

A varied clientele has been catered for by this lightly staffed project. It has proved possible for both relatively stable but dependent patients with past hospital stays of 20–30 years and the more actively ill, acute or new long-stay to live together successfully. Volatile residents and those whose main handicap is social withdrawal tend to complement each other in this setting, contrary to experience in group homes and in a large hostel elsewhere which lacked the same opportunities for privacy (Falloon and Marshall, 1985). The introduction of new residents is also facilitated. Since the project opened in May 1983 12 additional patients from the preparation houses have been successfully settled in vacancies, mainly from moves to independent accommodation, without the difficulties encountered in filling group home places.

The age range of the 5 women and 13 men who make up the current population is from 41 to 75 years. Almost two-thirds are suffering from schizophrenic illnesses, with markedly varied spectrums of positive and negative symptoms; others have severe affective disorders and conditions ranging from Korsakoff's syndrome to obsessional neurosis.

Unintrusive but readily available and effective support to the project from the multidisciplinary Rehabilitation Team, as described later, has been essential to cope successfully with this clientele.

Ready access to hospital places on the rare occasions they are needed is also essential and is facilitated by the Team's involvement. During the ten years of the project's life seven residents have had temporary readmissions. Two of these have had several admissions due to manic illnesses and have gained from the acceptance by management, staff and other residents that their homes in the project remain for them to return to without difficulty.

INTENSIVELY STAFFED PROJECTS

The group homes and 209 have operated without subsidy from the National Health Service. NHS funding for community projects was introduced for the first time in the late 1980s as part of a drive to close the large mental hospitals. As a result fully staffed projects became feasible, which were intended to cater for their residual populations.

There was unfortunately a general tendency to approach this new development without adequate recognition of aspects that had proved important for the success of unstaffed accommodation, including careful preparation prior to discharge from hospital, close attention to personal compatibilities and social networks, and most fundamentally the need for a varied range of accommodation to allow choice.

The model most widely adopted was simply the addition of care staff to the single group home despite the fact that the main problem in unstaffed homes, that physical and emotional closeness may be unhelpful for some patients, is not necessarily solved by the presence of staff on a 24 hour basis and may even be exacerbated. It is not easy for them to be supportive and facilitating within the confines of a small house without also being intrusive, and organizational requirements such as shift work tend to conflict with the intended informal, 'normal' milieu.

Subsequent experience of staffing in a number of houses has shown that it can in fact extend their benefits to an increased proportion of the more disabled patients, who relish their own small-scale homes with the extra support and companionship of staff, but it has also confirmed that this does not meet the needs of all patients.

Staffed accommodation which is more spacious, offers a wider choice of companions, and provides individual units which enable residents to withdraw when they need, on the 209 model, is also required.

Special projects

Wakeling Court, which opened in April 1989 as a joint Springboard Housing Association and Newham District Health Authority project, exemplifies this aspect, features of which have also been incorporated in other staffed schemes (Table 1).

The building presents as a continuation of the terraced houses of one of the main residential roads of the area, extending to the corner where it meets a road which is replete with shops, cafes, public houses and other amenities. This site and the surrounding neighbourhood meet many of the requirements for a 'humane environment' (Smith, 1976) and are likely to promote integration (Trute and Segal, 1976) and facilitate activities popular with long-term patients (Abrahamson and Brenner, 1978; Abrahamson and Ezekiel, 1984).

Space is emphasized throughout the project. There are 15 individual studio flats each of which comprises bedroom, sitting and kitchen areas and a toilet; five of them are specially equipped for deaf residents. There is also one self-contained flat and an attached house for a group of three who use all the other facilities. The main dining and sitting area is open plan but can be divided for particular activities. It extends into a terrace and garden, increasing the sense of space, light, and freedom to move around. The whole of this area is readily accessible from the flats and although also easily accessible from the street does not influence the frontage. A major difference from '209' is that the project is staffed around the clock. A total of 18 care staff operate a key worker system supervised by the project leader and deputy. The milieu remains housing in orientation but there is more structuring of the daily programme.

As well as the weekly tenants' meeting, there are currently keep-fit and relaxation, current affairs, women's, and communication groups as well as craft and recreational activities. Activities outside the project are also encouraged and a variety have been developed. However, the balance between organized activities and residents' freedom and independence is clearly important and the approach is flexible according to their varying needs and preferences at different times.

The main resident group was prepared for about a year in the Goodmayes Hospital rehabilitation ward and a further group came from the hospital's deaf unit which patients attend on a daily basis from long-stay wards. They have integrated well together and inter-group relationships have developed. Both sets are in general more disabled than the group home or '209' clientele although there is some overlap. They are almost entirely schizophrenic patients (89%) mainly from the 'old' long-stay group (63%), with an average length of continuous stay in Goodmayes of 19.6 years. Most of the 7 women and 12 men are in the 50–70 years age group (range 32–80). All have proved able to cope with their flats, with where needed the assistance of staff at a level which is negotiated individually. It has been remarkable to find improvements in wellbeing, appearance, and particularly conversation during the second year of the project's life. Prior to discharge from hospital five (26%) scored within the conventional potential for discharge category on the Rehabilitation Hall and Baker (REHAB) Scale (Hall and Baker, 1984), eight (42%) were in the intermediate and six (32%) in the most disabled categories. Repeat of the scale after one year in the project showed that nine (50%) now scored in the lowest, eight (44%) in the intermediate and one (6%) in the highest categories.

There have been two short readmissions to hospital since the project opened.

ASPECTS OF CARE

The evolution of this range of housing provision has been facilitated by, and has in turn promoted, developments in other aspects of long-term patient care.

The role of preparation

The value of adequate pre-discharge preparation has become increasingly clear as varied projects have been developed. Five preparation houses on the hospital campus, ranging in size from four to eight places, have been used since the first opened in the 1970s. Prospective residents referred from the wards are assessed by the multidisciplinary Rehabilitation Team, with particular emphasis on their own wishes.

A structured but flexible programme, to which they are gradually introduced before moving in, enables them to learn in a realistic fashion domestic skills including cooking, shopping, budgeting, laundry and cleaning, to their best ability. This is a slow process usually taking months, but may be a year or more in some cases as pre-set time limits are not imposed. Apart from their practical value, mastery of these activities promotes self-confidence and acts as a vehicle for the development of social and interpersonal skills and the testing of compatibilities for living together.

Carrying through the programmes at an appropriate pace has depended on the tact and commitment of the occupational therapy helpers who staff the houses on a daytime basis. They are supervised and supported by the Rehabilitation Team, which also provides specialist input directly to the residents.

The helpers' contribution has proved to be remarkable in developing warm, accepting milieus in the houses and acting as role models, as well as in the direct teaching of practical and social skills.

They have mainly been mature women whose personalities and life experiences seem to be crucial to their ability, with only modest formal training, to get the best out of very handicapped patients.

The preparation houses also provide residents with opportunities to learn more about alternatives to hospital and gradually clarify the sort of accommodation for which they wish to aim, which is not necessarily the same as they or staff initially envisaged. The eventual transition to the community is eased by intensified staff support at this critical stage. Residents are also free to end their involvement with the preparation houses and return to the ward at any time, which has in fact been the main reason for unsuccessful outcomes. They are given every opportunity to try again but are not pressed into doing so. A number have been successfully resettled after their second or third try.

A 12 place rehabilitation ward with 24 hour staffing was added to the houses in 1987 to deal with more disabled patients, and has since prepared most of the Wakeling Court and some of the staffed group home residents. Its milieu is essentially similar to the preparation houses but the programme provided by the nursing staff and the Rehabilitation Team emphasizes self-care, communication skills, and experience of the Community, whilst patients are not expected to reach so high a level of domestic skills as they will usually move on to accommodation where a high level of staff help is available. The ward has recently transferred to a large house for eight residents, with a smaller satellite house, on the hospital campus.

Assessments of the preparation houses

Rigid selection criteria for the houses are avoided. A study of 82 patients who had participated between 1976 and 1984 confirmed the wide spectrum involved (Peng, 1984).

Sixty (73%) had been successfully settled out of hospital in a range of accommodation including group homes, warden supported and independent flats, and the '209' project. Twenty-two (27%) went back to their wards, although more than one-third were later settled outside hospital after further involvement in the preparation houses or via the rehabilitation ward or other routes. The successful and unsuccessful groups were similar in age (average 54 and 56 years respectively, with a range of 25–73 years) and in diagnosis (59% and

58% schizophrenia; 41% and 42% affective and other disorders) but the unsuccessful group had significantly more previous admissions (mean 5.6 versus 4.6) and longer total lengths of admission (mean 14.4 versus 9.9 years).

In terms of patients' own views on the preparation houses, a questionnaire study (Larkin, 1989) indicated that 80% of the residents of the three houses surveyed considered themselves happy there. They summed them up as comfortable and homely and with more space for their possessions than the wards. A minority felt they had not enough free time to do what they wanted and appeared to dislike the element of responsibility for others.

Social networks: community care without community?

That 'warmly persuasive word community' (Williams, 1976) is notoriously difficult to define but at its heart is 'the fundamental theme of man together as opposed to man alone' (Scherer, 1972). The expectation that the mentally ill would become integrated within the community fuelled the idealism of the deinstitutionalization movement and social network considerations might be expected to be central to its practice.

It is therefore disturbing that the original concept of 'Community Care' has tended to become 'Care in the Community' (NETRHA, 1984), an apparently trivial change in nomenclature that underlines a trend to regard where care takes place as the main criterion (Acheson, 1989) rather than whether or not there is real community in Scherer's sense of the term.

This trend may have been fuelled by longstanding misapprehensions about the personal relationships of long-stay patients. The assumption that they function essentially as isolates was enshrined in the organization of mental hospitals during the custodial era, despite earlier emphasis on asylums as surrogate families (Scull, 1979). The most extreme view has been that long-stay schizophrenic patients are 'Ghostly figures who, like the crew of the Flying Dutchman, are able to walk through one another without leaving a trace' (Sommer and Osmond, 1963). More influentially, Barton (1959) in his seminal description of 'Institutional Neurosis' considered that whilst the possibility of one patient making a friend and confidant of another within a mental hospital would appear to be great 'it is surprising how infrequently it happens'. Similarly, in another influential text, Goffman (1968) suggested that the main affect between institutional patients was mutual antipathy, without any shared sense of solidarity.

Such misapprehensions were reflected in earlier studies of patients' attitudes to leaving hospital which ignored their possible wish to maintain relationships (Freeman *et al.*, 1965; Wing and Brown, 1970; Abrahamson and Brenner, 1983) and have still not been generally eradicated from resettlement policies.

Ward networks

A series of studies of social networks using the Goodmayes Network Assessment Questionnaire (GNAQ) has given a different picture of long-stay patients' relationships (Abrahamson and Ezekiel, 1984; Abrahamson *et al.*, 1989; Cotson *et al.*, 1990; Abrahamson, 1991). As with the similar Social Network Schedule (SNS) used elsewhere (Leff *et al.*, 1990) about two-thirds were able to respond adequately and the network sizes reported have also been comparable.

Mean sizes of 10–12 in the Goodmayes studies are considerably larger than those previously considered typical of psychotic patients (Pattison *et al.*, 1975), although there was wide individual variation with some very small networks of four or less and others of 25 or more. These long-stay patients consistently distinguished between acquaintances and the friends who on average formed one-third of the contacts; but ward staff tend considerably to underestimate the latter (Morrison, 1987).

The general picture was of networks containing a substantial number, though rarely all and frequently not a majority, of the residents on the same ward as the respondent. Wards are thus complex, overlapping series of social networks which provide an element of choice in the range and intensity of contacts, rather than the undifferentiated conglomerates which they may superficially appear to be.

Relationships with patients from other wards are also important and were about a quarter overall of the contacts reported. They were significantly more likely than own ward contacts to involve friendship, trust and confiding, possible because they are a freer expression of choice (Cotson *et al.*, 1990).

In some cases relationships had clearly been maintained for many years, despite being undermined by the usual hospital practice of moving patients around without regard to their networks.

Staff, either on or off the respondent's own ward, formed about one-third of the network constituents. Many patients clearly regarded staff members as friends and this has important implications for the relocation process and for the ethos and practice of care subsequently (Firth and Rapley, 1990).

There were few relationships with people outside hospital and these were almost always with ex-patients or staff, apart from an important component of relatives who provided about 10% of the total contacts and were significantly the most trusted.

It is essential that the practice of ignoring social networks in resettling long-stay patients is no longer perpetuated. They need to have a comparably complex range of relationships outside hospital if this aspect of the transition is not to bring loss rather than gain in terms of real community. Group home and flat residents have frequently mentioned relishing their new found freedom and independence yet missing the contacts they were used to in hospital: a disturbing point which has been confirmed by formal studies (Ryan, 1979; Keays, 1986; Goldie, 1988).

Expanding networks

A study of the social networks of patients resettled from the preparation houses into the 209 project (Abrahamson and Ezekiel, 1984) suggests that this style of preparation and accommodation has a role in expanding networks, and this has been confirmed by experience with later projects such as Wakeling Court.

Networks during the preparation period for 209, when patients maintained contacts within the main hospital as well as in the preparation houses, averaged 29 for schizophrenic patients and 30 for those with affective disorders, with as usual considerable individual variation. Networks were equally large in two reassessments during the first year after they had moved to 209, despite the loss of most hospital contacts, with a statistically non-significant trend to increase for the affective group where the average reached 39.

Nonetheless, a significant proportion of residents would have liked still more contacts. A quarter said they were sometimes lonely, compared to more than one-third when in hospital.

Network constituents

About half the constituents of the 209 networks were other residents and half were from outside the project. Most of the latter were current or ex-patients living in the community, with a small number of continuing hospital contacts who were clearly important to particular individuals. Relatives and in a few cases friends of relatives constituted 10% initially and later 17% of the total contacts. Only 2–3% were from the community at large.

A similar paucity of general community contacts is typical of group home residents but is not confined to patients in supported accommodation. It was also found amongst a local group of long-term outpatients living in their own homes, and in a survey of the clients of community psychiatric nurses (Burford, 1987). It is extensively documented in the mental handicap field (McConkey *et al.*, 1983; Landesman-Dwyer and Berkson, 1984; Firth and Short, 1987; Firth and Rapley, 1990).

The issue is more complex than the 'ghettoization' sometimes cited. In seeking more 'normal' social networks in the community for long-term patients it is important not to suggest that relationships with other mentally ill persons are somehow second class. To do so may be to discourage them from important personal experiences and mutual support (Estroff, 1981; Mandiberg and Telles, 1990) and overlooks the predominance of relationships between people with shared backgrounds in all walks of life. Experience of a local social club has emphasized how constructive relationships between long-term patients can be and the normality of their mutual help. They may form a springboard to contacts in the wider community by promoting confidence and providing opportunities (Segal and Aviram, 1978; Pascaris, 1991).

On the other hand, the lack of contacts in the general community underlines how far there is to go before genuine integration is achieved, and should not be glossed over. This remains perhaps the most critical issue to be faced if community care is fully to meet the high hopes originally held out for it. Wide ranging efforts are required to remove de facto constraints on patients' access to community resources, including the constraint of poverty—the very small personal incomes permitted by the 1984 Registered Homes Act are a particular anomaly, and to help them develop the complex social skills required (Firth and Rapley, 1990), if varied choices are to be genuinely available.

CLINICAL ASPECTS

Housing based long-term care requires a different clinical style from that traditional in hospital and similar settings. Most obviously, entering and leaving a house or flat or any part of the larger projects entails a process of social negotiation not usual for wards. The position of a guest in the patient's own home needs constantly to be borne in mind and potential intrusions on residents' lives, including assessment and monitoring, have to be particularly clearly justified. This was less ambiguous during the earlier group home phase when all staff input was on a visiting basis. With the advent of accommodation with care staff on site, it was thought essential to maintain unintrusiveness and respect for the residents' privacy, whilst preserving coordinated back-up from a multidisciplinary Rehabilitation Team.

For these reasons, whilst the Team meets regularly with staff within the larger projects such as 209 and Wakeling Court, to share problems and progress, such meetings are held outside the smaller projects. Specialist interventions are directed away from all the accommodation to more appropriate settings to avoid 'therapeutizing' the patients' homes. Exceptions are those which are available on a domiciliary basis in the general community, programmes designed specifically to modify behaviour within the residence itself, and the groups held in Wakeling Court because of the particular needs of its clientele.

Individual case reviews are carried out in the Rehabilitation Team house, not less than every three months for each resident. Their format, which is still evolving, has been influenced by an outpatient clinic designed to involve patients more fully than with conventional arrangements and to ensure continuity long-term (Abrahamson and Fellow-Smith, 1990). The resident is included throughout the review, rather than brought in after discussion amongst staff, except in exceptional circumstances. Residents can choose to limit the number of staff present or to brief privately a Team member to speak for them.

They also receive the normal general practitioner services, which now include health checks. Careful liaison is maintained with the Practices concerned by the medical members of the Rehabilitation Team as a high index of suspicion of physical disorders is essential with this population (Honig et al., 1989).

DISCUSSION

The relevance of some of the above themes to long-term patients' needs, including as already pointed out the role of housing itself, was well recognized early in the custodial era, yet these aspects were subsequently marginalized.

One response to this era's failures has been to recoil from every feature of the large institutions, to support this with a simplistic concept of normalization, and in consequence deny the need for any form of special accommodation for long-term patients. This is likely in practice to lead to partial deinstitutionalization, with patients who do not suit the stereotype of 'an ordinary house in an ordinary street' as the only acceptable community accommodation (Heginbotham, 1985) left behind in the remaining large hospitals.

At the other extreme is nostalgia for the asylums—or for an idealized memory of them. A revived role as the answer to current deficits in community care, especially those exposed to view by homelessness (Weller and Weller, 1988), has the appeal of simplicity, but this is an area where a simple solution is unlikely. Debate on long-term patients' need for asylum interpreted in more complex terms as a range of services (King's Fund, 1987) is welcome, but confusions about the concept remain and may also lead to an unsatisfactory form of partial deinstitutionalization (*Lancet*, 1987; Abrahamson, 1988).

Perhaps their own attitudes are the main reason it is important the pendulum does not swing back to leave patients in hospitals without choice. The three Goodmayes surveys and the earlier studies elsewhere, which together span more than 30 years, indicate that the proportion of long-stay patients with favourable attitudes to leaving hospital has not declined despite the discharge of many during these years. Their views continue to be moulded by realistic considerations, including increasing information about Community housing projects especially from those now living in them (Abrahamson et al., 1989).

The more disabled patients are clearly the most likely to be left behind (Levene et al., 1985; Carson, 1991; Fottrell, 1990; Holloway, 1991) although hospitals in fact often have less staff and poorer facilities than community projects, and no significant relationship between disability level and the wish to stay has been found in the Goodmayes studies. An effort has been made from the first local housing projects onwards to include as wide as possible a range of the Goodmayes population rather than only the more able. This has been facilitated by the preparation programme and emphasis on compatible groupings and aftercare and furthered by the design of the larger projects.

The gap between the disability levels of those moving out and those staying in hospital has narrowed, as evidenced by several surveys using the REHAB scale. In 1989 31% overall of long-stay ward patients fell within the traditional potential for resettlement category of the scale, 27% were in the intermediate range and 41% were in the most disabled category, compared to 26%, 42% and 32% respectively of the Wakeling Court population. A significant number of those in the most disabled sub-group in long-stay wards were patients with dementing rather than schizophrenic illnesses who may need specialist accommodation similar to that required by the majority of dementing patients who are in psychogeriatric wards (Manser, 1989).

For some in the most disabled category, some in the increasingly cited but poorly defined 'hard to place' category (Coid, 1991), and the less disabled who wish to stay in a neighbourhood they know well, remaining on a redeveloped hospital campus may be an appropriate option: the 'New Communities' approach (Jones, 1987).

This is very different from retaining them in hospitals as they now are. Major changes will be required to bring hospital accommodation in line with the best of the housing projects outside, and to counteract the 'alluring . . . but isolationist overtones of the mental health "campus" concept' (Turner, 1989) by bringing a range of general housing, shops and other amenities onto the sites. The overall aim should be to complement rather than substitute for provision outside.

The claim that a housing approach can be a cornerstone of deinstitutionalization is not meant to imply that it is an easy option. Much is required of housing management, rehabilitation teams, and especially project staff whose personal qualities have had a great deal to do with the success of the schemes. There is inevitably and rightly potential tension between a housing and a clinical ethos. In more than a decade since links were forged between the Rehabilitation Team and a major housing association this has proved to be largely creative because of mutual respect for each other's roles (Abrahamson, 1988; Start, 1989).

However, the situation is becoming more complex and problems are appearing which may be avoidable if past lessons are not overlooked. There is a temptation for some of the newer organizations in the field to assume that a commitment to normalization by itself ensures the right approach. There may be unwillingness to face the constraints on residents imposed by illness and disability and in consequence undervaluing of clinical and other specialist help. Paradoxically, this may be accompanied by quasi clinical practices of their own which imply the right ultimately to control important aspects of residents' lifestyles. The message to them—and to care staff—thus becomes contradictory: they are encouraged to regard themselves as tenants living normal lives in their own homes, yet are subjected to elaborate monitoring and other intrusions. These may be instituted in the name of responsibility to the Registration Authority (Registered Homes Act 1984) which adds its own input with equally little apparent awareness of the contradictions involved; with yet more demands, made of no other tenants in the community, from environmental health and safety officials.

The very real importance of care standards cannot obviate the need to think through their implications and for commonsense, professionalism, and research to find ways of combining personal freedoms with safety and continuing rehabilitation.

The end state for rehabilitation should not merely reflect the class norms and value preferences of those in authority (Jones et al., 1991), which they may benignly assume to be that of their clients, still less their wish to be safe from criticism. The challenge remains to promote circumstances that ameliorate constraints imposed by illness, disability and handicap and ensure that varied choices of lifestyle are genuinely available.

It is clear that many long-stay patients had potential for better lives that was obscured in the large institutions (Cutting et al., 1983). The next few years may determine whether the gains already made by Community Care are secured and creative solutions to its problems found, or institutionalization re-emerges either by a return to traditional hospitals or even within community provision. A long-term viewpoint is essential to ensure that history does not yet again repeat itself.

REFERENCES

Abrahamson, D. (1987) Chronic schizophrenia and long-term hospitalisation. *British Journal of Psychiatry*, **151**, 708.

Abrahamson, D. (1988) The need for asylum in society for the mentally ill or infirm. *Bulletin of the Royal College of Psychiatrists*, **12**, 76–77.

Abrahamson, D. (1991) The social networks of long-stay patients. *British Journal of Psychiatry*, **158**, 718–719.

Abrahamson, D. and Brenner, D. (1978) A study of 'old long-stay' patients in Goodmayes Hospital. *Final report of work carried out during tenure of a DHSS grant 1976–78.*

Abrahamson, D. and Brenner, D. (1982) Do long-stay psychiatric patients want to leave hospital? *Health Trends*, **14**, 95–97.

Abrahamson, D. and Ezekiel, A. (1984) The social networks of patients moving from hospital to the community. *Conference: Social Networks in Hospital and in the Community. The King's Fund Centre.*

Abrahamson, D. and Fellow-Smith, E. (1991) A combined group and individual long term out-patient clinic. *Psychiatric Bulletin*, **15**, 486–487.

Abrahamson, D., Swatton, J. and Wills, W. (1989) Do long-stay psychiatric patients want to leave hospital? *Health Trends*, **21**, 16–21.

Acheson (1985) 'That over used word Community!' *Health Trends*, **17**, 3.

Apte, R.Z. (1968) *Halfway Houses: A New Dilemma in Institutional Care.* G. Bell & Sons, London.

Barton, R. (1959) *Institutional Neurosis.* John Wright & Sons, Bristol.

Bucknill, J.C. (1858) Description of the new house at the Devon County Lunatic Asylum. *The Asylum Journal of Mental Science*, **4**, 318–328.

Burford, C. (1987) A survey of the social networks of the clients of community psychiatric nurses in Haringey. *Research Conference of the Team for Assessment of Psychiatric Services (TAPS).* London.

Carson, J.C., Shaw, L. and Wills, W. (1991) Which patients first: a study from the closure of a large mental hospital. *Health Trends*, **21**, 117–120.

Coid, J. (1991) Difficult to place psychiatric patients: the game of pass the parcel must stop. *British Medical Journal*, 302, 603–604.

Cotson, D., Croucher, P., Fernandex, P., Gallagher, A. and Lorenc, D. (1990) Goodmayes' continuing care ward survey: *Reports to Redbridge and Newham District Health Authorities*.

Cutting, J., Bleuler, M., Ciompi, L., Crow, J.T., Abrahamson, D. and Tantam, D. (1983) Schizophrenic deterioration. *British Journal of Psychiatry*, 142, 78–84.

Department of Health and Social Security (1975) *Better Services for the Mentally Ill*. HMSO, London.

Editorial (1987) The need for asylum for the mentally ill. *Lancet* 2, 546–547.

Estroff, S.E. (1981) *Making it Crazy: an Ethnography of Psychiatric Clients in an American Community*. University of California Press, London.

Falloon, I.R. and Marshall, G.N. (1983) Residential care and social behaviour: a study of rehabilitation needs. *Psychological Medicine*, 13, 341–347.

Firth, H. and Rapley, M. (1990) *From Acquaintance to Friendship: Issues and Strategies for People with Mental Handicap*. British Institute for Mental Handicap, Kidderminster.

Firth, H. and Short, D. (1987) A move from hospital to community: evaluation of community contacts. *Child: Care, Health & Development*, 13, 341–354.

Freeman, J., Mandelbrote, B. and Waldron, J. (1965) Attitudes to discharge amongst long-stay hospital patients and their relation to social and clinical factors. *British Journal of Social and Clinical Psychology*, 4, 270–274.

Goffman, E. (1968) *Asylums: Essays on the Social Situation of Mental Patients and Other Inmates*. Penguin Books, London.

Fottrell, E. (1990) Asylum for psychiatric patients in the 1990s. *Lancet* 335, 468.

Goldie, N. (1988) 'I hated it there but I miss the people': a study of what happened to a group of ex-long-stay patients from Clayburn Hospital. *Research paper 1, Health and Social Services Research Unit, Department of Social Services, South Bank Polytechnic, London*.

Hall, J.N. and Baker, R. (1984) *REHAB Rating Scale User's Manual*. Vine Publishing, Aberdeen.

Heginbotham, C. (1985) *Good Practices in Housing for People with*

Long-term Mental Illnesses. Good Practices in Mental Health, London.

Holloway, F. (1991) Elderly graduates and a hospital closure programme: experience of the Camberwell Resettlement Team. *Psychiatric Bulletin*, **15**, 321–323.

Honig, A., Pop, P., Tan, E.S., Philipsen, H. and Romme, M.A. (1989) Physical illness in chronic psychiatric patients from a community psychiatric unit: the implications for daily practice. *British Journal of Psychiatry*, **155**, 58–64.

Jones, D.W., Tomlinson, D. and Anderson, J. (1991) Community and asylum care: plus ca change. *Journal of the Royal Society of Medicine*, **84**, 252–254.

Jones, K. (1987) *Mental Health Closures: The way forward?* York: Institute of Advanced Architectural Studies.

Keays, M. (1986) Group Homes—the heart of community care today? *Dissertation for Certificate of Qualified Social Worker.*

King's Fund Forum (1987) *Consensus Statement: The need for asylum in society for the mentally ill or infirm.* King's Fund, London.

Landesman-Dwyer, S. and Berkson, G. (1984) Friendships and social behaviour. In: *Mental Retardation and Developmental Disabilities* (J. Wortis, ed.), Plenum Press, London.

Larkin, M. (1989) The role of the preparation house in rehabilitation: a study of residents' likes, dislikes and expectations. *Project report English National Board Course 242.*

Leff, J., O'Driscoll, C., Dayson, D., Wills, W. and Anderson, J. (1990) The structure of social network data obtained from long-stay patients. *British Journal of Psychiatry*, **157**, 848–852.

Levene, L.S., Donaldson, L.J. and Brandon, S. (1985) How likely is it that a district health authority can close its large mental hospitals? *British Journal of Psychiatry*, **147**, 150–155.

McConkey, R.M., Naughton, M. and Nugent, U. (1983) Have we met? Community contact of adults who are mentally handicapped. *Mental Handicap*, **11**, 57–59.

Mandiberg, J.M. and Telles, L. (1990) The Santa Clara County clustered apartment project. *Psychosocial Rehabilitation Journal*, **14**, 21–28.

Manser, M. (1989) The architecture of institutions for demented persons. *Interdisciplinary Topics in Gerontology*, **26**, 22–27.

Mental After Care Association (MACA) *Annual Report (1966).* London.

Morrison, F. (1987) The schizophrenic process and social networks on a continuing care ward. *Research dissertation for English National Board Course 945.*

North East Thames Regional Health Authority (NETRHA) (1984) *A New Philosophy of Care.* NETRHA, London.

Notes & News (1867) The asylum cottage at the Paris exhibition. *The Asylum Journal of Mental Science,* 13, 425–426.

Pascaris, A. (1991) Social recreation: a blind spot in rehabilitation? *Psychosocial Rehabilitation Journal,* 15, 43–54.

Pattison, E.M., Defransisco, D., Wood, P., Frazier, H. and Crowder, J. (1975) A psychosocial kinship model for family therapy. *American Journal of Psychiatry,* 132, 1246–1251.

Pritlove, J. (1985) *Group Homes: an Inside Story.* University of Sheffield Joint Unit for Social Services Research.

Ryan, P. (1979) Residential care for the mentally disabled. In: *Community Care for the Mentally Disabled* (J.K. Wing and R. Olsen, eds). Oxford University Press, Oxford.

Scherer, J. (1972) *Contemporary Community: Sociological Illusion or Reality?* Tavistock Publications, London.

Scull, A. (1979) *Museums of Madness.* Allen Lane, London.

Segal, S.P. and Aviram, U. (1978) *The Mentally Ill in Community Based Sheltered Care.* Wiley, New York.

Smith, C.J. (1976) Residential neighbourhoods as humane environments. *Environment and Planning,* A,8, 311–326.

Sommer, R. and Osmond, H. (1962) The schizophrenic no- society. *Psychiatry,* 25, 244–255.

Start, K. (1989) Models of residential care: the Springboard experience. *From Hospital to Community: A conference to celebrate a decade of cooperation in Care in the Community.* Springboard Housing Association, London.

Trute, B. and Segal, S.P. (1976) Census tract predictors and the social integration of sheltered care residents. *Social Psychiatry,* 11, 153–161.

Turner, T.H. (1989) The future of Britain's mental hospitals. *British Medical Journal,* 299, 1524–1525.

Weller, M.P.I. and Weller, B.G.A. (1988) Mental illness and social policy. *Medical Science and the Law,* 28, 47–53.

Williams, R. (1976) *Keywords.* Fontana/Croom Helm, London.

Wing, J.K. and Brown, G.W. (1970) *Institutionalism and Schizophrenia: A Comparative Study of Three Mental Hospitals 1960–1968.* Cambridge University Press, Cambridge.

World Health Organization (1979) *Schizophrenia, an International Follow-up Study.* John Wiley & Sons, Chichester.

13 COMMUNITY SERVICES FOR THE LONG-TERM MENTALLY ILL: A CASE EXAMPLE— THE CAMBRIDGE HEALTH DISTRICT

G. Shepherd, K. Singh and N. Mills

HISTORY AND BACKGROUND

The Cambridge Health District serves a population of approximately 270 000 people. The district is predominantly rural, with Cambridge city (population 110 000) in the centre. Cambridge and the surrounding area are quite prosperous and there are relatively low levels of unemployment and social deprivation. The economy of the city is heavily dependent on the University and other educational institutions with a strong bias towards service and 'high tech' industries. Outside the city agriculture predominates and the rural villages provide popular locations for London commuters. Cambridgeshire has one of the fastest growing populations in the country.

Fulbourn Hospital was founded in 1848 and still provides the

* The views expressed in this chapter are the personal views of the authors and should not be taken as necessarily representing those of the health authority or any other agency.

main location for inpatient care, although nowadays a wide variety of agencies are also involved in the provision of mental health services, including the local social services department, various independent ('voluntary') agencies, and charities. There is little private health care. The hospital is situated just on the edge of the city, about four miles from the centre, and an expensive, private housing estate has recently been built next to it, effectively joining the hospital to the city suburbs. In the 1950s, Fulbourn was at the forefront of the 'therapeutic community' movement under the direction of the then medical superintendent, Dr David Clark. He used the slogan of 'Activity, Freedom and Responsibility' to transform the old custodial institution and introduce a more socially oriented model of care with an emphasis on daily living skills, occupation, and the beginnings of a community based service (Clark, 1974). Conditions in the old institution prior to these changes have been vividly described in a series of interviews with Dr Clark (Barraclough, 1986a, 1986b).

Fulbourn thus began the process of resettling long-stay patients into the community more than thirty years ago and since 1955 the overall bed numbers have reduced from more than 1000 to just over 300 today. This includes a reduction of long-stay beds of more than 500. At present there are around 90 'acute' beds on the site, 120 long-stay, and 120 beds for the elderly mentally ill. There is a small (13 beds) 'acute' unit on the general hospital site (Addenbrookes) and future plans envisage expansion of services on this site with further acute beds, outpatient services, and possibly a day hospital. The general psychiatric service is organized around three, geographical 'sector' teams, each serving approximately 80 000 population, each with an acute admission ward of 28 beds, outpatient support and community nurses. These teams deal with all the routine psychiatric referrals from general practitioners and other community agencies and the follow-up of recently discharged patients. Most of the outpatients and day patients (including those recently discharged) are seen in various health authority premises in and around the city centre and in some local health centres working with the primary health care teams (GPs, etc.). In the last few years outpatient clinics and a 'Mental Health Centre' have been established in Ely, which is the only other sizeable town in the north of the district. There are further plans to 'resectorize' the city and rural areas so as to be able to develop more localized community mental health teams and possibly some kind of 'crisis intervention' service.

For many years there has been a separate service within the overall psychiatric provision which has specialized in the care of people with severe and long-term mental illness. This is known as the Cambridge Psychiatric Rehabilitation Service (CPRS). The CPRS was originally an essentially hospital based service, but over the years its links with a variety of community agencies have shifted the focus increasingly towards the community. The CPRS has provided a focus for the development of services for people with long-term mental health problems, although as the community services offered by the sector teams have developed so they have also taken on the care of a number of those with long-term problems. At present many of the community services are used by a mixture of 'CPRS' and 'sector team' clients. Currently the CPRS looks after approximately 120 long-stay patients in the hospital and a further 250 in the community.

LONG-STAY PATIENTS IN HOSPITAL

The CPRS has five 'continuing care' wards (approximately 90 beds) and these are occupied mainly by 'old' long-stay patients. Each ward pursues an active rehabilitation policy with the aim of maintaining functioning and providing a good quality of care, even if this does not eventually lead to discharge. Numbers in the continuing care wards have gradually reduced over the years as the more able patients have been resettled in the community and those now remaining represent the hard 'core' of the most disabled, dependent and institutionalized patients. Their average age (excluding the 'new' long-stay) is 63, with nearly 40% aged over 70, and their average length of stay is more than 20 years. Attempts have been made to rehouse as many as possible of these 'old' long-stay patients in domestic scale accommodation on or near the hospital site and currently more than 30 patients have been resettled in this way. Some of these developments have been achieved by using conversions of surplus staff accommodation already owned by the health authority and some through joint working with a local housing association. (These partnership arrangements will be described in more detail later.) There are plans to develop more of this kind of housing in the future, although we are now close to the limit of the numbers who may be cared for in such settings. Some are too physically frail and some of the younger, very disturbed psychotic patients seem to react badly to living in small, enclosed, domestic-scale, environments (see below). A small number of the current long-stay patients may still be able to live outside the hospital and there are currently plans to create another two small, 'high dependency' units with 24 hour staffing. We have tried to keep the needs of our existing long-stay population under constant review and we believe that there are now very few patients left in hospital who could manage without highly supervised (24 hour) care in the community.

The 'new' long-stay

There are two specialized units (n = 20 places) for so-called, 'new' long-stay inpatients. Both are modelled on the 'ward-in-a-house' approach (Bennett, 1980; Wykes, 1982) with relatively high levels of staffing—at least two nursing staff per shift at all times—and an integrated, multidisciplinary approach. The first is situated in a converted house situated next to the hospital entrance and has eight places. All the residents have spent at least one year continuously in hospital prior to referral and in each case there have been attempts to maintain them in a variety of community placements without success. They thus represent the most difficult of our younger, long-stay patients. Most have a diagnosis of schizophrenia with severe positive and negative symptoms which are resistant to conventional medications. Many also show other kinds of behavioural disturbance (e.g. violence to self or others, destruction to property, extreme sensitivity to changes in routines, etc.) which makes their management in the community difficult. In the long term some may eventually be resettled away from the hospital, but it is anticipated that this may take several years and there is no fixed upper limit on length of stay.

The second house has 12 places and has been designed to complement the long-term unit by providing 'medium-term' intensive rehabilitation for a similar group of new, long-stay patients. It is also modelled on the 'ward-in-a-house' philosophy, but has slightly lower staffing ratios and aims to deal with those patients who have the best chances of resettlement within two or three years.

It is our experience, along with others, in this field (e.g. Garety *et al.*, 1988), that among the new long-stay category there is a sub-group who can improve given long-term, intensive, rehabilitation of this kind. Thus, the term new long-*stay* may be something of a misnomer. Our impressions of these 'ward-in-a-house' developments are consistent with the published research findings and have been summarized in Shepherd (1991). He suggests that although such units can be effective in managing—and in some instances even improving—the functioning of the most difficult young, 'chronic' patients, they are not a panacea. It is difficult to maintain high quality care over long periods of time and requires a constant input in terms of staff training and support. A 'ward-in-a-house' is also not a cheap option, although its expense must be compared with the alternatives (i.e. poor care in the community with a large number of 'revolving door' admissions, or prolonged stay on an acute admission ward). Finally, it may not suit all patients and there are some 'new' long-stay who seem to function best where there is lots of space (i.e. on traditional wards), with low staffing input, and fairly 'loose', informal programmes. These are a minority—perhaps around 10%—but they can be a very significant minority since in the wrong kind of setting they can cause considerable disruption.

The CPRS also has a small (n = 12 beds) intake/assessment unit, which provides an admission facility for long-term patients from the community who are currently being followed up by community psychiatric nurses (CPNs) from the rehabilitation service. This is separate from the general sector team admission service and is thus able to provide continuity of care for long-term patients who suffer 'acute-on-chronic' relapses. Staff from the unit can make assessments in the community (usually together with one of the CPRS CPNs), arrange an admission if necessary, and maintain continuity of care through an extended period of follow-up after discharge. Many ex-patients continue to 'drop-in' to the unit after discharge, or are maintained as informal day patients, and this kind of prolonged support is encouraged. The unit is specifically aimed at 'revolving door' patients who require careful discharge planning if their position in the community is to be maintained. It also provides a preliminary screening of potential new long-stay inpatients and a specialized treatment service for 'difficult to treat' patients from other units in the hospital.

Day services for the long-term mentally ill within the hospital consist of an industrial unit ('Fulbourn Industries') with 50 places a day offering a variety of industrial and craft work (including horticulture and bicycle repairs). Most of the attenders at this unit have been coming for many years and there is a consensus that the role of 'industries' needs to be reviewed in line with the changing pattern of service provision. The Department of Employment also funds a small 'Employment Preparation Unit' for 10–12 people per day located alongside the main industrial workshop. This is an experimental venture aimed at providing assessment, short-term training, placement and support for people with mental health problems wishing to return to open employment.

There is also a lively day centre for long-term clients which is attended by both inpatients and day patients. This offers a variety of social and therapeutic activities and a hot meal each day. Transport is provided to and from the centre and it is well-attended. It also provides a base for the CPRS community nurse team (n = 5.5 whole time equivalent (WTE) + 1.0 WTE occupational therapist) who support more than 150 patients, many of whom regularly attend the day centre. This CPN team have been developing a 'case management' system based on the 'Research and Development for Psychiatry' (RDP) model (Clifford and Craig, 1988, see also Chapter 5).

The development of community provisions in Cambridge has been described in a number of papers (Bachrach, 1989; Shepherd, 1987, 1990a) and is the result of the efforts of people from a wide range of different agencies over several years. In the past, it was coordinated by a Joint Development Team (JDT) consisting of senior managers from health and social services and representatives from various voluntary agencies and user groups. The JDT established a number of 'sub-groups' to address specific areas of service development (e.g. sheltered housing, sheltered work, day care, etc.) and the function of these sub-groups was to monitor the current operation of each area of the service, to identify the needs in terms of new provisions, and to pass on these ideas to the main JDT for consideration for funding and implementation. The JDT then decided on priorities and allocated resources. The sub-groups thus involved staff 'on the ground' in monitoring the operation of the service and in identifying gaps in provision. They also encouraged a wide commitment to the process of service planning and development. This meant that there was a mechanism for coordinating strategic and operational planning and for involving all the relevant 'stakeholders' in the service (including representatives of users and their families). These mechanisms for joint planning are currently being reviewed in line with the recent government White Papers on NHS and community care reform which attempt to introduce 'purchaser' and 'provider' relationships into the planning and management of health and social services. Whether they will survive—and in what form—is therefore, at present, unclear.

CARE IN THE COMMUNITY

Residential provisions

There are more than 180 places (67 per 100 000) available in sheltered housing specifically for the long-term mentally ill. This figure increases to 300 places (110 per 100 000) if an estimate is included for the mentally ill catered for under 'Special Needs' provisions. The overall level compares with that for England as a whole of 26 places per 100 000 (Department of Health, 1988). The range of facilities includes 69 places (38%) in 6 hostels with 24 hour cover (sleeping night staff); 36 places (20%) in 11 group homes and 'bedsits' with daily staff visiting and one hot meal provided; and 76 places (42%) in 31 unstaffed group homes, 'bedsits', etc. In the 'Special Needs' provisions, most (n = 144) are in 6 direct access hostels; 14 places are in 'women only' provisions.

In terms of service providers, more than 80% of the facilities are operated by the 'independent' sector (i.e. non-profit making, housing agencies or charities). The housing agency generally provides the house and the basic staffing input, while the health authority provides professional support, training and back-up from the CPNs or the 'Community Support Team' (see below). There are usually joint management agreements with regard to the assessment and selection of new residents. Just over half (53%) of the sheltered housing for the mentally ill is managed by one housing association (Granta Housing Society) and there are particularly close working relationships between the CPRS and Granta. We have generally found it very helpful to work extensively with one housing agency as regular face-to-face contact helps build a good atmosphere of trust and cooperation. At a national level, there is generally a much greater contribution from local authorities (47%) and the private sector (32%) to residential care and much less of a contribution from the independent sector (21%). The lack of involvement of the private sector in residential provisions for the mentally ill in Cambridge undoubtedly partly reflects the success of non-profit, independent agencies in meeting the needs of the mentally ill. It is also probably partly attributable to special features of the local housing market (e.g. the influence of the tourist trade, foreign language schools, etc.).

Despite this rather well-developed range of housing options, we are still aware of a number of unresolved problems and difficulties.

Do we have the right balance of different kinds of facilities?

A good range of facilities, with different levels of supervision, is consistent with various recommendations in the literature (e.g. Thornicroft and Bebbington, 1989; Wing and Furlong, 1986). It certainly increases choice and helps maximize flexibility when it comes to finding a suitable placement for a given individual. However, there is still a gap with regard to the availability of accommodation with high levels of supervision and waking night cover that could offer placements in the community for some of our most disabled 'new' long-stay. Clearly, there are problems with regard to the care of very severely disturbed young patients in community settings, but we feel that this is an issue we would like to tackle in the future. There has also been a problem in the past with regard to a shortage of *permanent* as opposed to *transitional* places, especially in highly supervised accommodation. (This has reduced recently with the opening of two new 24 hour cover hostels by Granta and the National Schizophrenia Fellowship.) In our experience there is often a tendency to underestimate the need for highly supervised, permanent homes and a tendency to overestimate the capacity of the long-term mentally ill to improve their level of functioning and 'progress' on to less supervised accommodation. Such misplaced optimism can lead to underprovision of permanent housing with high levels of supervision.

How to provide adequate professional back-up and support for staff?

In such a diverse and complicated network of services the problems of providing adequate professional back-up and support to the direct care staff, many of whom are not trained, is a central issue. Most of the providing agencies (including the voluntary sector) invest some time and effort in staff training, but there is still a need for a system of 'in vivo' training and support. This has resulted in the establishment of a small, specialized, 'Community Support Team' (CST) consisting of a full-time psychologist, a full-time occupational therapist, and a part-time psychiatrist. Their role it is to visit the sheltered housing on a regular basis and provide the direct care staff with professional advice on the management of difficult individuals. They also help them with access to the various hospital and local authority resources (e.g. inpatient care, day services, social work help) and are sometimes an important source of non-specific help and emotional support. The CST works closely with the CPNs and social workers from the relevant sector teams who are supporting the individual clients, but their work is primarily facilitative. Thus, they do not provide a service directly, but instead they try to help others improve the effectiveness of their day-to-day contact with residents. Inevitably, members of the team have begun to build up a small, personal 'caseload' and sometimes do get drawn in to providing practical help or emotional support for individual clients.

Our experience with the Community Support Team has convinced us of the value of providing mobile, easily accessible, professional support. As Donald Dick pointed out some years ago, it is still the case that while the majority of patients spend most of their time in the community the majority of professionals spend most of their time in the hospitals (Dick, 1984). This balance has to be changed and the CST is a step in that direction. But, supporting others in their work is not easy. It is not just about delivering 'training packages' or 'learning modules'. It means working along-side staff and helping them solve their problems in the settings where they actually occur. The CST aims to build up relationships of trust and confidence based on a respect for the skills and contribution of non-professional staff and wherever possible they aim to validate staff in their own ways of working, rather than imposing 'solutions' from outside. One of the main functions of the CST is probably to help staff manage their anxieties and not to resort to 'institutional' solutions as ways of coping with fear and insecurity (of course, similar processes also go on in traditional institutions). To achieve this successfully requires complex and subtle skills and the outcomes may often be rather vague and difficult to quantify, but it is crucially important. If staff are not well trained and supported, then the danger that they will recreate new 'institutions' in the community is considerable.

What kind of training do residential care staff need?

This leads us to the general question of what kind of training residential care staff need. There is no simple answer to this, but clearly a balance has to be struck between giving staff enough clinical information to make them aware when they should be asking for professional help, while at the same time not 'overprofessionalizing' them and destroying their natural ability to relate to the clients as people. We have found certain specific items of clinical information to be very important (e.g. the nature and implications of 'negative' symptoms, the importance of medication, the possibility of detecting 'early warning' signs of impending relapse, etc.) and there are parallels here in working with family carers (Smith and Birchwood, 1990). Many of the same processes are evident, e.g. 'blaming' the patient for negative symptoms, not understanding why medication is important when symptoms are in remission, not recognizing that relapse is predictable and may even be preventable, among family *and* non-family carers.

One of the most important tasks is to help carers be realistic in terms of their expectations for change and 'improvement'. There is a general tendency in psychiatric services to confuse our own needs with the needs of the patient and to project our wishes and desires onto them, expecting too much (or too little) as a result. Frustration of these expectations can then lead to high 'EE' (expressed emotion), particularly in terms of criticism, just as between relatives and patients. We therefore place particular emphasis on helping staff understand their reactions to difficult behaviour and not blaming patients for not living up to their expectations. Clear and detailed feedback on staff performance is often very helpful in this process.

Liaison with the hospital

One of the most striking aspects of working in a community-oriented service is how little staff in hospital know of life outside the institution and *vice versa*. We have found it necessary to spend a considerable amount of time and energy simply interpreting and explaining these two different worlds to one another. From outside the hospital, 'Fulbourn' often appears a huge, monolithic organization with very peculiar rules and customs. Staff in the community often do not understand the hospital hierarchy, the difference between a junior registrar and a consultant, the difference between a student nurse and a qualified member of staff. They do not understand how ward rounds work, how decisions are made, why some people seem to be summarily discharged with little or no follow-up, while others are refused admission. In many respects they share the same frustration and bewilderment as family carers (and some professionals!) and they need to be given clear and intelligible information about who is responsible and accountable, both in hospital and in the community. It is desirable that they are provided with a stable figure who understands their perspective and who can communicate between the world of the hospital and the world outside. Whether CPNs provide this link, or whether it is done through something like the Community Support team is open to debate, but somebody certainly has to do it.

Intensive 'home-based support—a gap in the service?

Community services in Cambridge are quite well-developed, but they do essentially consist of a rather large, 'static', network of facilities. A major gap in the service is the mobile, intensive, 'home-based' support described by Stein and Test and others (e.g. Stein and Test, 1985; Olfson, 1990; Hoult, 1986). These teams complement attempts to treat acute crises in the community, by offering ongoing, intensive support for the most severely disabled patients, usually on a domiciliary basis. In our service, the CPNs and the CST attempt to meet this need, but there is a demand for a more multidisciplinary input and one that can provide 24 hour, 7-day a week, availability. Specialized teams providing this kind of intensive 'case management' service thus represent a priority development for the future.

Table 1 Summary of day care provisions

Name	Number of daily attenders (total clients)	Type of facility	Operated by
Cambridge Day Clinic	20–25 (120+)	Comprehensive range of psychiatric treatments and 'case management' service for recently discharged inpatients. Aims to prevent readmission	Health authority
St Columba Centre	10–15 (50–60)	Specialized group psychotherapy plus social support	Voluntary organization (funded by grants from health authority and social services)
'Gemini' social club	10–15 (40–50)	A social club for the long-term mentally ill in the community. Offers food, activity and support. Programme determined by members	Local social services dept
'Nova' Work Centre	10–15 (15–20)	Sheltered work, allied with social club. Long-term term attenders from the hospital	Health authority
Castle Project Workshop	20–25 (30–35)	High quality sheltered work. Furniture restoring toy making, Mentally ill integrated with long-term unemployed. Small (n = 8), independent, business	Richmond Fellowship (voluntary organization) Funded by grants from health authority and social services
Hester Adrian Workshop	15–20 (same)	Traditional sheltered workshop. Sub-contract packing and assembly. Mixed disabilities	Local social services dept
Ely Mental Health Centre	15–20 (35–40)	Social and therapeutic activities, plus out-patient clinics	Joint health/ and social services
'Rural' day care	5–10 (15–20)	Mobile staff team. General social support	Health and social services

Let us turn now to the provision of day care and other kinds of community supports.

Day care and community support

There are 100–130 places (37–50 per 100 000) available each day in a number of different projects specifically for those with mental health needs (Table 1). If one includes the day care provided on the Fulbourn site (approximately 40 places per 100 000) then the total day care provision in the district is close to the national average of 60–65 places per 100 000 (Department of Health, 1988). However, these national figures include 35 places per 100 000 provided by health authorities mostly in the form of day 'hospitals', about half of which are located on hospital sites. In Cambridge, almost three-quarters of the day care provision, is located away from the hospital site and the direct contribution of the local authority is much smaller (23% v. 37%), whereas the contribution of the voluntary sector is relatively larger (20% v. 5%). The Cambridge service is also marked by a relatively strong emphasis on work-oriented activities and about half of the day places in the community are provided in different kinds of work projects. As indicated, the voluntary sector is very active, supporting some services financially, and acting as a direct service provider in other instances. For example, one of the best work projects (the 'Castle Project') is managed by the Richmond Fellowship and the local MIND group (CMWA) runs social evenings, coffee mornings and a 'Befriending' scheme which offers support to nearly a hundred people. The local National Schizophrenia Fellowship (NSF) runs regular meetings, holds support groups and has a local 'helpline'. In addition to these specific facilities, there are also a range of daytime activities (e.g. adult education classes, church groups, 'job club', etc.) which are used by people with mental health problems alongside members of the general public.

We have tried to create a balanced range of day provisions with multiple opportunities for work and other kinds of structured activities, and a similarly wide range of social supports. As in residential care, we have also tried to develop a partnership between health, social services, and the voluntary sector. Just as in residential care, a number of problems and issues have emerged.

The problem of engagement

Most day care and community services face problems in engaging the clients they wish to provide services for. This is a paradoxical situation and raises all sorts of theoretical and practical dilemmas. For example, should services make an effort to engage people who do not seem to want to attend? If 'yes', how? If 'no', why not? Are there certain kinds of clients who are always going to be difficult to engage? If so, why is this? If efforts are going to be made to engage people who do not seem to want to attend for day care, then should this 'outreach' be done by day care staff, or should it be handed on to CPNs who work exclusively in the community? In our own experience, a certain amount of outreach work can be done by day staff, but this can begin to interfere with their other responsibilities. There must therefore be good links between the day care staff and CPNs or other specialist teams, especially over the engagement and 'handover' of difficult clients. Moving a service into the community also does not necessarily guarantee an increase in its availability (indeed, sometimes the converse is true) and there can be very simple problems affecting access such as shortage of money, or poor public transport.

Who goes where? 'streaming' or 'mixing'?

A range of different day care options allows the possibility of tailoring individual 'packages' of care to meet individual needs. It is thus common for clients to make use of more than one facility as part of their weekly programme. However, this diversity of provision can also create a 'streaming' effect whereby groups of low functioning, low energy clients tend to concentrate in one setting, or around one activity (e.g. the 'drop-in'). This can restrict the range of activities that can be taken on in a given setting and make it difficult to pursue a philosophy of active user involvement. These problems can be overcome with patience and perseverance, but our experience suggests that there may be advantages in not having a *too* well differentiated system which creates very homogeneous groups. There are advantages in preserving groups with fairly mixed abilities, although clearly there are also limits to this strategy.

Physical facilities and social interaction

Social support is one of the primary aims of any community service and the physical characteristics of particular facilities can have a profound effect on the kinds of social interactions that take place in them. The majority of our long-term attenders are suffering from schizophrenia and many experience difficulties in social situations where there are high levels of interpersonal demands. At the same time, others complain of loneliness and the need for close, emotional support and stable, confiding relationships. Community services therefore need to be able to provide both these different kinds of social support and also to balance opportunities for social contact with opportunities for social withdrawal (Mitchell and Birley, 1983). Buildings should contain places to 'hide', as well as places to be together. The nature of the physical space may also affect patterns of staff–client interaction. For example, if there are large and comfortable offices, staff are more likely to spend time together, rather than with the clients. This may be appropriate if staff need a lot of time for confidential discussion, but it may interfere with attempts to facilitate joint staff/user 'ownership' of the project. It is also worth recalling that Linn et al. (1979) found that the number of rooms devoted to group therapy was *inversely* associated with a favourable outcome in day care for people with schizophrenia in the community. Various kinds of work and structured activities (e.g. the 'clubhouse' model, see below) seemed much more useful. All these factors need to be taken into account in the selection and design of buildings.

Sheltered work

We do not believe that sheltered work need necessarily be boring (Shepherd, 1989; Mills, 1991). Apart from the financial gains that work can bring—and for people on very low incomes even small rewards can be significant—work also offers social status and an identity which is an alternative to the patient role. Work can provide social contacts and support, a means of structuring one's time, a sense of personal achievement and mastery, and offers a criterion of recovery from illness. Despite high levels of unemployment, work therefore remains one of the most powerful 'medicines' in psychiatry (and it is relatively free from side effects!). In

Cambridge one of the most interesting examples of work projects is to be found in the 'Castle Project' (Grove, 1989). This is owned and managed by the Richmond Fellowship and is situated in a small business estate off one of the main streets near the centre of town.

From the outside it looks like any of the other 'starter units' on the site, but from the inside one can see that its employees and the way that it operates are rather special. The Castle Project concentrates mainly on woodworking—furniture restoration, toy making, and the manufacture of a range of craft products (bookends, ornamental clocks, recycled compost bins, etc.) which it sells direct to the public. At a time of increasing mechanization, when traditional workshops are worried about how they are going to continue to find subcontracts for packing and assembly, the 'Castle Project' provides a service to the public and produces quality goods for sale. Workers need have little prior knowledge of woodworking skills when they begin to attend, but with encouragement from staff they can soon develop skills, and a pride in their work, and a confidence in themselves. Much of this comes from the energy and creativity of the workshop staff and the manager who is herself a talented artist and designer. All the staff are employed primarily for their technical skills and not as 'therapists', or mental health workers. Every attempt is also made to consult the workers and involve them in decisions about how the project will be run and there is a continued emphasis on maintaining, as far as possible, the attitudes and expectations of an 'ordinary' small business.

A 'Placement Officer' is attached to the workshop whose role it is to find opportunities for the workers who wish to move on to open employment. She works with local factories and offices to negotiate part-time placements and provides liaison and support for both the worker and the employer. This scheme works well because of the quality of the assessment and preparation that is possible in the realistic work atmosphere of the main workshop prior to placement. There is also a continuity of support and good links have now been built up between the unit and local businesses (some of whom are represented on the project's own Management Committee). The latest venture is to set up a small, cooperative business, offering a 'print finishing' service. This is attached to the main workshop and is intended to be financially self-sufficient, providing permanent, paid employment for up to eight people. This exciting development underlines the importance of involving staff who have real technical and commercial skills and the advantages of a location which offers day-to-day contact with the local business community. It is a long way from the traditional, hospital based, 'industrial therapy' (IT) unit.

The 'clubhouse' model

In the development of community support for people with long-term mental health problems in Cambridge we have tried to use some of the principles outlined by Beard and his colleagues based on their work in 'Fountain House' in New York (Beard *et al.*, 1982). More than forty years ago they developed the 'clubhouse' model which was radically different, both in terms of its underlying philosophy and its working practices, from traditional day centres. People who attend a clubhouse are not *patients*, or *clients*, they are *members*. The members take on specific responsibilities for running the clubhouse and there are deliberately not enough staff to meet all the needs that the clubhouse creates for itself. Members are thus made to feel that they are really needed in order that the club can function and they are, in fact, integral to its success. In New York, 'Fountain House' members run a cafe and restaurant which serves over three hundred hot meals a day, they keep records of members' attendance, help organize 'work placements', and ensure that other members are informed of events taking place inside and outside the clubhouse. There is a 'mix' of clients, with the more capable members working alongside those with more severe difficulties. Each member has an opportunity to work and to contribute, but no-one is forced. The principles of voluntarism, choice and commitment are thus seen as more important than the principle of activity by itself.

In Cambridge, we have tried to introduce elements of the clubhouse model into a number of our day facilities, particularly the 'Gemini' social club (with its strong emphasis on user involvement) and the Cambridge Day Clinic (with its canteen run by users and its emphasis on 'self-help' work projects). We see the shift from 'teaching patients cooking skills' to 'helping people become important and valued workers within the context of cooperative work' as being central. It is not just a shift from being passive 'patients' to being active 'users'. It is also a shift from an emphasis on simple skills acquisition to trying to foster a sense of status, giving people a positive social role, and trying to improve their confidence and self-esteem. Creating a valued social role therefore entails much more than just improving instrumental competence. It depends upon the social 'structure' of the situation and the 'message' that this conveys, both to the client and to the outside world regarding the status of those participating (of the concept of 'normalization'; see Wolfensberger, 1972). In the UK we have tended to separate the activities of work and social support (e.g. in 'drop-ins' and sheltered workshops) but there may be merit in trying to combine the two since this can then offer the possibility of meaningful activity, within a valued social context. This seems to us to be one of the key ingredients of effective social support.

Dependency and the 'drop-in'

This brings us to issues of 'dependency' and 'institutionalization' in community settings. The so-called 'negative' symptoms of schizophrenia are often just as prevalent outside, as inside, the institution and the tendency for people with long-term mental health problems to become dependent on an artificial system of social supports is well documented. But, some degree of dependency is probably inevitable. It is a predictable consequence of not having access to the 'normal' range of social supports (e.g. jobs, families, friendships). 'Dependency' should therefore not be seen as wrong *in principle* and we should beware of the dangers of expecting people to achieve unrealistic levels of independence. If clients make stable and important relationships in a particular setting and are reluctant to leave, then this is not necessarily 'wrong' (indeed, it may have been one of the reasons for attending in the first place) but their needs in terms of support must be continually reviewed and the question asked, 'Could these needs be better met elsewhere?' (e.g. in a non-psychiatric setting). Dependency is not an all-or-nothing phenomenon and people may become partly dependent on one set of supports, while still receiving other kinds of support in other places. Thus, the problem is often not dependency per se, but how to help people 'diversify' their sources of support and identify the right kinds of support that will best meet their needs. This implies a rather different task (Harris *et al.*, 1986).

'Dependency' is a particularly important issue in relation to the concept of the 'drop-in'. This is a popular feature of many day services and can provide a useful focus for social interaction and communication. However, without also having the opportunity to participate in more structured activities, the 'drop-in' can simply exacerbate problems of apathy and lack of motivation. The 'drop-in' room at the day clinic is typical—a large room with armchairs placed around the edge, some tables with magazines and games like chess and scrabble (generally unused). A radio provides background music, punctuating the passing day with news broadcasts, not too loud to stop people talking if they wish, but not too quiet to make the usual silence hang too heavily. Coffee and tea are freely available on a 'do-it-yourself' basis upstairs and people may drop in for five minutes, two hours, or sometimes all day. It is an environment with very little structure and very few demands. Clients may not be encouraged to develop autonomy or to use their initiative and are at risk of becoming even more passive, 'institutionalized', and withdrawn. To counteract this, we have tried to make the 'drop-in' a focus for the user-led activities and a 'clearing house' for information about what is going on in the centre and elsewhere. There is also an expectation that everyone will become involved in at least one 'social' and one 'therapeutic' activity. The social activities have included going on outings, fundraising for a holiday, running a jumble sale and a market stall, social evenings, going as a group to the cinema, or the pub, organizing a barbecue, etc. The therapeutic activities have included a supportive group for women, art therapy, music therapy, anxiety management and psychotherapy. We have tried to use activity and social pressure as antidotes to 'dependency' and 'institutionalization', but it is sometimes a struggle. A completely unstructured 'drop-in' makes this struggle much harder.

Staffing issues

Staff are at the heart of any good service and working in community settings can pose special problems for staff. For example, it can be extremely anxiety-provoking going home at night worrying whether a particular client will be safe until morning. It is much easier going home at night from a hospital, where there are plenty of staff around to look after difficult, dangerous, or worrying patients. (Of course, patients aren't necessarily 'safe' in hospital, but that is how it *feels*.) Working in the community therefore requires staff to make many more judgements about the risk of harm to the patient or to her/his family and these judgements are inherently stressful. Coping with this stress demands staff who are calm and confident in their ability to make decisions. It also requires good teamwork, effective leadership, and strong mechanisms for staff support. These are all important in inpatient settings, but in the community they are vital.

Regarding key staff characteristics, just as in residential care, one of the most difficult problems is finding staff who know enough about the realities of severe mental illness so as not to be naive and unrealistic in their expectations, but yet who are also not so 'indoctrinated' by psychiatric services that they have lost their ability to see 'patients' as 'people'. A particular issue concerns the extent to which staff are able to help clients take on responsibilities for themselves. There needs to be an unobtrusive structure where tasks and roles are clearly defined, but where the participation of clients remains essential. This requires a very subtle kind of staff influence, particularly with the least motivated clients, and the temptation for staff to feel that 'in the end, it's just a lot easier if I do it myself' is sometimes difficult to resist.

Another staff problem that can occur concerns the 'boundaries' between staff and clients. When you are living and working alongside people in a relaxed, informal atmosphere, it can be hard—especially for inexperienced staff—to find the right balance between the need to treat clients as 'people' and the necessity not to step entirely outside their professional roles. This line is never very clear and there are dangers of a kind of false 'equality' which can lead to patronizing, even exploitative, relationships. Crossing the boundaries of responsible professional conduct can obviously have potentially serious consequences for both the staff member and the client. Senior staff therefore need to be aware of these potentially difficult situations arising.

A 'mixed economy' in day care? Power and responsibility

Much of what we have said about day care and community support revolves around themes of involvement and responsibility. These are reflected in the activities that are offered in different settings and who takes responsibility for leading and organizing them. For 'therapeutic' activities it tends to be the staff who are 'in charge', whereas in non-therapy, or 'life skills', activities there is more room for greater involvement of clients and greater equalization of power and authority.

So, can you have a 'mixed economy' of staff-led and user-led activities? Is it possible to combine 'therapy' with the principle of 'user involvement', or does the one inevitably interfere with, and confuse, the other? These are difficult questions. A confusion of 'ideologies' can cause stress and tension for both staff and clients and can be very difficult to live with, but sometimes there is no choice. (For example, the Day Clinic has to struggle with both 'therapeutic' and 'user-led' approaches because of the nature of its client group and their needs; 'Gemini', by contrast, can operate solely with a 'user-led' philosophy.) These fundamental questions of philosophy are particularly important when one is trying to set up a new venture and, generally speaking, it is much easier to *dis*empower people, than it is to *em*power them. Once a particular facility has developed a specific kind of 'culture', this can be very difficult to change.

The needs of carers

The needs of relatives are becoming increasingly clearly recognized and the role of families as 'partners' in the care of the long-term mentally ill is now an accepted principle in the development of services (Kuipers and Bebbington, 1985). To what extent is it possible to address the needs of carers and clients *together* in day settings and to what extent do their needs come into conflict? We have certainly encountered some instances where there is an apparent 'conflict of interests' between clients and their carers and where clients are adamant that they do *not* wish their families to be involved in any way in their care. This is a difficult area, but we do try to maintain a 'family approach' (Bennett *et al.*, 1976) and include relatives in the initial assessment and address their needs, as well as the clients', as part of the ongoing programme of care. But we also believe that families may require a specialized service, specifically tailored to meet their individual needs, as described by Smith and Birchwood (1990) and we are in the process of considering how to develop such a service locally.

COORDINATION CASE MANAGEMENT

The range of residential and community services outlined above implies a considerable need for coordination of services. Case management (Intagliata, 1982; Kanter, 1989) has emerged as a possible solution to these problems and, if the recent White Paper *Caring for People* (Department of Health, 1989) is to be taken at face value, then it is to form the 'cornerstone' of community care in the future. Case management is an important and useful idea, but it has a number of problems which have yet to be addressed (Shepherd, 1990b). Firstly, there remains considerable confusion as to what is actually meant by the term 'case management'. Is it simply a bureaucratic, managerial exercise concerned with the efficient allocation of resources, or, does it depend on an ongoing relationship with the client, like a special form of problem-solving psychotherapy, where the aim is to advocate for the client and ensure that their needs are met without paying too much attention to resource constraints? Health and social services seem to be developing very different models ('care programming' v. 'care management') and it is unclear whether the roles of 'purchaser' and 'provider' can be split in this way. Different models of case management obviously have very different implications with respect to training and practice and these have to be addressed before attempts are made to put a 'system' into place. Secondly, case management will not provide a magic solution to the problems of coordination and cooperation between the different agencies providing care. It provides a focus for their solution, but it still requires good joint working and cooperation 'on the ground' both *within* and *between* agencies (e.g. between CPNs and inpatient teams, between health services and the 'independent sector', etc.) if these are to be resolved in practice. Finally, case managers can never be a substitute for the range of services we have discussed here. Case management is primarily a device for coordinating service inputs and for ensuring continuity of care; it is not a remedy for failing to provide an adequate range of sheltered housing, day care and community supports.

In Cambridge, we have some experience with case management approaches. The Cambridge Day Clinic is involved in a national project, coordinated by 'Research and Development for Psychiatry' (RDP), which is aimed at establishing and evaluating case management systems for the long-term mentally ill in a number of different health districts (Clifford and Craig, 1988). As indicated earlier, the CPRS CPNs are also experimenting with their own version of case management based on the RDP system. The most recent policy guidance from the Department of Health (1990) has also provoked a district-wide debate on the concepts of case management, care management, care programmes, etc. As we have struggled to understand and implement these ideas, a number of additional practical and technical problems have emerged. For example, what kind of instrumentation and record-keeping system do you need? What are the optimal sizes of caseloads? How do you identify those people who most need case management and those who do not? How do you counter professional resistance to adopting case management approaches? (e.g. from CPNs and social workers who are worried about job security; or psychologists and occupational therapists who are concerned about the possible loss of professional specialization that case management entails). But, despite these problems we remain convinced that case management *is* an important idea. Services must identify clear points of responsibility, i.e.*people*, who can be held accountable for the coordination and maintenance of care for those with long-term needs. This is the central challenge of case management approaches. If it can be achieved, then this will be a very considerable step forward.

CONCLUSIONS

Despite some of the difficulties which exist at a national level, the services described in Cambridge show what can be achieved, over a long period of time, by a small, but committed group of people. As envisaged in some of the original planning documents (e.g. Department of Health and Social Security, 1975; Department of Health, 1985) a range of hostels, group homes, workshops, day services, and other community supports have been developed through the cooperation of a number of different agencies. Many of the functions of the hospital, in terms of long-term care, have now been replaced by community facilities, although it is clear that there is a continuing need for acute beds and highly staffed, highly professional, care for a small number of the 'old' and 'new' long-stay patients. Of course, Cambridge is not 'typical' and it is certainly not alone in having developed good quality community services. Nottingham (Howat et al., 1988) and Exeter (Beardshaw and Morgan, 1990) also have well-developed services and there are probably many more which are less well-known. But, on the basis of our experience, we would now like to try to identify some of the ingredients of successful 'community care'.

Firstly, a group of committed people must exist who are prepared to work actively on behalf of this specific client group. Resources have to be clearly targeted on the needs of the long-term mentally ill and there must be a clear-headed recognition that they will not be well served by vague appeals to 'prevention'. Secondly, there must be a willingness to work with a wide variety of different agencies and a recognition that no single agency can be expected to provide all services by itself. One then has to grapple with the problems of inter-agency cooperation at both an operational and a managerial level and this requires patience, openness, and a respect for what other people can contribute. Thirdly, there must be effective mechanisms for coordinating and monitoring care and for integrating administrative and financial structures at a local level. Fourthly, there is the question of money. The problem is often not so much an absolute shortage of money, but rather a relative shortage in the 'right' place in the system and the difficulty of transferring resources from one system to another (Mangen, 1988; Mechanic and Aiken, 1987). However, the importance of money can be overstated: ideas, enthusiasm, motivation, etc. are all just as important as money and you cannot change a service simply by an injection of resources. (Neither can you change one without it and this also has to be acknowledged.) Fifthly, one must address the problems of staff and staff training. Staff and informal carers are at the heart of any good service and it cannot work without them. For many reasons, it is often difficult to foster a positive attitude towards working with the long-term mentally ill and they may be seen as difficult, 'unrewarding', 'depressing', etc. Staff must therefore be helped to set realistic goals and to understand the reality of chronic psychiatric disability. They must not become too despondent if the patients do not—and cannot—meet *their* expectations, but they must also notice change when it does occur. One of the most important ingredients of any training programme is probably the opportunity to meet and observe colleagues in other settings who are working with similar problems.

This brings us to the last ingredient of all. In our 'quick fix' culture there are few people who are prepared to put in the considerable investment of time and effort necessary to build a service up—and even fewer managers and planners who are prepared to wait around for the results. This means that, despite the many theoretical descriptions of 'model programmes', there are relatively few good, working examples. Without being able to *see* what effective community services actually look like it is difficult to convince sceptical professionals (and managers) of their value and impossible to train new staff. Perhaps the most important ingredient in developing community services is therefore time itself. In Cambridge, we have been extremely fortunate in having a District and a Regional Health Authority who were not prepared to force a short-term closure date on the hospital. Rather, they were prepared to support the development of community services and allow the hospital to shrink as a *consequence*, not a *cause* of community care policies. As the House of Commons Select Committee observed, 'Any fool can close a mental hospital: it takes time and trouble to do it properly and compassionately' (House of Commons, 1985, para. 40). These are wise words. They are not an excuse for inaction, nor for laziness. They are a recommendation to proceed slowly, to be open to criticism, and to the possibility of learning from one's mistakes. These are the characteristics that mark out a really successful service. Good services are not assembled from a ready made 'kit', they 'grow', and like all organic things, they sometimes turn out not quite how you expected. Community care thus *can* work, but it is not easy. However, the evidence is overwhelming that good community services are preferred over traditional hospital systems by both patients and their families alike. Creating good community care is therefore a considerable challenge, but it is one that is well worth trying to meet.

REFERENCES

Bachrach, L.L. (1989) Some reflections from abroad. *Hospital and Community Psychiatry*, **40**, 573–574.
Barraclough, B. (1986a) In conversation with David Clark: Part I. *Bulletin of the Royal College of Psychiatry*, **10**, 42–49.

Barraclough, B. (1986b) In conversation with David Clark: Part II. *Bulletin of the Royal College of Psychiatry*, 10, 70–75.

Beard, J., Propst, R.N. and Malamud, T.J. (1982) The Fountain House model of psychiatric rehabilitation. *Psychosocial Rehabilitation Journal*, 5, 47–59.

Beardshaw, V. and Morgan, E. (1990) *Community Care Works*. MIND Publications, London.

Bennett, D.H. (1980) The chronic psychiatric patient today. *Journal of the Royal Society of Medicine*, 73, 301–303.

Benett, D.H., Fox, C., Jowell, T. and Skinner, A.C.R. (1976) Towards a family approach in a psychiatric day hospital. *British Journal of Psychiatry*, 129, 73–81.

Clark, D. (1974) *Social Therapy in Psychiatry*. Penguin Books, London.

Clifford, P. and Craig, T. (1988) *Case Management Systems for the Long-Term Mentally Ill: A Proposed Inter-Agency Initiative*. NUPRD, London.

Department of Health and Social Security (1975) *Better Services for the Mentally Ill*. Cmnd. 6233, HMSO, London.

Department of Health (1985) *Mental Illness: Policies for Prevention, Treatment, Rehabilitation and Care*. Cmnd. 9674, HMSO, London.

Department of Health (1988) *Residential Accommodation for Mentally Ill and Mentally Handicapped People: Number of Local Authority, Voluntary and Private Homes and Places at 31 March 1988 England*. Government Statistical Service, London.

Department of Health (1989) *Caring for People: Community Care in the Next Decade and Beyond*. HMSO, London.

Department of Health (1990) *Community Care in the Next Decade and Beyond: Policy Guidance*. HMSO, London.

Dick, D.H. (1984) Services in the net. In: *Psychiatric Services in the Community* (J. Reed and G. Lomas, eds). Croom Helm, London.

Garety, P.A., Afele, H.K. and Isaacs, D.A. (1988) A hostel-ward for new long-stay psychiatric patients: the careers of the first 10 years' residents. *Bulletin of the Royal College of Psychiatrists*, 12, 183–186.

Grove, B. (1989) Integration into the working world. *Psychiatric Bulletin*, 13, 28–29.

Harris, M., Bergman, H.C. and Bachrach, L. (1986) Individualised network planning for chronic psychiatric patients. *Psychiatric Quarterly*, 58, 51–56.

Hoult, J. (1986) Community care of the acutely mentally ill. *British Journal of Psychiatry*, **149**, 137–144.

House of Commons (1985) *Second Report from the Social Services Select Committee on Community Care*. HMSO, London.

Howat, J., Bares, P., Pidgeon, J. and Shepperson, G. (1988) The development of residential accommodation in the community. In: *Community Care in Practice* (A. Lavender and F. Holloway, eds). Wiley, Chichester.

Intagliata J. (1982) Improving the quality of community care for the chronically mentally disabled: the role of case management. *Schizophrenia Bulletin*, **8**, 655–674.

Kanter, J. (1989) Clinical case management: definition, principles, components. *Hospital and Community Psychiatry*, **40**, 361–368.

Kuipers, L. and Bebbington, P. (1985) Relatives as a resource in the management of schizophrenia. *British Journal of Psychiatry*, **147**, 465–470.

Linn, M.W., Caffey, E.M., Klett, J., Hogarty, G.E. and Lamb, H.R. (1979) Day treatment and psychotropic drugs in the aftercare of schizophrenic patients. *Archives of General Psychiatry*, **36**, 1055–1066.

Mangen, S. (1988) Implementing community care: an international assessment. In: *Community Care in Practice* (A. Lavender and F. Holloway, eds). Wiley, Chichester.

Mechanic, D. and Aiken, L. (1987) Improving the care of patients with chronic mental illness. *New England Journal of Medicine*, **317**, 1634–1638.

Mills, N. (1991) The structure of work environments in psychiatric rehabilitation. *Psychiatric Bulletin*, **15**, 69–72.

Mitchell, S. and Birley, J.L.T. (1983) The use of ward support by psychiatric patients in the community. *British Journal of Psychiatry*, **142**, 9–15.

Olfson, M. (1990) Assertive community treatment: an evaluation of the experimental evidence. *Hospital and Community Psychiatry*, **41**, 634–641.

Shepherd, G. (1987) What Makes the Cambridge Service Work? In: *An International Perspective on Community Services and Rehabilitation for Persons with Chronic Mental Illnesses* (M. Jansen, ed.). World Rehabilitation Fund, New York.

Shepherd, G. (1989) The value of work in the 1980's. *Psychiatric Bulletin*, **13**, 231–233.

Shepherd, G. (1990a) Need in the community: A district model. In: *Community Care—People Leaving Long-stay Hospitals* (S. Sharkey and S. Barna, eds). Routledge, London.

Shepherd, G. (1990b) Case management. *Health Trends*, 2, 59–61.

Shepherd, G. (1991) Psychiatric rehabilitation for the 1990's. In: *Theory and Practice of Psychiatric Rehabilitation* (F.N. Watts and D.H. Bennett, eds). Wiley, Chichester.

Smith, J. and Birchwood, M. (1990) Relatives and patients as partners in the management of schizophrenia: the development of a service model. *British Journal of Psychiatry*, 156, 654–660.

Stein, L.I. and Test, M.A. (1985) *The Training in Community Living Model: A Decade of Experience*. Jossey Bass, San Francisco.

Thornicroft, G. and Bebbington, P. (1989) Deinstitutionalisation— from hospital closure to service development. *British Journal of Psychiatry*, 155, 739–753.

Wolfensberger, W. (1972) *The Principle of Normalization in Human Services*. National Institute of Mental Retardation, Toronto.

Wing, J.K. and Furlong, R. (1986) A haven for the severely disabled within the context of a comprehensive psychiatric community service. *British Journal of Psychiatry*, 149, 449–457.

Wykes, T. (1982) A hostel-ward for 'new' long-stay patients: An evaluative study of a 'ward-in-a-house'. In: *Long Term Community Care: Experience in a London Borough, Psychological Medicine Monograph Supplement 2*. Cambridge University Press, Cambridge.

14 THE INFLUENCE OF NORMALIZATION ON PSYCHIATRIC SERVICES

J. Carson, T. Glynn and J. Gopaulen

DEVELOPMENT OF THE PRINCIPLE

This chapter sets out to provide an outline of the concept of normalization and its relevance for the care of the mentally ill. We begin by tracing the development of the concept, and we outline its current status. We then describe our own attempts to apply the principle to one of our residential facilities. Finally we consider some of the strengths and limitations of the model and its possible future role in guiding service developments in community care.

The term normalization is most closely associated with one person, Wolf Wolfensberger. However, as Perrin and Nirje (1985), point out, the concept was first developed and articulated by Nirje, making its initial appearance in print in 1969. Nirje's early definition of normalization was, 'making available to all mentally retarded people patterns of life and conditions of everyday living which are as close as possible to the regular circumstances and ways of life of society'. The key principle was that people with learning difficulties should be given the opportunity to live a life as close in nature to that of others, with the same rights and responsibilities. They take particular issue with Wolfensberger for having deviated from these early ideas. One of Wolfensberger's early attempts to define the concept was that it constituted, 'the utilization of means which are as culturally normative as possible in order to establish and/or maintain personal behaviours and characteristics which are as culturally normative as possible' (Wolfensberger, 1972). It is interesting to note how different this definition is from Nirje's. Despite this criticism Tyne (1987) mentions that, 'Wolfensberger's has been the major intellectual contribution to thinking about normalization both in North America and internationally'.

The bulk of the work that has been conducted in the normalization area has been in the learning difficulties field. Yet Wolfensberger himself highlighted the value of this approach for psychiatric services as far back as 1970. In an early paper (Wolfensberger, 1970), he stressed that psychiatric services should be run in such a way as to assist patients to achieve maximum integration into society. To achieve this he put forward a number of service goals. He claimed that residential or other psychiatric facilities should not congregate more than 25 to 50 patients together. He stressed the crucial role of work in normal settings and criticized many activities providing daytime occupation for patients. He stated that, 'recreational therapy . . . as well as the euphemistically labelled occupational therapy . . . may debilitate and demoralise'. In a subsequent paper (Wolfensberger, 1972), he continued to stress the prominence that should be given to work, but also made a number of controversial remarks that undoubtedly would not have endeared him to the psychiatric establishment. He claimed that many of the top professionals were themselves mentally disturbed, and that as a whole mental health workers were 'readily derided' by others. He also somewhat prophetically anticipated that his ideas would be met with greater resistance by those in the mental health field than those in the learning difficulties area. Indeed it is only now some 20 years later that some of his ideas are beginning to have an effect on mental health services (Ramon and Giannichedda, 1988).

Perhaps the greatest impetus to the acceptance of normalization ideas has come from the move towards community care (Shepherd, 1988). The ensuing widespread resettlement of long-stay patients into the community has led many workers to consider what sort of theoretical model they should adopt. The almost simultaneous demise of the therapeutic community and the token economy as models of working with the chronically mentally ill had left somewhat of a vacuum. Even some of the most influential work on alternatives to psychiatric hospitalization, the Training in

Community Living Model (Stein and Test, 1978, 1985), lacked a strong theoretical underpinning. For many people normalization was the model that should fill this gap (Braisby et al., 1988).

Early attempts to apply Wolfensberger's work in the UK focused on people with learning difficulties. They were strongly influenced by the Community and Mental Handicap Educational and Research Association (CMHERA) (O'Brien and Tyne, 1981). It was not until much later that a concerted attempt was made to apply the theory towards the care of the mentally ill (Braisby et al., 1988). These authors claimed that the goal of a mental health service could be briefly stated as, 'facilitating an individual's personal and social integration . . . while they live, work and relax in the least restrictive or protective environment possible'. What marks their approach as different is that it is one of the first attempts to operationalize some aspects of normalization thinking to the tasks facing resettlement workers. They suggest several new methods of working with patients. Among these is that staff adopt a 'getting to know you', framework originally devised by Brost et al. (1982). Other authors have used this approach towards work with elderly persons (Thomas and Rose, 1986; Thomas et al., 1990). The 'Getting to know you' approach to assessment is fundamentally different to a lot of work previously conducted with long-stay populations (Hall, 1980; Baker and Hall, 1988). The traditional approach towards assessment epitomized by the development of the REHAB Scale (Baker and Hall 1983) has been to rely on standardized nurse behaviour rating scales. Rather than interview chronic patients themselves many researchers have relied on nurse observations. In the 'Getting to know you' approach, the resettlement worker spends a considerable amount of time trying to build up a comprehensive picture of a chronic patient's lifestyle. They aim to answer a number of questions such as, 'What is this person's life like?', 'How did this person come to be here?'. The methodology adopted is of a time intensive, qualitative, single case approach. By its nature, the assessment involves a major experiential component for the worker, designed often to highlight the poverty of institutional environments.

When patients are transferred to the community Braisby and his colleagues further advocate that they be moved into houses or flats containing only a very small group of residents. Housing they argue should be dispersed, and not concentrated near to other devalued groups. This dispersed housing model has been very influential in some of the new community care developments. The Forest Community Project established by MIND in Waltham Forest was based on these ideas. The dispersed housing model is not without its disadvantages. It might for instance weaken patients' social networks by placing them in very small groups in different localities. Similarly it undoubtedly leads to greater staff travelling time and more managerial problems. The model may not be the most appropriate one for many of the patients currently remaining in the large asylums. Several studies have clearly demonstrated the severe dependency levels of current inpatient populations (Carson *et al.*, 1989a; Webb and Clifford, 1988; Croucher *et al.*, 1989).

THE CURRENT STATUS OF NORMALIZATION

Several reviewers have been critical of the concept of normalization. Baldwin (1985) cites the numerous different definitions of the term as being confusing, including its recent reformulation as 'social role valorization' (Wolfensberger, 1983). Baldwin also takes issue with the fact that the model is based on several untested assumptions, such as the supposed critical role of unconsciousness, which we will return to later. More recently, Rapley (1990) has criticized clinical psychologists for their, 'near total and unconditional acceptance of the principle'. He also bemoans the lack of empirical investigation in this area. Other authors such as Race (1987) claim that ideas around normalization are far more deep-rooted and complex than people imagine. This presumably makes them harder to scrutinize. Clifford (1986) draws our attention towards problems in applying the principles to people with mental illness. He claims that normalization advocates shift the blame for the chronically institutionalized to an 'inhumane system' and 'poor care'. In doing this they are underestimating the serious nature of psychiatric disturbance and this in turn hinders the formation of meaningful social integration. Robertson (personal communication) echoes this when he states that 'problems arise when normalization becomes tantamount to a denial of problems'.

Brechin and Swain (1988) take particular issue with the whole notion of ordinary housing, holidays and valued social roles. They feel that this sounds perilously close to a marketing strategy, and that the individual might be compelled to adopt a middle class value system in order to be accepted. This is a theme taken up by Szivos and Griffiths (1990) who state that, 'normalisation practices which encourage passing and assimilation to mainstream values, perpetuate a cycle of negativity valuing disability, and make it harder for the individual to come to terms with his or her disability'. They further suggest that consciousness raising for disadvantaged groups may be a more acceptable paradigm in that these groups would then develop a stronger and more positive group identity by 'acknowledging and owning their stigma'.

Most of the empirical studies that have been conducted to date on normalization have been carried out in the United States and Canada. Blake (1986) looked at 100 ex-psychiatric patients living in boarding houses in New Jersey. He claimed that rather than being empowered as consumers, the reality was that many of them had become, 'depersonalised as commodities: instead of gaining additional freedoms they may be abandoned'. Mesibov (1976) argues that the concept is not readily amenable to confirmation or refutation, and that the evaluation instruments devised, Program Analysis of Service Systems (PASS) and Program Analysis of Service Systems Implementation of Normalization Goals (PASSING), mistakenly focus on service systems, rather than on specific individuals. Trainor and Boydell (1986), in a study conducted in Toronto, looked at the proportion of generic services that supported chronic psychiatric patients in the community. They found that it was only in the vocational or educational area that generic agencies had made a serious attempt to try and meet the needs of psychiatric patients. In contrast to this, there was little evidence of the successful uptake of services in the income maintenance, housing or social recreational spheres. Generic services they concluded are not therefore meeting the needs of the mentally ill. They suggest the need for specialist rather than generic services.

Some support for normalization principles comes from the research of Hull and Thompson (1981a). They conducted an extensive study of 157 special residential facilities for the mentally ill. They found support for the idea that size of facility is important. The larger the residence the less normalizing the environment. Independent living facilities scored higher on normalization criteria even when social competence is controlled. There was also some evidence to suggest that facilities located in more middle class areas had higher scores on environmental normalization, and tended to provide more potentially integrating services and resources. In a subsequent paper (Hull and Thompson, 1981b), they conclude that facilities that score highest on normalization criteria actually encourage the development of more independent functioning in ex-patients. Patients living independently showed more awareness and more utilization of community facilities than those living in board and care homes. As was pointed out earlier, there are a dearth of empirical studies in this field.

THE TOMSWOOD HILL PROJECT

The Tomswood Hill Project is located within the grounds of Claybury Hospital on the outskirts of London. The project was our second attempt to apply the principles of normalization to an element of our residential care service. The first project we estab-lished, the Fencepiece Road Project, was taken over by another health authority. The Tomswood Hill Project was set up to cater for a much more disabled resident population than in the first project.

The project consists of a group of four ordinary three bedroomed houses. These were previously used for staff accommodation. In April 1988, these were taken over by the then rehabilitation area of the hospital after being redecorated and upgraded. The philosophy of the project was to conduct rehabilitation training in a domestic setting based on normalization principles. The fact that the project was located on the edge of the hospital campus would be seen by many to violate some of the tenets of normalization. The project could be seen to suffer from 'deviancy image juxtaposition'. In ordinary terms, this means that setting it up next to another facility with a very negative public image would reflect badly on the project.

There are nine residents in the project's three houses, with three per house. The fourth house serves as a staff base, but is also used for training and social purposes. The houses are semi-detached and grouped together in a row, allowing easy access for both staff and residents. At the project's inception, there were four men and five women with an average of 50.9 years, ranging from 34 to 76. Eight of the residents were diagnosed as suffering from chronic schizophrenia, with one having a unipolar depressive disorder. The mean length of hospitalization was 17.25 years, with a range from one to 42 years. On the Baker and Hall (1983) REHAB Scale, the average Total General Behaviour Score for this group was 48, though individual scores ranged from 0 to 97. Most of the residents fell into the moderately handicapped category, and would in the normal course of events have been unlikely to be considered for placement in such a scheme.

The initial work of setting up the project houses was completed within a month. At first only the project manager and two other staff were appointed, with the remaining staff being released from their previous duties nearer the commencement of the project. Regular informal meetings were arranged for the future residents and staff so that people could get to know each other. Residents were selected from wards in the hospital's continuing care sector allocated to Waltham Forest Health Authority.

To prepare the staff team, the project manager attended a course on PASS-3 (Program Analysis of Service Systems), based on the work of Wolfensberger and Glenn (1975). Collaboratively the staff team developed the principles of the type of service that this new project should offer. In many ways this was radically different from the service then being offered within the hospital because of the differences in approach and resources. To give an impression of how the Project is run, we will discuss the service drawing on the seven core themes of normalization as described by Wolfensberger.

1. The role of the (un)consciousness

This theme states that most people function with a high degree of unconsciousness. In human services, staff are said to be unconscious of 'the nature of the plight of devalued, handicapped, poor or needy people' (Wolfensberger and Thomas, 1983). Normalization aims to heighten the awareness of staff to their unconscious actions. To do this, staff are all given instruction about the theory. This is also backed up by group discussions of individual values and by participation in an exercise called 'Lifestyles' (Brown et al., 1984). It is usually found that many of the opportunities that staff value for themselves are not generally available to people with mental health problems, especially people on long-stay wards. Another awareness raising activity, 'What is a home', is used to help reinforce an appreciation of the project houses as being the residents' homes. The effect that such an approach has on nursing staff is perhaps best gauged by some of the comments from student nurses who have done placements in Tomswood Hill. One commented, 'it is so nice to see these patients as people'. Another stated, 'I don't really think of these residents as patients any more but as people living next door who we can help'.

2. The relevance of role expectancy

This theme states that where a group of people has certain expectations of another group, they will create conditions that will confirm their expectations. People with mental health problems tend to be seen in a very negative light. How does the mental health service see its own consumers? Does it try and develop social roles for people, does it encourage positive role expectations? In Tomswood Hill positive role expectancies are conveyed in three main ways. Firstly, residents live in individual houses with their own bedrooms and individual possessions. Secondly, a range of activities are offered to enhance residents' functional living skills. Residents are offered at least two hours' structured activity each day. These activities include menu planning, shopping, cooking, self-medication, personal self-care, care of clothing and relaxation. Thirdly, staff are educated about their use of language and labels. Residents are seen as people with mental health problems, and not as 'diagnoses'. If a resident is diagnosed as suffering from schizophrenia, they are seen as a person with a mental health problem and not as a schizophrenic.

3. The conservatism corollary

This theme argues that the more devalued a person or a group is, then the more important it is to add value to that group. At the very least the service should not do anything to further devalue the image of the person or group in society.

Residents go out individually or in a very small group so as not to draw excessive attention to themselves. Use is made of public transport or taxis rather than hospital transport. Staff make a conscious effort with residents to enhance appearance and appropriate dressing, to present a positive image in whatever aspect of daily living is being undertaken.

4. The developmental model

The essence of this theme is to encourage the development of 'personal competency enhancement'. It is really to do with offering people the chance to try things rather than feeling 'they won't be able to do that!'. The project staff aim to foster a 'let's try' approach amongst residents. The project is also an area where personal independence can be encouraged in a realistic way as the service is provided in ordinary housing.

5. The power of imitation

Normalization requires that imitation can be used in a positive way. The models available to many long-stay patients are often people with similar handicaps. To use imitation positively means providing residents with positive valued role models. The variability of even this small resident group partly achieves this. Individual residents are drawn from several hospital wards. No distinction is made between the desirability or dependency level of an individual so as to group them with others who are similar. Ages vary as do the genders within the house groups. Having an enthusiastic committed staff team also conveys a positive message to residents.

6. The dynamics of social imagery

The social image of people with mental health problems is fairly negative. This core theme suggests that everything possible should be done to enhance the social image of residents. The nature of the project itself goes some way to achieving this. None of the houses is marked as any different from the surrounding houses. The houses can only be seen as ordinary houses where people live. The staff team are encouraged through the previously mentioned awareness activities to see the residents as individuals who need varying degrees of guidance and support to live as comfortably as possible. It is hoped that this will better prepare individuals for the transition to other community living projects.

7. The importance of personal social integration

As has already been pointed out, people with mental health problems tend to be labelled and may be segregated. This theme suggests that individuals be supported, encouraged and given opportunities to take part in normal everyday community activities. Residents of Tomswood Hill wherever possible use community facilities and not the adjoining hospital campus. As well as local shops, hairdressers and sports facilities, residents have chosen to utilize community dental, chiropody and ophthalmic services.

The normalization approach does not always rest easily with nursing care. While individuals are encouraged to make their own choices and as much autonomy as possible is given, there is sometimes a tension created by this. For example, if it is a resident's choice not to eat, how long should nursing staff go before intervening if the person's health is at risk? Project staff try to offer appropriate levels of support and assistance, while also allowing room for individual development and growth. It is important to keep in mind the phrase 'as much as possible', and strive towards this.

NORMALIZATION AND HOSPITAL-HOSTELS

In this chapter, we have described a model of rehabilitation based on the notion of ordinary housing. The rehabilitation literature does not cite this as one of the most progressive developments in the residential field. Rather the most popular new rehabilitation facility is the hospital-hostel, which typically caters for between 12 and 20 residents. As Shepherd (1991) points out these units attempt to combine the best in hospital care, having for instance professional staffing, with some of the best features of community care, such as a non-institutional appearance. While there are now several descriptions of these units and how they work (Garety et al., 1988; Gibbons and Butler, 1987; Goldberg et al., 1985) few authors have tried to link them with the concepts of normalization. Indeed some would argue that the alternative term for these facilities, the so-called 'ward-in-a-house', reveals their true nature. Some advocates of a normalization approach would state that they violate normalization principles simply by virtue of their size

(Braisby et al., 1988). Despite this criticism these units do at least attempt to train rehabilitation skills within a domestic setting, unlike the typical rehabilitation ward. How do these facilities compare with facilities run along normalization lines?

It is perhaps not surprising, given the general dearth of empirical literature on normalization, that few authors have compared traditional rehabilitation services with services based on a normalization philosophy. In one of the few published studies, Brugha et al. (1988) did attempt to look at their day services using a normalization measure, PASSING, and comparing it with the MRC Needs for Care Schedule. Recently we have conducted a study at Claybury comparing our two intensive rehabilitation wards with the Tomswood Hill Project. In a sense this is a comparison between a more traditional and a more progressive approach to rehabilitation. Along with another colleague, Fidelma Dowling, we compared both sets of facilities using a range of measures which included REHAB, staff and consumer satisfaction measures, a management practices questionnaire, a normalization measure PASS–3 and a recently developed quality of life assessment, the Life Experiences Checklist (Ager, 1990). While we are still in the process of analysing all the data, already it is apparent that the Tomswood Hill Project has performed better on several measures, particularly the Life Experiences Checklist. This checklist covers five areas, Home, Leisure, Relationships, Freedom and Opportunities. Our initial results suggest that living in the project leads to an improved quality of life for residents. It might also be the case that residents in hospital–hostels would show similar improvements relative to people living on rehabilitation wards. Indeed as Shepherd (1991) points out, this also turns out to be the case. This brings us back to the original point of the need for a comparison of facilities run along normalization lines, with the best in current rehabilitation practice, the hospital-hostel. Such a study is eagerly anticipated.

CONCLUDING COMMENTS

It is interesting to reflect on the notion that some 20 years after publication of Wolfensberger's first paper on the application of normalization ideas in psychiatry, that the movement has still only had limited impact on Britain's psychiatric services. While Renshaw (1987) could claim that the 'philosophy of normalisation is behind much of the current thinking in service development in the UK', a more cautious appraisal by Ramon (1988) was that for the time being normalization does not offer 'a coherent and comprehensive model for practitioners who would like to carry it out'. Indeed a similar sentiment moved Professor Liberman to comment that it was 'an ideology in search of a technology'. No doubt part of the failure for its uptake will be blamed on the dominance of the medical model in psychiatry. Baldwin (1989) has identified other reasons for its failure to become established not least of which has been the behaviour of some of the movement's advocates, which he criticizes for their adopting 'neologistic speech patterns, proselytising and over-zealousness'. In a similar vein Emerson (1990) criticized the '"either you're with us or agin us" mentality which has stifled any attempts to debate or question the received wisdom of normalisation'.

Similarly one might ask the question whether the approach is a feasible one to implement with people who have long-term mental health problems. For instance two of the objectives towards helping devalued people, those of image and competency enhancement, are exceptionally difficult to put into practice. Physical integration is much easier to achieve than social integration. In an earlier paper we demonstrated the difficulties of successfully building competency enhancement (Carson et al., 1989b). It would, however, be wrong to assume from the above that normalization has little relevance for people with mental health problems. Our own experience with the Tomswood Hill Project has taught us that there are valuable lessons to be learned from the approach. Paradoxically one of the most significant findings we have noted is that psychiatric rehabilitation is best carried out within a domestic rather than a ward setting. While this is also the message that has come from the hospital-hostel type projects such as 111 Denmark Hill (Garety and Morris, 1984) and Douglas House (Goldberg et al., 1985), none of these has used the three person house model that we have with separate adjacent accommodation for staff. It is ironic that having learned this, we were too late to implement it in our first two new community residential units which were planned in advance of this work. Normalization may well prove to be the dominant theoretical force behind the community care movements in the future and while agreeing that psychiatric services have much to benefit from it we should follow Emerson's (1990) caution and 'examine more closely the actual impact of the practices advocated by normalisation on the lives of service users, communities and society'.

REFERENCES

Ager, A. (1990) *The Life Experiences Checklist Manual.* NFER-Nelson, Windsor.

Baker, R. and Hall, J. (1983) *REHAB: Rehabilitation Evaluation Hall and Baker.* Vine Publishing, Aberdeen.

Baker, R. and Hall, J. (1988) REHAB: a new assessment instrument for chronic psychiatric patients. *Schizophrenia Bulletin,* **14,** 97–111.

Baldwin, S. (1985) Sheep in wolf's clothing: impact of normalisation teaching on human services and service providers. *International Journal of Rehabilitation Research,* **8**(2), 131–142.

Baldwin, S. (1989) Applied behaviour analysis and normalisation: new carts for old horses? A commentary. *Behavioural Psychotherapy,* **17,** 305–308.

Blake, R. (1986) Normalisation and boarding homes: an examination of paradoxes. *Social Work in Health Care,* **11**(2), 75–86.

Braisby, D., Echlin, R., Hill, S. and Smith, H. (1988) *Changing Futures. Housing and Support Services for People Discharged from Psychiatric Hospitals.* King Edward's Hospital Fund, London.

Brechin, S. and Swain, J. (1988) Professional/Client relationships: creating a working alliance with people with learning difficulties. *Disability, Handicap and Society,* **3**(3), 213–226.

Brost, M., Johnson, T., Wagner, L. and Deprey, R. (1982) Getting to Know You—One Approach to Service Assessment and Planning for Individuals with Disabilities. Wisconsin Coalition for Advocacy, Madison.

Brown, H., Alcoe, J. and Hope, R. (1984) *Lifestyles: For People Who Have Mental Illness.* East Sussex County Council, Brighton.

Brugha, T., Holloway, F. and Wainwright, A. (1988) Day care in an inner city setting. In: *Community Care in Practice.* (A. Lavender and F. Holloway, eds). Wiley, Chichester.

Carson, J., Shaw, E. and Wills, W. (1989a) Which patients first—a study from the closure of the large psychiatric hospital. *Health Trends*, 21, 117–120.

Carson, J., McAlpin, B., Glynn, T. and Shaw, E. (1989b) The Role of Normalisation in the Community Care of the Mentally Ill, Unpublished paper. Claybury Hospital.

Clifford, P. (1986) Why I haven't joined the normies: some doubts about normalisation. *South East Thames Rehabilitation Interest Group Newsletter*.

Croucher, P., Abrahamson, D. and Cotson, D. (1989) Restandardising REHAB: a cross validation study. Paper given at British Psychological Society Symposium on 'Using REHAB in Rehabilitation and Resettlement'. Available from Claybury Hospital.

Emerson, E. (1990) Consciousness raising, science and normalisation. *Clinical Psychology Forum*, 30, December, 36–40.

Garety, P. and Morris, B. (1984) A new unit for long stay psychiatric patients, organisation, attitudes and quality of care. *Psychological Medicine*, 14, 183–192.

Garety, P., Afele, H. and Isaacs, D. (1988) A hostel ward for new long stay psychiatric patients: the careers of the first 10 years' residents. *Bulletin of the Royal College of Psychiatrists*, 12, 183–186.

Gibbons, J. and Butler, J. (1987) Quality of life for new long stay psychiatric inpatients: the effects of moving to a hostel. *British Journal of Psychiatry*, 151, 347–354.

Goldberg, D., Bridges, K., Cooper, W., Hyde, C., Sterling, C. and Wyatt, R. (1985) Douglas House: A new type of hostel ward for chronic psychiatric patients. *British Journal of Psychiatry*, 147, 383–388.

Hall, J. (1980) Ward Rating Scales for long stay patients: a review. *Psychological Medicine*, 10, 277–288.

Hull, J. and Thompson, J. (1981a) Factors which contribute to normalisation in residential facilities for the mentally ill. *Community Mental Health Journal*, 17(2), 107–113.

Hull, J. and Thompson, J. (1981b) Predicting adaptive functioning among mentally ill persons in community settings. *American Journal of Community Psychology*, 9(3), 247–268.

Mesibov, G. (1976) Alternatives to the principle of normalisation. *Mental Retardation*, 14(5), 30–32.

O'Brien, J. and Tyne, A. (1981) *The Principle of Normalisation: A Foundation for Effective Services.* CMHERA, London.

Perrin, B. and Nirje, B. (1985) Setting the record straight: a critique of some frequent misconceptions of the normalisation principle. *Australia and New Zealand Journal of Developmental Disabilities,* 11(2), 69–74.

Race, D. (1987) Normalisation: theory and practice. In: *Reassessing Community Care.* (N. Malin, ed.). Croom Helm, Beckenham.

Ramon, S. (1988) Towards normalisation: polarisation and change. In: *Psychiatry in Transition: The British and Italian Experiences.* (S. Ramon and M. Giannichedda, eds). Pluto Press, London.

Ramon, S. and Gianichedda, M. (1988) *Psychiatry in Transition: The British and Italian Experiences.* Pluto Press, London.

Rapley, M. (1990) Is normalisation a scientific theory? *Clinical Psychology Forum,* No. 29, October, 16–20.

Renshaw, J. (1987) New initiatives in community care. In: *Clinical Psychology Research and Developments* (H. Dent, ed.). Croom Helm, Beckenham.

Shepherd, G. (1988) Current issues in community care. Paper presented at Second Annual One Day Conference on Psychiatric Rehabilitation, Oxford, 13 December.

Shepherd, G. (1991) Psychiatric rehabilitation for the 1990s. Foreword. In: *Theory and Practice of Psychiatric Rehabilitation* (F. Watts and D. Bennett) 2nd edn. Wiley, Chichester.

Stein, L. and Test, M. (eds) (1978) *Alternatives to Mental Hospital Treatment.* Plenum Press, New York.

Stein, L. and Test, M. (eds) (1985) *The Training in Community Living Model: A Decade of Experience.* Jossey Bass, San Francisco.

Szivos, S. and Griffiths, E. (1990) Consciousness Raising and Social Identity Theory: A Challenge to Normalisation. Forum, 28, *Clinical Psychology,* August, 11–15.

Thomas, D. and Rose, N. (1986) Getting to Know You. A Reflection and Review of an Individualised Approach to Service Planning. North Manchester Health Authority.

Thomas, D., Holt, V., Illingworth, M., Maddocks, N. and Robinson, E. (1990) Designing services with people who are elderly. In: *Community Care—People Leaving Long Stay Hospitals* (S. Sharkey and S. Barna, eds). Routledge, London.

Trainor, J. and Boydell, K. (1986) *The Politics of Normalisation.* Canada's Mental Health, March, 19–24.

Tyne, A. (1987) Shaping community services: the impact of an idea. In: *Reassessing Community Care* (N. Malin, ed.). Croom Helm, London.

Webb, Y. and Clifford, P. (1988) *Warley Hospital Patients Needs Survey*. National Unit for Psychiatric Research and Development, London.

Wolfensberger, W. (1970) The principle of normalisation and its implications to psychiatric services. *American Journal of Psychiatry*, 127(3), 291–297.

Wolfensberger, W. (1972) *The Principle of Normalisation in Human Services*. NIMR, Toronto.

Wolfensberger, W. (1983) Social role valorisation: a proposed new term for the principle of normalisation. *Mental Retardation*, 21(6), 234–239.

Wolfensberger, W. and Glenn, L. (1975) *Program Analysis of Service Systems: PASS*. NIMR, Toronto.

Wolfensberger, W. and Thomas, S. (1983) *Program Analysis of Service Systems' Implementation of Normalisation Goals. PASSING*. NIMR, Toronto.

15 AN AMERICAN PERSPECTIVE: CRISES IN SERVICES FOR PEOPLE WITH SERIOUS MENTAL ILLNESSES*

E.F. Torrey

In the US, the modern era in public services for people with serious mental illnesses began immediately following World War II with the realization that such illnesses were common and that state mental hospitals were, on the best of days, remarkably untherapeutic and, on the worst of days, snake pits. The response of the federal government was to create a National Institute of Mental Health to which it gave responsibility for research on mental illnesses and the training of increased numbers of psychiatrists, psychologists, psychiatric social workers and psychiatric nurses.

Services for people with serious mental illnesses remained the exclusive responsibility of state government until 1963, when Congress passed President John F. Kennedy's Community Mental Health Centers (CMHC) Act. In describing what the legislation would accomplish, the President said that 'reliance on the cold mercy of custodial isolation will be supplanted by the open warmth of community concern and capability' (Kennedy, 1963). Following passage of the CMHC Act, people with serious mental illnesses

* An earlier version of this chapter was written by the author for E.F. Torrey, K. Erdman, S.M. Wolfe and L.M. Flynn, eds *Care of the Seriously Mentally Ill* Washington DC Public Citizen Health Research Group and National Alliance for the Mentally Ill, 1990

were made eligible for several other federal programmes including Supplemental Security Income (SSI), Social Security Disability Income (SSDI), Medicaid and Medicare. Prior to 1963, then, states had almost total fiscal responsibility for the care of their mentally ill residents; after 1963 an increasing proportion of this fiscal burden shifted from the states to the federal government. Today, the federal share of the approximately $24 billion annual public cost of services to people with mental illnesses is 50% or approximately $12 billion.

The CMHC Act and subsequent efforts of federal and state governments to improve care for people with mental illnesses seemed reasonable at the time and clearly were motivated by the best of intentions. These efforts coincided with the introduction of antipsychotic medication, which became widely available by the late 1950s, thereby making deinstitutionalization of people with mental illnesses feasible. In the 30-year period from 1955 to 1984, the number of patients in public mental hospitals was reduced from 552 150 to 118 647, a reduction of just under 80%. Hundreds of thousands of mentally ill individuals who previously had been held in custodial state mental hospitals were discharged to what was supposed to be community care. The federally funded CMHCs, support programmes such as SSI and SSDI, and increased numbers of mental health professionals were all going to work with state governments to provide care for these individuals. That was the way it was supposed to happen.

When one surveys the current scene in the US, it is clear that whatever was supposed to happen did not happen and that deinstitutionalization has been a disaster. Despite the approximately $24 billion per year in public funds being spent on services for people with mental illnesses, despite almost $3 billion in federal funds spent to create Community Mental Health Centres, despite over $2 billion in federal funds and uncounted additional billions in state funds spent to train more mental health professionals, services for people with serious mental illnesses in the United States in 1993 are the shame of the nation. The road to hell truly is lined with good intentions; the gateposts on this road are painfully evident.

1. There are now more than twice as many people with schizophrenia and manic-depressive psychosis living in public shelters and on the streets as there are in public mental hospitals

Estimates of the total number of homeless individuals in the US have ranged from 250 000 to 3 million. In probably the best study done to date, the Urban Institute in Washington, DC in 1988 estimated that the total number was between 567 000 and 600 000. In March 1990, the United States Bureau of the Census undertook an exhaustive count of the homeless population and reported 230 000 such individuals.

There are many causes of homelessness. Most surveys have found that between 30 and 40% of single homeless people are alcoholics or drug addicts; some of these people use shelters and soup kitchens because they have spent their own funds for alcohol and drugs. Another important cause of homelessness is the reduced availability of low-income housing as inner cities have become gentrified and as federal support for low-income housing has eroded drastically (particularly in the 1980s). There are also some homeless people who have no job skills and no family support and use shelters as places to try and get their lives together.

The most controversial segment of the homeless population is the group with serious mental illnesses such as schizophrenia and manic-depressive psychosis. The question of what percentage of the homeless this group constitutes has unfortunately become a political football with liberals arguing that it is a small percentage (and that cuts in social programmes and housing are the cause of most homelessness), while conservatives contend that mentally ill people make up a large percentage (and thus that state mental health authorities, not the failure of social programmes and housing, are to blame). Many of the studies concerning this question have been tainted by such political preconceptions, with widely varying results.

Increasingly, however, there is a consensus that approximately 25–30% of single homeless adults living in shelters are seriously mentally ill. Studies done in the mid-1980s in Boston (Bassuk *et al.*, 1984), Philadelphia (Arce *et al.*, 1983) and Washington (Torrey *et al.*, 1985) reported that between 36 and 39% of adult shelter residents had schizophrenia. With the influx of large numbers of crack users into city shelters in many urban areas the overall percentage of homeless persons with schizophrenia has probably decreased. A 1988 study in Los Angeles found that 28% of homeless people in shelters had schizophrenia, manic-depressive psychosis or major depression (Roegel *et al.*, 1988); this survey, however, failed to include the 15% of shelter residents who refused to cooperate, among whom there were certainly many with paranoid schizophrenia. Another 1988 California study of three counties reported that 30% of homeless people in shelters had a severe mental disorder (Vernoz et al., 1988). A 1989 study of homeless people in Baltimore shelters found that 31% of men and 41% of women had schizophrenia, manic-depressive psychosis, or major depression (New York Times, 1989), while another 1989 study in New York reported that 17% of shelter residents had 'a definite or probable history of psychosis' and another 8% 'a possible history of psychosis' (Susser et al., 1989).

For homeless individuals not living in shelters but rather in parks, alleys, abandoned buildings, doorways, subway tunnels, etc., the percentage with serious mental illness appears to be even higher than 25–30%. A study of individuals living on heating grates and on the streets of New York City estimated 'that 60% exhibit evidence of schizophrenia as manifested by disorganized behaviour and chronic delusional thinking' (Cohen et al., 1984). In Los Angeles, a 1988 study of homeless persons (two-thirds of whom slept in places other than shelters) found that 40% had psychotic symptoms (Gelberg et al., 1988). By contrast, a study of homeless individuals living on grates and sleeping in doorways in Washington, DC found that only 29% had a history of psychiatric hospitalization as reported by the individual (Greene, 1989).

Taking all available data into consideration, it would appear that approximately 30% of single adult homeless individuals living either in shelters or on the streets are seriously mentally ill, mostly with schizophrenia and manic-depressive psychosis. If the total number of homeless adults is conservatively estimated to be only 500 000, then the number of seriously mentally ill homeless would be approximately 150 000 individuals. By comparison, the most recent data available on patients in the nation's 286 state and county psychiatric hospitals reveals that there are just over 68 000 patients with schizophrenia and manic-depressive psychosis. There are, then, more than twice as many people with schizophrenia and manic-depressive psychosis living in public shelters and on the streets as there are in public mental hospitals.

Common sense says that many of the homeless people with serious mental illnesses must be the same people who were discharged from state mental hospitals, and several studies have shown that this is so. A study carried out at the Central Ohio Psychiatric Hospital in 1985 followed 132 patients for six months after their discharge and found that within that period 36% of the discharged patients had become homeless (Belcher, 1988a). The truly alarming aspect of this study, however, is that the 132 discharged patients were not the sickest people being discharged from that hospital; another 61 discharged patients 'were not medically cleared by hospital staff to participate in the study because of the severity of their psychotic behaviour' (Belcher, 1988b), and it seems likely that an even higher proportion of this group presumably became homeless. In Massachusetts a 1983 study of 187 patients discharged from a public psychiatric hospital found that 27% had been homeless at least occasionally within the previous six months (Drake et al., 1989). And in Los Angeles, a 1988 study of 53 homeless mentally ill individuals living on the streets, on beaches or in parks reported that 79% had been previously hospitalized in state mental hospitals or on the psychiatric wards of general hospitals (Lamb and Lamb, 1990).

> The man called himself Joe No Name and was living in a doorway in Philadelphia. He admitted that he had been in a psychiatric hospital many times. An observer visited him regularly over six months, trying to gain his trust and persuade him to accept help. On one occasion Joe 'reached out and asked if I would touch the tip of his finger so he could see if I was real or "just part of the electric current in the wires above."' He refused to go to a shelter because 'to go inside would mean instant death'. One night he suddenly disappeared and was not seen again. (Eisenhuth, 1983)

Having approximately 150 000 seriously mentally ill individuals living in public shelters and on the streets in 1990 in the United States, the wealthiest nation in the world, is quite an extraordinary and unacceptable state of affairs. It was, in fact, the existence of large numbers of seriously mentally ill individuals in the nation's poorhouses in the 1820s and 1830s which led to the building of state mental hospitals as a 'humane' alternative. We have, in essence, returned to where we began 170 years ago; at no time in the intervening years have there been as many seriously mentally ill individuals, most receiving no treatment, living in the community.

> Mark X living under a subway platform in downtown Philadelphia. He smeared his feces and picked constantly at large open sores, stopping only to respond briefly to voices ... He was truly regressed, and often survived only by reaching out to the tracks a

DIMENSIONS OF COMMUNITY MENTAL HEALTH CARE

few feet from his hiding place to pick crumbs or crusts discarded by passengers on the platform above. Many times large rats would outrace Mark for the food ... There were many days when he seemed almost catatonic. His occasional attempts to respond [to a volunteer trying to make contact] were usually interrupted by the deafening rumble of the steel wheels of subway cars ... He was removed from under the subway platform when private subway police were hired to 'clear the bums out'. Attempts to get Mark X committed for treatment to a psychiatric hospital failed. (Eisenhuth, 1983)

Staying alive on the streets or in public shelters when one's mind is working normally is extremely difficult. When the mind cannot think clearly because of schizophrenia or manic-depressive psychosis it is a living hell.

- 'I know one woman who has been raped 17 times', says an official of the Central City Hospitality House in San Francisco (Cooper, 1988). Infectious diseases, tuberculosis and untreated medical problems are endemic.
- In New York City 'a homeless man, attacked by seven teenagers, was thrown over a wall and dropped about 50 feet into Riverside Park early yesterday leaving him with a fractured leg and back injuries' (New York Times, 1986).
- In Massachusetts, a homeless man and woman were savagely beaten to death. Such vulnerable people, editorialized a newspaper (Cape Cod Times, 1984), 'are the natural prey of anyone looking for some loose change, a pack of cigarettes, a bottle. They are rabbits forced to live in company with dogs.'

Phyllis Iannotta, age 67, had been diagnosed with paranoid schizophrenia and hospitalized. Following her discharge no follow-up or aftercare took place and she became a shopping bag lady on the streets of New York. In 1981 she was raped and stabbed to death in a parking lot on West 40th Street. In her bag was found two sweaters, a ball of yarn, an empty box of Sloan's linament, a vial of perfume, a can of Friskies turkey-and-giblet cat food, and a plastic spoon. (Herbert, 1985)

There have been a few tentative beginnings at solving the problem of homelessness among people with mental illness. The federal McKinney Act funds included $35 million in 1989 for mental health services for the homeless. The National Institute of Mental Health elevated the problem to 'priority' status in 1989 and allocated $4.5 million for research and demonstration grants. But most of the care for people who are homeless and mentally ill continues to come largely on a voluntary basis from the private sector, especially the community groups, churches and synagogues that operate 90% of public shelters and soup kitchens. These are the so-called 'thousand points of light', individuals who are doing their best to fill the holes left by the breakdown in public psychiatric services and by the failures of American psychiatry, psychology and social work. The crisis of homelessness among people with mental illnesses will continue until such time as public psychiatric services are improved. The private sector is doing more than its share; as the *US News and World Report* recently noted, 'it is difficult to see ... how the thousand points of light can put out much more wattage' (Whitman, 1989).

2. There are now more people with schizophrenia and manic-depressive psychosis in prisons and jails than in mental hospitals

According to the United States Department of Justice, on any given day in 1989 there were 1 042 136 individuals in the nation's prisons and jails (56 000 in federal prisons, 644 000 in state prisons, and 341 636 in local jails). Studies to ascertain how many of the prisoners have serious mental illnesses have shown varying results; a 1989 review of these studies concluded that '10 to 15 per cent of prison populations ... need the services usually associated with severe or chronic mental illness' (Jemelka *et al.*, 1989). This review defined chronic mental illness as including 'schizophrenia, unipolar and bipolar depression, or organic syndromes with psychotic features'.

On the lower end of the scale, a study in Chicago's jail found that only 6.4% of prisoners had schizophrenia, mania or major depression (Teplin, 1990). A study of a prison in Maryland reported that 9.5% of the inmates met diagnostic criteria for schizophrenia and another 3.1% had a major depressive disorder (Swetz *et al.*). In Philadelphia, 11% of all admissions to the city jail were said to have a diagnosis of schizophrenia (Acker and Fine, 1989). In the State of Washington, 10.3% of prisoners were diagnosed with schizophrenia, schizotypal disorder, or manic-depressive psychosis (Jemelka *et al.*, 1989), while in Michigan's prisons, '20 per cent of the state's 19 000 convicts suffered from severe mental impairment meaning delusions, hallucinations, and loss of contact with reality' (Luke, 1987). The Los Angeles County Jail presently holds 24 000 inmates on any given day and, according to professionals who have worked there, approximately 15% of them have serious mental illnesses. That means that there are approximately 3600 seriously mentally ill individuals in that jail, which is 700 more than the largest mental hospital in the United States. The Los Angeles County Jail is, *de facto*, the largest mental hospital in this country.

Given all the data it seems reasonable to conclude that approximately 10% of inmates in prisons and jails, or approximately 100 000 individuals, suffer from schizophrenia or manic-depressive psychosis. For comparison, there are approximately 68 000 patients with schizophrenia and manic-depressive psychosis in the nation's public mental hospitals. *Thus, there appear to be approximately 100 000 individuals with schizophrenia and manic-depressive psychosis in prisons and jails compared with approximately 68 000 in public mental hospitals.*

> In 1987 a 29-year-old woman, arrested for breaking an antenna off a car, gave birth to a baby in a cell of the Erie County Holding Center, a county jail in Buffalo. Nobody, including the woman, was aware that she had been eight months pregnant. She was known to be seriously psychotic and, at the time of the birth, screamed loudly to the guards to get the 'animal' out of her clothing. By the time the guards retrieved the baby it was dead. At the time the jail was estimated to be holding more seriously mentally ill persons, approximately ninety, than was the psychiatric unit of the Erie County Medical Center. (Erie Alliance for the Mentally Ill, 1987)

There is a consensus that the percentage of inmates with serious mental illnesses in the nation's prisons and jails has 'increased slowly and gradually in the last 20 years and will probably continue to increase' (Jemelka *et al.*, 1989). These are, of course, the same years during which the state mental hospitals were discharging patients wholesale without providing aftercare for most of them. The cause-and-effect relationship between these two trends is self-evident and was illustrated by another aspect of the previously mentioned 1985 study from Ohio. In that study, 33 individuals with schizophrenia and manic-depressive psychosis who had been discharged from the state mental hospital were located six months later. During the six months, 21 of the 33 individuals (64%) had been arrested and jailed (Belcher, 1988c). Most arrests did not involve violence but were for misdemeanours such as 'threatening behaviour' in public and 'walking in the community without clothes'. Prior to their discharge from the hospital these individuals had had an average of 12.5 hospital admissions in the preceding five years and had a history of not taking their medications once they left the hospital. According to the author of the study, 'the jail was an asylum of last resort, where they received little or no mental health treatment and were quickly released' to begin another cycle of streets–hospital–streets–jail.

> George Wooten, age 32, was booked into the Denver County Jail in 1984 for his one hundredth time. He had been diagnosed with schizophrenia at age 17 and developed a fondness for sniffing paint, after which he creates 'a disturbance' and the police arrest him. According to a newspaper account: 'Eight years ago the officers might have taken Wooten to a community mental health center, a place that was supposed to help the chronically mentally ill. But now they don't bother . . . Police have become cynical about the whole approach. They have learned that "two hours later [those arrested] are back on the street . . . the circle of sending the person to a mental health center doesn't work."' (Kilzer, 1984)

Prisons and jails were not created to be mental hospitals. And yet, because of the failure of public psychiatric services, prisons and jails have become *de facto* shelters of last resort for psychiatrically ill individuals. In Buffalo, when police took mentally ill individuals to the emergency unit of the local mental health centre, psychiatrists refused to admit the persons 43% of the time (Egri *et al.*, 1985). The police then charged such persons with misdemeanours and put them in jail just to get them off the streets, often for their own safety. In Oregon, a study of seriously mentally ill individuals in prisons and jails found that 'in about half the cases a failed attempt at commitment had preceded the arrest' (McFarland *et al.*, 1989). The person's family had sought help for them by trying to get them admitted to a psychiatric hospital but were turned down, often because no beds were available or because the person did not meet stringent state laws for dangerousness to self or others. The person then commits a minor crime such as trespassing, shoplifting or disorderly conduct and ends up in jail rather than in a psychiatric hospital. In many communities public officials representing mental health and corrections spend much time and effort shuttling mentally ill individuals back and forth between the two systems. As a recent reviewer summarized the situation: 'With both agencies exhibiting a "he's yours" posture, the mentally ill offender falls through a crack, if not a gaping hole, in the system of care for the mentally ill' (Jemelka *et al.*, 1989).

> Timothy Waldrop, 24 years old and who had been voted the friendliest boy in his high school graduating class, had been treated for schizophrenia for several years. He was arrested for armed robbery and sentenced to five years in the Georgia state prison. In prison his antipsychotic medication was stopped; 'a few days later Waldrop gouged out his left eye with his fingers.' Despite resuming his medication he then cut his scrotum with a razor and, while in restraints, 'punctured his right eye with a fingernail leaving himself totally blind'. (Plott, 1985)

In states like Kentucky and Montana, county jails are used (sometimes for several days) to hold mentally ill individuals awaiting transportation to a mental hospital; such individuals have not been charged with any crimes.

The quality of care that mentally ill inmates receive in prisons and jails varies greatly. There are a few programmes that provide good psychiatric care and that have been cited as models for the rest of the country; the King County Jail in Seattle, Washington, the Boulder County Jail in Boulder, Colorado and the jail diversion programme in Norristown, Pennsylvania, are examples of such programmes. Much more common, however, are prisons and jails where mentally ill inmates are neglected or abused. In Arizona's maximum security prison, for example, mentally ill prisoners may be 'chained naked to bed posts and left there 20 hours a day for up to three days at a time' according to a 1989 report in the *Arizona Republic*. 'Prison officials said the procedure is part of standard mental-health practice to keep "self-abusive and suicidal" inmates from hurting themselves' (Van Der Werf, 1989).

A major problem in providing care for mentally ill inmates of prisons and jails is the inability of psychiatrists to give them medication because of stringent laws designed to protect prisoners from involuntary medication. Such laws do indeed protect non-mentally ill prisoners from the abuse of a 'Clockwork Orange' system of chemical mind control. But the laws also make it difficult or impossible to medicate blatantly psychotic inmates who, because of their brain disease, have no insight into their illnesses or need for medication. In Kentucky, for example, the *Lexington Herald-Leader* described an inmate with paranoid schizophrenia who had refused to come out of his cell 'for years' (Nance, 1989). 'He refuses to take psychotropic drugs, which probably could reduce his delusions, possibly even eliminate them. But courts almost never allow prisons or mental hospitals to force medication.'

3. Increasing episodes of violence by seriously mentally ill individuals are a consequence of not receiving treatment

Mentally ill individuals are inherently no more violent than non-mentally ill persons. When they are treated, in fact, studies suggest that their arrest rate is *lower* than that of the average citizen. The wards of a well-run mental hospital are much safer on any given day than the streets of most cities.

When individuals with serious mental illnesses such as schizophrenia and manic-depressive psychosis are *not* treated, however, they will occasionally commit acts of violence. These acts may be in direct response to imagined threats (e.g. a belief that another person is going to kill him so he strikes first), delusional thinking (e.g. that another person is really the Devil in disguise), or auditory hallucinations (e.g. voices commanding the person to hurt another). The violent acts, in short, are usually part and parcel of the person's illness.

The mass exodus of people with serious mental illnesses from public mental hospitals in the last three decades has placed literally hundreds of thousands into the community. The majority receive little or no treatment once they leave the hospital. As noted above, approximately 150 000 mentally ill individuals are living in public shelters or on the streets; another 100 000 are in prisons and jails, most of them charged with misdemeanours. Another several hundred thousand—nobody knows the precise number—are living with their families or by themselves. *The majority of all of these are receiving little or no psychiatric treatment because most public psychiatric services have broken down completely.* Occasional episodes of violence then became inevitable.

Herbert Mullin, a young Californian diagnosed with paranoid schizophrenia, was admitted to facilities for the mentally ill five times. At least twice he was labeled as potentially dangerous because of his illness, yet he was released without continuing treatment or aftercare. In a period of four months he randomly murdered thirteen individuals in order to avert, in his delusional thinking, an earthquake along the San Andreas Fault.

Following his conviction, the foreman of the jury wrote a letter to then-Governor Ronald Reagan saying that 'I hold the state executive and state legislative offices as responsible for these . . . lives as I do the defendant himself—none of this need ever have happened.' (Lunde and Morgan, 1980)

It is clear that episodes of violence by individuals with untreated serious mental illnesses are on the increase. One only has to listen to daily news reports to become aware of frequent stories about acts of violence committed by individuals identified as former mental patients. Since 1965 there have been eight separate studies documenting the rise in violent acts by untreated psychiatric patients. In one of the studies, for example, psychiatric patients in a New York City hospital in 1975 were compared with those in 1982; the latter group had had significantly more encounters with the criminal justice system and almost twice as many episodes of violence towards persons (Karras and Otis, 1987).

Juan Gonzalez, age 43, took a sword with him in July 1986 aboard the Staten Island ferry where he proceeded to randomly kill two and wound nine other passengers. He had been staying in a public shelter and had been observed saying repeatedly: 'I'm going to kill. God told me so. Jesus wants me to kill.' He was taken to a university hospital, diagnosed with paranoid schizophrenia, and released after two days of observation. Two days later he committed the crime. (Sullivan, 1986)

Most such episodes need not happen if the public system of psychiatric care is operating as it should. Men like Juan Gonzalez do not arrive from outer space; most such individuals have been treated in psychiatric hospitals on multiple occasions but then released with no aftercare or follow-up. Jorge Delgado, who walked naked into St Patrick's Cathedral in New York in 1988 and killed an elderly man, had been hospitalized psychiatrically seven times; in the six months preceding his act of violence he had been evaluated twice by psychiatrists who found no reason to commit him involuntarily for treatment.

Lois E. Lang, 44 years old, walked into the corporate headquarters of a financial firm in New York City in November, 1985 and shot to death the elderly president of the firm and a receptionist. Three months previously Ms Lang had been arrested for at least the fifth time, diagnosed with paranoid schizophrenia, and released from the hospital after fourteen days. At the time of the killings Ms Lang was homeless and said to have a delusion that she was part-owner of the firm and was owed money. (Raab, 1985)

While it is not possible to predict dangerousness with a high degree of accuracy, it *is* possible to pick out those untreated mentally ill individuals who are most likely to become violent. Recent studies have shown that the four most important predictors of dangerousness in mentally ill individuals are: (1) neurological abnormalities such as noted on examination; (2) paranoid symptoms; (3) refusal to take medications; and (4) a history of violent behaviour (Krakowski *et al.*, 1989; Smith, 1989; Hafner, 1986). The last factor is by far the most accurate predictor of future violence and yet *most mentally ill individuals with histories of violence are released to the community without aftercare or follow-up*.

This fact was frighteningly well-illustrated in a 1983 study carried out by Dr Richard Lamb in Los Angeles. He followed up 85 mentally ill men who had been arrested and found incompetent to stand trial. Of the 85 men, 92% had been arrested on felony charges (murder, attempted murder, rape, armed robbery, assault with a deadly weapon), 68% had previous arrests for felonies, and 86% had previous psychiatric hospitalizations. Despite this record of psychiatric illness and felonies, two years after their arrest, 54 of the 85 men had been released and, for 34 of them (40%), *no plan whatsoever had been made for aftercare or follow-up* (Lamb, 1987).

Sylvia Seegrist, age 25, walked into a shopping center near Philadelphia in 1985 and randomly shot ten people, killing two. She had been hospitalized for schizophrenia twelve times in the previous ten years, clearly labeled as potentially dangerous (she had tried to strangle her mother and had stabbed a psychologist), and had told psychiatric professionals repeatedly that 'she felt like getting a gun and killing people'. Yet she had been released with no follow-up or assurance that she would take the medicine which controlled the symptoms of her illness. (Seegrist, 1986)

Such situations are deplorable, needlessly endangering both the individual who is mentally ill, the person's family members who are frequent victims, and the community at large. It is further evidence of the breakdown in public psychiatric services; when the public fully recognizes the needless dangers which this breakdown in services entails it will demand that services for people with mental illnesses be improved.

4. Mental health professionals have abandoned the public sector and patients with serious mental illnesses

In 1945, during Congressional hearings that led to the creation of the National Institute of Mental Health (NIMH), it was said that there were only about 3000 psychiatrists in the United States and that many of them were not fully trained. Although half of the 3000 were employed in the public sector—mostly in state mental hospitals caring for individuals with serious mental illnesses—it was said to be very difficult to recruit psychiatrists for rural state hospitals such as Montana State Hospital or Wyoming State Hospital, each of which had only two psychiatrists on staff. The answer, everyone agreed, was to train more psychiatrists, and the fiscal reponsibility for doing so was given to NIMH.

Federally funded training for mental health professionals began in 1948 with a $1.4 million programme. The money was given directly to university departments of psychiatry, psychology and psychiatric social work to support faculty salaries and pay stipends to some students. A small programme was also implemented to support psychiatric nursing. By 1969 the NIMH training funds had reached $118.7 million per year and by the early 1980s, when the programme was phased down, they had totalled over $2 billion. Most states supplemented the federal training funds. Virtually every mental health professional trained in the United States since 1948 has had the majority of his or her training costs subsidized by public—federal and state—funds.

From the point of view of numbers alone, the subsidized training of mental health professionals has been a huge success. Psychiatrists have increased from 3000 to 40 000, psychologists from 4200 to 70 000, and psychiatric social workers from 2000 to approximately 80 000. The total increase in these three professions has been more than twenty-fold, during a period in which the population of the United States increased less than two-fold.

From the point of view of individuals with serious mental

illnesses, however, the publicly subsidized training of mental health professionals has been an abysmal failure. The reason, quite simply, is that once psychiatrists, psychologists and psychiatric social workers were trained, almost all of them abandoned the public sector for the monetary rewards of private practice. No payback obligation was included with the subsidized training, despite assurances from federal officials during the original 1945 Congressional hearings that a payback would be built into the programme; specifically, Dr Robert Felix testified that 'I would think that a reasonable requirement of these men [sic] would be that they would spend at least one year in public service for every year they spent in training at public or state expense' (Torrey, 1988). However, this payback obligation was not implemented until 35 years later when federal training funds had been almost phased out.

What kind of patients do psychiatrists, psychologists and psychiatric social workers see in their private practices? This question was answered by a 1980 survey of mental health professionals in private practice, which found that only 6% of patients seen by psychiatrists and 3% of patients seen by psychologists had ever been hospitalized for mental illness (Taube *et al.*, 1984). The authors of another recent survey (Knesper and Pagnucco, 1987) summarized it as follows: 'The [psychiatrists, psychologists, and psychiatric social workers] appeared to spend much of their time treating conditions that many people would consider minor.'

And what has happened to individuals with serious mental illnesses who must rely on the public sector? Increasingly such individuals are seen by no psychiatrist at all. At the Wyoming State Hospital, for example, in 1987 *for almost a year there was no regular psychiatrist on the hospital staff at all*. In 1947, when there were 3000 psychiatrists in the United States, the hospital had two full-time psychiatrists, but in 1987, with 40 000 psychiatrists in the nation (and 15 in the state of Wyoming), it had none. The Montana State Hospital, which had two full-time psychiatrists in the late 1940s, still had only two full-time psychiatrists in the late 1980s despite the fact that there were 37 elsewhere in the state. Both hospitals had to resort to private firms that hire out psychiatrists for exorbitant sums—the current rate is approximately $180 000 per year—and that are popularly referred to as 'rent-a-shrink' companies. The director of one such firm noted in 1988: 'Business is booming. We're getting requests all the time from rural areas'

(Worthington, 1988). Under such programmes it is common for a new psychiatrist to take over the wards of a state hospital as frequently as every two weeks; the consequences for the continuity and quality of patient care are obvious.

It should be noted that many of these jobs for mental health professionals in the public sector pay decent salaries. A perusal of advertisements placed in 1990 in the newspaper of the American Psychiatric Association revealed annual salaries for public-sector psychiatrists ranging from $100 000 to $120 000, with liberal leave policy (up to six weeks vacation) and fringe benefits. A few, such as Wyoming State Hospital, even offer free housing. Despite this, most mental health professionals opt for the private sector where monetary rewards are higher and the patients are easier to treat.

In addition to 'rent-a-shrink' companies, the other way in which public-sector psychiatric facilities have filled psychiatric vacancies in the United States has been to import foreign-trained physicians. This practice became widespread in the 1970s, and it is currently estimated that approximately two-thirds of the psychiatrists in public psychiatric hospitals and clinics in the United States are foreign medical graduates. Some of these are as competent as any American medical graduate, but there is evidence from licensing examination results that many others are not (Torrey, 1988). The overreliance on foreign medical graduates in public mental health facilities also raises moral issues; one of the world's wealthiest nations is importing psychiatrists from poorer countries to fill public-sector jobs that American-trained psychiatrists have abandoned. By 1986, in fact, there were more than twice as many Indian, Pakistani and Egyptian psychiatrists in the United States as there were in India, Pakistan and Egypt (Torrey, 1988). We should be grateful to foreign medical graduates for keeping American public psychiatric services from collapsing entirely, but we should also remember that they are needed because of the refusal of most American psychiatrists to work in the public sector.

The worst news of all, however, is that finding mental health professionals to treat patients with serious mental illnesses in public facilities is becoming increasingly difficult. The primary reason for this is the explosive growth in the 1980s of for-profit psychiatric hospitals which hire away at higher salaries the few professionals remaining in the public system. These hospitals, the majority of which are owned by the Hospital Corporation of America,

National Medical Enterprises, Community Psychiatric Centers, and Charter Medical Corporation, have proliferated rapidly, especially in those states which have abandoned 'certificate-of-need' laws limiting the building of new hospitals.

The profit margin of these for-profit psychiatric hospitals is very high. A major reason for this is that they accept few seriously mentally ill patients. Instead, they fill their beds with substance abusers (especially alcoholics) and teenagers who are unhappy for one reason or another. In fact, these for-profit hospitals have invented a new disease—teenagism—which coincidentally lasts only as long as the family's medical insurance benefits. Through aggressive advertising these hospitals convince parents that teenage problems are best treated by psychiatric hospitalization. 'If you have a child who is out of control', the advertisement reads, 'send him to us'. John E. Halasz, MD, Medical Director of Chicago's Institute for Juvenile Research, called the rapidly rising hospitalization of teenagers 'a racket' (Pickney, 1989). But it is a profitable racket and in 1989 the *Wall Street Journal* said that the four major hospital chains 'plan to build at least 45 more psychiatric hospitals in the next three years' (Schiffman, 1989). The staff for these hospitals, like those built in recent years, will be drawn heavily from psychiatrists, psychologists, psychiatric social workers and psychiatric nurses remaining in public-sector positions. Some of these for-profit hospitals are even starting to specialize in specific teenage problems, such as Hartgrove Hospital in Chicago, which recently set up 'one of the nation's first treatment programs to wean teenagers from Satanism' (*Washington Post*, 1989).

5. Most Community Mental Health Centers have been abysmal failures

In 1963, Congress passed legislation setting up Community Mental Health Centers (CMHCs) with federal construction and staffing grants. The purpose of the CMHCs was clearly outlined by Mr Boisfeuillit Jones, Special Assistant to DHEW Secretary Celebrezze: 'The basic purpose of the "President's" program is to redirect the focus of treatment of the mentally ill from state mental hospitals into community mental health centers.'

Since 1967 a total of 575 CMHCs have received federal construction grants ($294.7 million) and 697 CMHCs received staffing and operations grants ($2364.6 million); the total CMHC programme has thus cost $2.7 billion. CMHCs that received construction grants legally obligated themselves to provide five basic services for 20 years.

Using the federal Freedom of Information Act, the Health Research Group obtained from the National Institute of Mental Health CMHC data including site visit reports carried out on contract by Continuing Medical Education, Inc. A report issued in March 1990 by the Health Research Group and the National Alliance for the Mentally Ill (Torrey *et al.*, 1990) documents the magnitude of the CMHC failure:

- Some CMHCs took federal funds but 'never materialized', i.e. never even began delivering services. Others simply disappeared or went out of business. Still others are being used for completely different purposes (e.g. offices for private physical therapists).
- Some CMHCs were used as private hospitals or are being run illegally by for-profit corporations such as the Hospital Corporation of America.
- Some CMHCs built swimming pools and tennis courts with the construction funds, and hired lifeguards, swimming instructors, and gardeners with the staffing grants. One CMHC used federal construction funds to build both a swimming pool and a chapel, the latter presumably constructed so that seriously mentally ill individuals who were not receiving services could at least pray.
- Some CMHCs, once in operation, requested and received federal NIMH permission to reduce their public psychiatric beds at the same time as state and local authorities said more beds were needed.
- Many CMHCs have failed to provide 'a reasonable volume of services to persons unable to pay therefor' as specified by law.
- Overall, it is estimated that approximately 140 out of the 575 CMHCs, or 25%, are seriously out of compliance and subject to recovery of federal funds. The amount to be recovered is estimated to be $50–100 million. Approximately another 140 CMHCs are technically out of compliance.
- Only approximately 30 of the 575 that received construction funds (5%) are operating as Congress originally intended: 'to redirect the focus of treatment of the mentally ill from state mental hospitals into community mental health centers'.

It is important to note that a small number of federally funded CMHCs developed into excellent programmes and provide quality services to individuals with serious mental illnesses. These programmes further accentuate the contrast with the vast majority of CMHCs which did not develop along such lines.

Defenders of CMHCs argue that they *are* seeing large numbers of individuals with serious mental illnesses. They point to a 1988 survey carried out by the National Council of Community Health Centers, the Washington lobbying office for CMHCs, which claimed that 'the proportion of clients on a typical community mental health agency caseload who are seriously mentally ill averages 45 per cent' (National Council of Community Mental Health Centers, 1988, 1990). What they fail to point out is that in this survey 'serious mental illness' was defined as including everything under the sun, such as 'passive–aggressive personality disorders' which, according to the American Psychiatric Association, is a diagnosis applied to individuals who procrastinate and dawdle and are stubborn, forgetful and intentionally inefficient. This, says the National Council of CMHCs, is 'serious mental illness'. A much more accurate analysis of the patients seen in CMHCs, published by the National Institute of Mental Health in 1988, showed that *only 9% of individuals being treated by CMHCs had either 'schizophrenia' or 'other psychotic disorders'* (Windle et al., 1988). By contrast, 20% were diagnosed as having 'social maladjustment' or 'no mental disorder'.

Representative of many CMHCs is the Park Center in Fort Wayne, Indiana, previously known as the Fort Wayne CMHC, which received $12.7 million in federal funds between 1977 and 1981 and which still operates with predominantly state and federal funds. Instead of providing services for individuals with schizophrenia and manic-depressive psychosis, it advertised itself in a 1989 brochure as follows:

Every year we help thousands of people face the challenges of our complex world. Most people who come to Park Center feel a need for help with a life adjustment problem. Counseling services are for those experiencing:
- Unhappy relationships
- Inability to communicate effectively
- Anxiety
- Depression

- Indecision
- Procrastination
- Poor job performance
- Parenting problems
- Alcohol problems

High stress levels adversely affect work and family life. Counseling services help people reduce conflicts and strengthen relationships. At Park Center, *We Help You Face the World.*

Individuals with serious mental illnesses do not have a 'life adjustment problem' but rather a primary brain disease. They do not need 'counselling' alone as much as they need medication, vocational rehabilitation and decent housing. They do not need to 'face the world' but rather to become part of the world.

An example of one of the many CMHCs that failed abysmally in its primary function to provide services for seriously mentally ill people is the Hancock County CMHC in Ellsworth, Maine. In 1976 the Hancock County Mental Health Association received a $100 000 federal construction grant to build a free-standing, one storey CMHC to serve the residents of Hancock County. The CMHC was affiliated with the respected Community Counseling Center in Bangor, in whose catchment area it was situated. From 1977 to 1983 the Hancock County CMHC provided outpatient services, emergency services, and consultation and education, but not inpatient services or partial hospitalization.

In 1983 the Hancock County Mental Health Association essentially evicted the CMHC from the federally subsidized building and began renting the offices out for profit to private service providers such as privately operated physical therapy services. NIMH became aware of this violation of federal regulations in June 1983 during a site visit by an NIMH official. The building has been used for non-CMHC purposes continuously since 1983 in clear violation of the law. An August 1988 site visit report for NIMH noted that 'none of the five essential services is being provided by the grantee either in the federally-constructed space or in any other location . . . The grantee is out of compliance.'

Officials of the Community Counseling Center in Bangor tried repeatedly to bring the situation to the attention of state and federal officials. In 1989, NIMH finally referred the case to the DHHS Office of the General Counsel to initiate recovery action; no action had been taken by early 1990. The President of the Community Counseling Center wrote to the Director of NIMH as follows:

The stewardship of the taxpayers' dollars is important. No federal agency should take over six years to act on blatant violations of federal regulations. I sincerely hope that the situation in Ellsworth, Maine is an isolated example of NIMH mismanagement and is not indicative of a widespread pattern of ineptitude and failure to ensure that buildings built with federal construction grant funds are properly used. (Letter of 12 December 1989)

The Health Research Group and the National Alliance for the Mentally Ill's CMHC report included a detailed account of the Hancock County CMHC. Following the report's release, the *Bangor Daily News* questioned the chairman of the Hancock County Mental Health Association, Robert Keteyian, who responded as follows:

> ... Keteyian agreed that his Association was not in compliance with federal regulations, adding that his group had notified the National Institute of Mental Health in writing that it was not in compliance on numerous occasions. 'We wondered why they never responded,' he said.
>
> Placing several 'for-profit' tenants in the building along with a few non-profit organizations, Keteyian said, was just a way to help pay the mortgage. (Higgins, 1990)

6. The funding of public services for individuals with serious mental illness is chaotic

One need only visit an emergency room in any large city hospital to witness the disaster of public psychiatric services for people with serious mental illnesses. In one emergency room in New York City, individuals with schizophrenia and manic-depressive psychosis 'were handcuffed to the armrests of wheelchairs Friday morning as they waited for beds ... Sometimes patients have to sleep in shifts [in the waiting area] because there is not enough room' (Barbanel, 1988). Mental health administrators in the city blame state authorities for the lack of public psychiatric beds, while the state maintains that it is the city's responsibility. What neither says publicly is that they are playing a game of shift-the-fiscal-burden; the losers in this game are inevitably individuals with serious mental illnesses.

The funding of public services for people with mental illnesses in the United States is an incredible pastiche of federal, state and local sources with no overall coordination and with individual pieces that are often at odds with each other. Federal dollars, comprising approximately 50% of the total, include Medicaid, Medicare, Supplemental Security Income (SSI), Social Security Disability Insurance (SSDI), block grants and housing programmes of various kinds. State and local funds for people with serious mental illnesses come from a variety of departments including mental health, social services, housing, vocal rehabilitation and corrections. To run a department of mental health at the state or local level one needs to be primarily an accountant to keep track of the many sources of funds and what they can be used for. This chaotic funding system has grown piecemeal over the 25 years since Medicaid and Medicare were enacted; new programmes have been added incrementally, with virtually no attempt made to fit the funding pieces together into a coherent whole. The system of funding public services for people with mental illnesses in the United States is, in short, more thought-disordered than most of the individuals the system is intended to serve.

At the federal level the funding programmes strongly favour hospitalization for people with mental illnesses despite an official policy of deinstitutionalization. Dr Rohn S. Friedman has called this contradiction a 'psychiatric chimera—an official policy of deinstitutionalization grafted onto an everyday practice of hospitalization' (Friedman, 1985). Federal Medicaid and Medicare will pay for the institutionalization of a mentally ill individual on the psychiatric ward of a general hospital or in a nursing home, but will usually not pay for maintaining the same individual in a state mental hospital. For this reason states shut down wards of state hospitals, even when the beds are clearly needed, to try and force psychiatric admissions into general hospitals or nursing homes where the federal government will cover the majority of costs. States publicly rationalize their action as promoting community living and a less restrictive environment for patients, but these rationalizations are often a thin veneer covering an underlying economic imperative. This was clearly demonstrated by economist William Gronfein who published an analysis of data on deinstitutionalization from 1973 to 1975 and concluded that 'Medicaid payments are very strongly associated with the amount of deinstitutionalization in the early 1970s' (Gronfein, 1985). While the states, cities and federal governments are playing this fiscal tug-of-war, mentally ill individuals needing hospitalization get caught in the middle, handcuffed to an emergency room wheelchair while the search for a bed continues.

The consequences of chaotic funding for public psychiatric care can also be seen in services other than hospital beds. Elderly individuals with serious mental illnesses who require an injection of antipsychotic medication must come to a clinic to receive it because federal Medicare will not reimburse a nurse to give the same injection at home. Individuals with serious mental illness who are able to work part-time often will not do so because of losing their SSI and therefore Medicaid eligibility. Outreach programmes to treat and rehabilitate homeless mentally ill individuals are not carried out because such programmes are usually not reimbursable through federal Medicaid. There are no fiscal incentives to promote continuity of care and to prevent hospitalizations. In fact, from the state's point of view, it has been pointed out that 'it is often cheaper for the patient to go to the hospital than to stay out' (Friedman, 1985) if hospitalization costs are covered by federal Medicaid funds.

Another aspect of the chaotic funding of services for people with serious mental illnesses is the failure to implement and use service models that have proved effective. An example is the Louisville Homecare Project, carried out between 1961 and 1964, which showed that 77% of psychiatric admissions could be averted by using public health nurses to give medication in clients' homes (Torrey, 1990). The use of crisis homes in Southwest Denver was another experimental programme demonstrating that hospitalization rates could be reduced dramatically (Torrey, 1990). Both of these programmes were allowed to die because the effective mechanism of providing service—using public health nurses and crisis homes—was not reimbursable by federal Medicaid. The same is true for many model rehabilitation programmes that have proved to be effective for mentally ill individuals, but which are rarely replicated because they do not fit existing federal reimbursement schemes; an example is the Fairweather Lodge, a group of mentally ill individuals who live together and operate a community business (Torrey, 1990).

In all of these cases states are reluctant to use a service delivery system, no matter how effective it is, if federal programmes such as Medicaid will not reimburse them for it. As Dr Charles Kiesler (1982) has pointed out, 'Quite unintentionally, Medicaid has become the largest single mental health program in the country'. As early as 1978, President Carter's Commission on Mental Health concluded that 'the level and type of care given to the chronically mentally disabled is frequently based on what services are fundable and not what services are needed or appropriate' (Task Panel, 1978). This means that demonstration programmes can demonstrate and model programmes can model, but if their results, however praise-worthy, are contrary to the existing system of economic incentives then such programmes will be neither extended nor replicated. Demonstration programmes will continue to be mere tinkerings with the status quo, demonstrating the deficiencies of the present without significantly influencing the future.

7. An undetermined portion of public funds for the care of the seriously mentally ill is literally being stolen

Public programmes serving people with serious mental illnesses are not generally thought of as likely venues for theft or other criminal activity. And yet such programmes spend approximately $25 billion each year, much of it on contracts with non-profit corporations, with remarkably little auditing or oversight of these expenditures. It is a situation ready-made for theft, which is usually not labelled as such; rather, among mental health professionals, as in other white-collar circles, it is euphemistically called 'misappropriation of public funds'.

There are many forms of theft from publicly funded programmes for the mentally ill. Petty theft of personal property from mentally ill patients occurs commonly in psychiatric hospitals, made easy by the fact that other patients can be blamed and the victims themselves are often so confused that they cannot assist in pinpointing when the property was taken. Another common form of petty theft in programmes for people with mental illnesses is some mental health professionals' practice of seeing private patients during the same time as they are being paid to see public patients; this has become widespread and implicitly condoned as it has become increasingly difficult to recruit mental health professionals to public-sector jobs. This is in essence the theft of time, the cost of which adds up very quickly since such professionals are comparatively well paid.

We can only guess how frequently larger 'misappropriation of public funds' occurs in the delivery system of public psychiatric services. In the few instances when it has been looked for, it has often been found, sometimes glaringly obvious and undetected for years by officials who were performing virtually no oversight function. Some recent examples follow.

*Timpanogos Community Mental Health Center (Provo, Utah)**

The Timpanogos Community Mental Health Center was established in 1967 with federal construction and staffing grants from the National Institute of Mental Health. Its function was to deliver psychiatric services to mentally ill residents of three counties in the Provo region. By 1988, it had an annual budget of approximately $8 million. In 1976, former state legislator Glen Brown was hired by the board of Timpanogos CMHC to be executive director. As such he had authority to contract for specialty services. Brown, Director of Specialty Programmes and psychologist Carl V. Smith, and business manager Craig W. Stephens then proceeded to set up contracts under which they paid themselves for the same work more than once.

According to a 1988 investigation of the Utah Legislative Auditor General, as reported in the *Deseret News*, 'In 1987 alone, for example, Smith earned $728 503.72 in total compensation, including salary, contract earnings and car and credit card allowances. Stephens earned $501 461 followed by Brown with $149 065 . . . In essence, these employees were paying themselves repeatedly to perform their regular duties.' The investigation also revealed that 'five employees were appropriated as much as $41 000 each per year in car allowances' and that 'five of the eight top center employees were given American Express credit cards for virtually unlimited use'. The total amount received by Brown, Smith and Stephens was estimated to be approximately $3.6 million between 1983 and 1988.

During these same years, budget cutbacks at Timpanogos CMHC forced repeated reductions in services for the mentally ill. Waiting lists became longer; patients discharged from Utah State Hospital had to wait nine weeks for an appointment at the CMHC

---

* Data on the Timpanogos CMHC case was taken from 'An Expenditure Review of the Timpanogos Community Mental Health Center', Report by the Utah Legislative Auditor General, April 1988; 'An Investigative and Prosecution Report by the Office of the Utah Attorney General', September 18, 1989; and by news accounts of the case in the *Deseret News*.

to receive medications. The CHMC facilities also deteriorated; according to a news account, 'Some tables are held up with bricks. Chairs have books stashed under them for proper balance. A lunchroom couch sags to the floor because its springs are broken.'

In October 1988 the Utah Attorney General filed criminal charges consisting of 117 felony counts against Brown, Smith and Stephens. Each pleaded guilty to five felony counts, are serving two years in the Utah State Prison, and will be paroled in August 1991. In addition, the court ordered that Brown make restitution of $255 000, Smith make restitution of $1 702 792, and Stephens make restitution of $1 400 994. Since 1989 Timpanogos CMHC has had a highly-regarded new director and has made excellent progress in getting its programmes back in order.

Tarrant County Mental Health–Mental Retardation Services (Fort Worth, Texas)*

Tarrant County Mental Health–Mental Retardation Services (TCMHMR), serving the Fort Worth area, is one of 35 regional public programmes under the Texas Department of Mental Health and Mental Retardation. It has an annual budget of approximately $20 million, of which 50% are state funds, 10% Tarrant County funds, and the remainder federal, insurance, and fee-for-service funds. It has a staff of 680 employees and is run by a nine-member Board of Directors appointed by the Tarrant County commissioners. The Board of Directors sets agency policies and appoints the TCMHMR programme's executive director, who, from 1979 until his resignation in 1989, was Loyd Kilpatrick, a former high school football coach and assistant director of a State Center for Human Development.

Services for people with mental illnesses in Tarrant County have been deplorable. Compared with other states, Texas ranked 46th in 1990) in per capita funding for mental illness services, and

---

* Data on the Tarrant County Mental Health–Mental Retardation Services case was taken from news stories in the *Fort Worth Star-Telegram* by Carolyn Poirot, Stan Jones and Bob Mahlburg between October 1988 and March 1989, and from a letter of 10 May, 1990 from Tarrant County District Attorney Tim Curry to the Board of Trustees of TCMHMR Services.

within Texas, Tarrant County ranks 34th among the 35 regions. The new county psychiatric inpatient unit is half empty because funds are not available to staff it. Patients discharged from the state hospital at Wichita Falls often must wait several weeks to be seen for outpatient services. Supervised housing for mentally ill individuals is virtually non-existent, and rehabilitation programmes are available for only a fraction of those who need it. County officials estimate that there are between 300 and 400 mentally ill individuals among the 2700 inmates in the county jail who are receiving no psychiatric services and untreated mentally ill individuals are strikingly evident among the homeless population in Fort Worth.

Despite these deplorable services in a grossly underfunded public programme for the mentally ill, Executive Director Kilpatrick benefited handsomely from the programme. According to a series of articles in the *Fort Worth Star-Telegram* based on outstanding investigative reporting, Kilpatrick's annual salary when he was hired in 1979 was $33 000, but by 1989 it had risen to $200 937 including retirement benefits and a leased automobile; that was more than twice the salary of the Texas governor. The chairman of the board that approved Kilpatrick's salary and benefits, Roger Williams, owns car dealerships from which TCMHMR purchased most of its vehicles, a fleet which increased from four vehicles when Kilpatrick was hired in 1979 to 47 vehicles when he resigned in 1989. The purchases were theoretically made using closed bids but, according to the *Star-Telegram*, 'at least two agency employees said Kilpatrick told them that sealed bids were opened early so Williams could underbid them'. Bid records showed that 'at least six of Williams' low bids were within $50 of the next lowest bid'. The bank deposits of TCMHMR were also directed to a bank of which Williams was a director without soliciting bids for the business.

In October 1989, as the *Star-Telegram* series was being published, Loyd Kilpatrick abruptly resigned from TCMHMR 'for what he called health reasons'. Williams and the board thereupon gave Kilpatrick an additional $214 000 in severance pay plus 'the 1989 Chevrolet Suburban that the agency was leasing for him'. Texas state auditors examined TCMHMR's books and reported that the agency 'may have misappropriated as much as $500 000' over 10 years and TCMHMR was ordered to repay $200 000 to the Texas Department of Mental Health and Mental Retardation. On

15 March 1990, a grand jury indicted Kilpatrick on four counts of felony theft. In June 1990, a new executive director, said to be highly regarded, was appointed to head TCMHMR and changes were made on the board of the agency.

Harris County Mental Health–Mental Retardation Authority (Houston, Texas)*

Harris County Mental Health–Mental Retardation Authority (MHMRA) is responsible for public psychiatric services for 2.7 million people living in Houston. Its 1988 budget was $41.8 million of which $13.3 million came from county taxes, $14.7 million from state taxes, and the remainder from federal taxes and other sources. According to the newspapers it was headquartered in 'the posh Weslayan Tower' where rent as of 1990 was $9000 per month. Houston ranks with Los Angeles and Miami as cities having the worst public psychiatric services in the nation. In 1987, 6098 patients applied for admission to the eight-bed psychiatric emergency unit at Ben Taub Hospital. Even since the opening of the Harris County Psychiatric Center in 1988 there have been long waiting lists at both the hospital and at the six outpatient clinics staffed by the Department of Psychiatry of Baylor College of Medicine on contract with MHMRA. The large number of untreated mentally ill homeless living at the Star of Hope Mission and beneath the San Jacinto River Bridge is a barometer of the gross inadequacy of Houston's public psychiatric services.

On 5 April 1990, four men were indicted in Harris County for 'engaging in organized criminal activity' and allegedly sharing $700 000 in proceeds from the 1985 sale of a mental health clinic building to MHMRA for $2 million; the building had an appraised value of $1.3 million and prosecutors 'would only say that the defendants kept money they allegedly overcharged the authority'. Indicted were Eugene Williams, who had been the Director of MHMRA for 12 years until he was fired in 1989; Dr George L.

---

* Data on the Harris County Mental Health–Mental Retardation Authority case was taken from news stories in the *Houston Chronicle* by Pete Slover, Stephen Johnson, Jo Ann Zuniga and R.A. Dyer, and in the *Houston Post* by John Mecklin, Brenda Sapino, Robert Stanton, Katherine Kerr, and Peter Brewton between July 1988 and April 1990.

Adams, a psychiatrist who had been a Professor of Psychiatry at Baylor College of Medicine until his 1988 appointment as Professor of Psychiatry at Dartmouth Medical School; John P. Chambers, a 'psychotherapist' and President of Discovery Center, Inc.; and Joe F. Wheat, a lawyer. Bail for each of the indicted men was set at $1.4 million.

Williams had also been indicted in 1989 along with the MHMRA business manager and 'accused of stealing $800 000 in deferred income annuities'; however, a district judge threw out that indictment 'saying he found insufficient evidence that the men's annuity plans were illegal'. Williams' annual salary and benefits ranged from $105 108 to $108 581 between 1985 and 1987.

Dr Adams, as Baylor's director of community and social psychiatry programmes, 'helped negotiate the school's contract' with MHMRA; the contract totalled $1.76 million annually. In addition to being employed by Baylor, Dr Adams was also employed by MHMRA on a separate contract of $33 600 per year 'as a management consultant'. MHMRA Director Williams, in addition to his employment by MHMRA, was employed part-time by the Department of Psychiatry at Baylor College of Medicine and was said to teach 'a seminar on mental health administration'. The wife of the Chairman of the MHMRA Board was also employed 'as a part-time clinical assistant professor of psychiatry at Baylor' and 'reportedly had worked for Adams'.

John P. Chambers' organization, Discovery Center Inc., had received a $66 000 annual contract from 1984 to 1986 to provide some staff for MHMRA clinics through the Baylor contract. Chambers' wife was employed by MHMRA as a social worker. Chambers was President of the land company which sold the clinic building to MHMRA for $2 million in 1985, the transaction on which the April 1990 indictment was based. Chambers was also said to be under investigation for the sale of at least two other properties to MHMRA; *in one of them a building with an appraised value of $1.5 million was purchased by Chambers and his brother for $2.1 million and sold four hours later to MHMRA for $3.3 million.*

Commenting on the land deals, Harris County Judge Jon Lindsay said in 1988: 'The county got ripped off, MHMRA got ripped off, the people who need the services got ripped off.' District Attorney John B. Holmes stated that MHMRA 'was operated in a way that apparently made it easy to steal'.

In September 1988, Eugene Williams was fired as Director of MHMRA. Three months later Dr Jan Duker, a highly respected psychologist and former state mental health commissioner, was appointed to the position and said that one of her top priorities would be 're-establishing credibility' for MHMRA. Several replacements were also made on the MHMRA board and in early 1990 Dr Duker moved MHMRA headquarters from the expensive leased space to a building already owned by the agency.

New York Psychotherapy and Counseling Center (Queens, NY)

The New York Psychotherapy and Counseling Center (NYPCC) was incorporated as a not-for-profit agency in 1974. The purpose of the corporation was to provide outpatient psychiatric services at six clinics in Queens and Brooklyn for mentally ill residents of adult homes. Most of these residents had been previously hospitalized in state psychiatric hospitals. Approximately 95% of the income of NYPCC was derived from Medicaid payments for outpatient psychiatric services, usually at a rate of $53 for a 30-minute individual visit. The executive director of NYPCC was Rabbi Isidore Klein, whose son served as assistant executive director. Two psychiatrists, Jack Schnee and Harold Finn, were medical co-directors.

In December 1989, the New York State Commission on Quality of Care for the Mentally Disabled released a report entitled 'Profit-Making in Not-for-Profit Corporations: A Challenge to Regulators'. It claimed that 'NYPCC was only nominally a not-for-profit corporation. In reality, it functioned as a profit-making corporation for its key officers rather than solely for a public purpose.' Among the specific allegations of the report were that NYPCC had used 'improper Medicaid billings of $1.4 million by reporting group therapy services at their clinics as individual services for which higher reimbursement is paid, and by operation of an unlicensed clinic'. The report also alleged that Rabbi Klein, Dr Schnee and Dr Finn, the three senior executives, were paid 'in excess of $150 000/year each, in addition to generous tax-deferred compensation, insurance, and luxury cars for personal and private use'. Finally, the report alleges that Rabbi Klein, Dr Schnee and Dr Finn created a limited partnership owned by themselves and their children that purchased real estate, which they then leased to

NYPCC; this led to 'profit-making of $720 000 over a three-year period through less-then-arm's length property transactions with family-owned businesses, one of which realized a 4917 per cent return on a $10 000 investment.'

In summarizing these findings the report noted that 'there is virtually no scrutiny by State licensing and funding agencies of how money is actually spent by the not-for-profit agencies'. Referring to NYPCC, the Commission noted that 'although these and other irregularities in the agency's operations were called to the attention of senior state OMH [Office of Mental Health] officials in October 1988, no enforcement action has been taken by OMH either directly or by referrals to other appropriate state agencies, despite their commitment to do so, and despite repeated inquiries from the Commission in subsequent months'. Finally, on 7 December 1989, the Commissioner of Mental Health agreed to refer the Commission report to the office of the New York State Attorney General's Office; as of June 1990, no action had been taken.

The report on NYPCC is similar to another report the Commission released three years earlier entitled *Profit Making in Not-for-Profit Care: A Review of the Operations and Financial Practices of Brooklyn Psychosocial Rehabilitation Institute, Inc.* (New York State Commission, 1986). In that report, Dr Karl Easton, a psychiatrist who was the founder and medical director of Brooklyn Psychosocial Rehabilitation Institute (BPRI), was said to have 'violated Federal and State tax laws'. The report also stated that a treatment centre run by BPRI 'fraudulently billed the Medicaid program for over $1.4 million in 1985 alone'. Furthermore, through a series of interlocking corporations controlled by the Easton family, 'actual rents paid [since 1980] have totalled $2.7 million, which represents almost entirely profit on the landlord's initial cash investment of $150 000 and $30 000 in the properties leased to BPRI . . . The net return to the Eastons on their investment to the Boerum Hill Residence and adjacent apartments has ranged *from 180 to 420 per cent annually since 1980.* The return on The Lafayette Center has been *from 150 to 237 per cent each year since mid-1979.'* New York State subsequently revoked BPRI's operating certificate and sued it for recovery of funds which it claimed had been wrongfully diverted; as of June 1990 the case had not been settled.

These cases illustrate that it is relatively easy to steal funds from public programmes for people with serious mental illnesses. The Tarrant County case came to light only after it had been investigated by newspaper reporters. The New York cases were uncovered by an independent state agency, the New York State Commission on Quality of Care. The Utah case was made public by the State Legislative Auditor General. In none of these states did the state department of mental health play any role in uncovering the misuse of funds despite the fact that it funded the largest share of these programmes. There appears to be an assumption that administrators and professionals working in public programmes for people with mental illnesses are dedicated individuals who do not steal. This is true for the vast majority of such individuals, but the number of exceptions will not be known until such programmes are subjected to much closer fiscal scrutiny than has heretofore been the case.

8. Guidelines for programmes for people with mental illnesses at both the federal and state level are often made by administrators who themselves have had no experience in this field

The actual care of people with mental illnesses in the United States takes place in hundreds of hospitals and thousands of outpatient clinics and rehabilitation programmes. Decisions about how such care should be provided, however, is often determined by guidelines established by federal and state administrators in such programmes as Supplemental Security Income (SSI), Social Security Disability Income (SSDI), Medicaid, Medicare, Community Support Programs (CSP), Housing and Urban Development (HUD) programmes, Protection and Advocacy (P and A) programmes, and special grant programmes such as the Stewart B. McKinney Homeless Assistance Act. These guidelines determine which services will be funded or reimbursed by the federal or state governments and which services will not; since federal and state funds comprise approximately 90% of the funds supporting public mental illness services, the guidelines in effect determine both what care will be given and how it will be given.

One of the biggest frustrations for professionals working hands-on with mentally ill people in hospitals and clinics is trying to tailor their treatment decisions to meet federal and state guidelines. For example, for an elderly individual with schizophrenia who needs an injection every three weeks, a home visit by a nurse to give the injection is not reimbursable by Medicare, but a visit to a clinic for the injection is reimbursable. In a rural area with no public transportation, the difference between these services often is critical. Most professionals who provide direct service to mentally ill individuals have long suspected that many administrators who set the guidelines for federal and state reimbursement have had no personal experience providing direct services to people with mental illnesses and do not know what they are talking about. In most cases this turns out to be precisely the case.

At the federal level, for example, crucial decisions regarding Medicaid reimbursement for services to people with mental illnesses are made in the sprawling headquarters of the Social Security Administration in Baltimore. Since Medicaid is the single largest source of public funds for mental illness service in the United States, it might be expected that the government's theoretical think-tank on such matters, the National Institute of Mental Health (NIMH), would have expertise to contribute and input into Medicaid decisions. In fact, NIMH has virtually no input to the Medicaid funding decisions made by the Social Security Administration.

NIMH itself is virtually devoid of professionals who have had practical, hands-on experience working with seriously mentally ill individuals in the public sector beyond the brief, and in some cases ephemeral, exposure received during their professional training, which often took place a decade or two earlier. Despite having administered the $3 billion CMHC programme over 22 years, as well as the multi-million dollar Community Support Program (CSP) over the past 13 years, NIMH has almost no professional staff who can speak from experience in treating individuals with serious mental illnesses in the public sector.

To illustrate this point, information was obtained under the federal Freedom of Information Act on the training and experience of NIMH staff members in charge of guidelines and funding for the CSP, which gives grants to states to develop and coordinate services for people with mental illnesses (currently $24.3 million per year), and the Protection and Advocacy Program, which funds pro- grammes protecting the rights of mentally ill people (currently $14.0 million per year). Of the seven professional staff members assigned to these two programmes, only one appears to have ever had any employment experience working with mentally ill individuals, and that experience consisted of administrative duties in a CMHC half-time for eight months. The two individuals in charge of these programmes have had no experience whatsoever in serving people with mental illnesses; one of them has a Bachelors degree and 21 years' experience as an administrator of psycho-pharmacology research grants, while the other has a Masters degree in Public Administration, four months' experience evaluating personnel usage in a town police and fire department, and seven years' experience in various administrative capacities at NIMH.

The situation at the state level is only modestly better than at the federal level. The most important official in determining policies that affect state programmes for people with mental illnesses is the director of the state department of mental health. As of May 1990, only about 20% of such directors had ever had any clinical experience in treating people with mental illnesses. With respect to professional background, the group of state mental health directors currently includes 2 psychiatrists, 13 psychologists, 8 social workers, 2 lawyers, 1 director with a degree in education, 2 directors with degrees in public administration, and 23 directors without advanced degrees but with administrative experience in state government. Only a handful of them have extensive experience working with people with mental illnesses.

I do not argue that training as a mental health professional qualifies an individual to administer programmes for people with mental illnesses; indeed, many mental health professionals are notoriously poor administrators. Conversely, amongst the most highly respected state directors of mental health have been lawyers and public administrators. I do argue that, all other things being equal, it is highly desirable for federal and state officials who are setting policies and guidelines for the treatment of people with mental illnesses to have had some clinical experience working with such people. Such a background should be the rule, not the exception. This should not preclude gifted administrators with a special interest in mentally ill people from being appointed to such positions, but such administrators should then undertake to get first-hand experience working with people with mental illnesses.

In probably no other area of federal or state government—including education, corrections, social services and transportation—has the primary responsibility for programmes been turned over to administrators who themselves have had so little academic training or practical experience in the relevant field. Public programmes for people with serious mental illnesses are unique in the degree to which responsibility for them has been assigned to individuals who do not know what they are talking about. Good intentions are not a sufficient qualification for important positions in this field.

REFERENCES

Acker, C. and Fine, M.J. (1989) Families under siege: A mental health crisis. *Philadelphia Inquirer*, September 10.

Arce, A.A., Tadlock, M., Vergare, M.J. *et al.* (1983) A psychiatric profile of street people admitted to an emergency shelter. *Hospital and Community Psychiatry*, **34**, 812–817.

Barbanel, J. (1988) System to treat mental patients is overburdened. *New York Times*, February 22, p. A–1.

Bassuk, E.L., Rubin, L. and Lauriat, A. (1984) Is homelessness a mental health problem? *American Journal of Psychiatry*, **141** 1546–1550.

Belcher, J.R. (1988a) Rights versus needs of homeless mentally ill persons. *Social Work*, **33**, 398–402.

Belcher, J.R. (1988b) Defining the service needs of homeless mentally ill persons. *Hospital and Community Psychiatry*, **39**, 1203–1206.

Belcher, J.R. (1988c) Are jails replacing the mental health asylum for the homeless mentally ill? *Community Mental Health Journal*, **24**, 185–194.

Cape Cod Times (1984) A ferocious crime against the helpless. July 22.

Cohen, N.L., Putnam, J.F. and Sullivan, A.M. (1984) The mentally ill homeless: isolation and adaptation. *Hospital and Community Psychiatry*, **35**, 922–924.

Cooper, C. (1988) Brutal lives of homeless S.F. women. *San Francisco Examiner*, December 18, p. A–1.

Drake, R. E., Wallach, M. A. and Hoffman, J.S. (1989) Housing instability and homelessness among aftercare patients of an urban state hospital. *Hospital and Community Psychiatry*, **40**, 46–51.

Egri, G., Keitner, L. and Harwood, T.B. (1985) Not mad enough, not bad enough: Where should they go? Erie County Forensic Mental Health Service, Buffalo, mimeo.

Eisenhuth, B. (1983) Profiles of the street people. *Hospital and Community Psychiatry*, **34**, 814.

Erie Alliance for the Mentally Ill (1987) For some mentally ill, road to treatment begins in jail, *Newsletter*, Buffalo, March.

Friedman, R.S. (1985) Resistance to alternatives to hospitalization. *Psychiatric Clinics of North America*, **8**, 471–482.

Gelberg, L., Linn, L.S. and Leake, B.D. (1988) Mental health, alcohol and drug use, and criminal history among homeless adults. *American Journal of Psychiatry*, **145**, 191–196.

Greene, M.S. (1989) Data challenge ideas on D.C. street people. *Washington Post* May 21, p. 1.

Gronfein, W. (1985) Incentives and interventions in mental health policy: A comparison of the Medicaid and community mental health programs. *Journal of Health and Social Behavior*, **26**, 192–206.

Hafner, H. (1986) The risk of violence in psychotics. *Integrative Psychiatry*, **4**, 138–142.

Herbert, W. (1985) Lost lives of the homeless. *Washington Post*, October 19, p. G–4.

Higgins, A.J. (1990) Hancock County health center fails federal standards, Nader group charges. *Bangor Daily News*, March 24.

Jemelka, R., Trupin, E. and Chiles, J. A. (1989) The mentally ill in prisons: A review. *Hospital and Community Psychiatry*, **40**, 481–490.

Karras, A. and Otis, D.B. (1987) A comparison of inpatients in an urban state hospital in 1975 and 1982. *Hospital and Community Psychiatry*, **38**, 963–967.

Kennedy, J.F. (1963) Special message to Congress on mental illness and mental retardation, February 6.

Kiesler, C.A. (1982) Mental hospitals and alternative care. *American Psychologist*, **37**, 349–360.

Kilzer, L. (1984) Jails as a 'halfway house' or long-term commitment? *Denver Post*, June 3.

Knesper, D.J. and Pagnucco, D.J. (1987) Estimated distribution of effort by providers of mental health services to U.S. adults in 1982 and 1983. *American Journal of Psychiatry*, **144**, 883–888.

Krakowski, M.I., Convit, A., Jaeger, J. *et al.* (1989) Neurological impairment in violent schizophrenic inpatients. *American Journal of Psychiatry*, **146**, 849–853.

Lamb, H.R. (1987) Incompetency to stand trial: Appropriateness and outcome. *Archives of General Psychiatry*, 44, 754–758.

Lamb, H.R. and Lamb, D.M. (1990) Factors contributing to homelessness among the chronically and severely mentally ill. *Hospital and Community Psychiatry*, 41, 301–305.

Luke, P. (1987) 67% of inmates need some mental help, survey shows. *Grand Rapids Press*, September 4.

Lunde, D.T. and Morgan, J. (1980) *The Die Song*. W.W. Norton, New York. p. 313.

McFarland, B.H., Faulkner, L.R. and Bloom J.D. *et al.* (1989) Chronic mental illness and the criminal justice system. *Hospital and Community Psychiatry*, 40, 718–724.

Nance, K. (1989) Program for prisoners shackled by lack of funds. *Lexington Herald-Leader*, June 25.

National Council of Community Mental Health Centers (1988) *Services for the Seriously Mentally Ill: A Survey of Community Mental Health Agencies*. Washington.

National Council of Community Mental Health Centers (1990) *Some Facts about Community Mental Health Centers*. Washington.

New York State Commission on Quality of Care for the Mentally Disabled. (1986) *Profit-Making in Not-for-Profit Care: A Review of the Operations and Financial Practices of the Brooklyn Psychosocial Rehabilitation Institute, Inc.* Albany, New York, November.

New York State Commission on Quality of Care for the Mentally Disabled. (1988–89) *Annual Report*, p. 16.

New York State Commission on Quality of Care for the Mentally Disabled. (1989) *Profit-Making in Not-for-Profit Corporations: A Challenge to Regulators*. Albany, New York, December.

New York Times (1986) Homeless man is assaulted. October 6, p. B–5.

New York Times (1989) September 10, p. 36.

Pickney, D.S. (1989) Youth psychiatric hospitalization is up dramatically. *AMA News*, March 10, p. 46.

Plott, M. (1985) Man who blinded self is moved from prison, *Atlanta Constitution*, March 8.

Raab, S. (1985) Deak murder suspect has been found paranoid. *New York Times*, November 21, p. B–3.

Roegel, P., Burnam, M. A. and Farr, R. K. (1988) The prevalence of specific psychiatric disorders among homeless individuals in the inner city of Los Angeles. *Archives of General Psychiatry*, **45**, 1085–1092.

Schiffman, J.R. (1989) Teenagers end up in psychiatric hospitals in alarming numbers. *Wall Street Journal*, February 3, p. 1.

Seegrist, R.S. (1986) What happened to Sylvia. *Philadelphia Inquirer Magazine*, August 24.

Smith, L.D. (1989) Medication refusal and the rehospitalized mentally ill inmate. *Hospital and Community Psychiatry*, **40**, 491–496.

Sullivan, R. (1986) City inquiry in ferry slashing criticizes hospital for release. *New York Times*, July 12, p. A–1.

Susser, E., Struening, E.L. and Conover, S. (1989) Psychiatric problems in homeless men. *Archives of General Psychiatry*, **46**, 845–850.

Swetz, A., Salive, M.E., Stough, T. *et al.* The prevalence of mental illness in a state correctional institution for men. Mimeo.

Task Panel. (1978) *Reports Submitted to the President's Commission on Mental Health*, Vol. II. US Government Printing Office, Washington, p. 369.

Taube, C.A., Burns, B.J. and Kessler, L. (1984) Patients of psychiatrists and psychologists in office-based practice: 1980. *American Psychologist*, **39**, 1435–1447.

Teplin, L.A. (1990) The prevalence of severe mental disorder among male urban jail detainees: Comparison with the Epidemiologic Catchment Area Program. *American Journal of Public Health*, **80**, 663–669.

Torrey, E.F. (1988) *Nowhere to Go: The Tragic Odyssey of the Homeless Mentally Ill*. Harper & Row, New York. pp. 72, 171, 172.

Torrey, E.F. (1990) Economic barriers to widespread implementation of model programs for the seriously mentally ill. *Hospital and Community Psychiatry*, **41**, 526–531.

Torrey, E.F., Bargmann, E. and Wolfe, S.M. (1985) *Washington's grate society: Schizophrenics in the Shelters and on the Street*. Health Research Group, Washington.

Torrey, E.F., Wolfe, S. M. and Flynn, L.M. (1990) Fiscal misappropriations in programs for the mentally ill: A report on illegality and failure of the federal construction grant program for Community Mental Health Centers. Health Research Group and National Alliance for the Mentally Ill, March, mimeo.

Van Der Werf, M. (1989) Nude inmates bound to 'rack' for hours; practice defended. *Arizona Republic*, April 27.

Vernoz, G., Burnam, M.A. and McGlynn, E.A. *et al.* (1988) *Review of California's Program for the Homeless Mentally Ill.* Rand Corporation, Santa Monica.

Washington Post (1989) Psychiatrists to 'treat' Satanism. September 7, p. C–6.

Whitman, D. (1989) Shattering myths about the homeless. *US News and World Report*, March 20, p. 28.

Windle, C., Poppen, P.J. and Thompson, J.W. *et al.* (1988) Types of patients served by various providers of outpatient care in CMHCs. *American Journal of Psychiatry*, **145**, 457–463.

Worthington, R. (1988) Psychiatrist shortage in rural US. *San Francisco Sunday Examiner and Chronicle*, November 27, p. A–1.

16 COMMUNITY CARE: USERS' PERSPECTIVES

D. Ross, P. Campbell and A. Neeter

INTRODUCTION

We write this chapter as people who have been in receipt of psychiatric services for a very long time—for two of us it is more than half our lifetimes. We write it too as members of a discussion and pressure group—Camden Mental Health Consortium—which is made up mostly of service users. In what follows we have drawn to a degree on our own personal experiences, but we have drawn more heavily on discussions that have taken place in Consortium over several years and on the arguments that have been formulated as a result.

You will find in this chapter no scholarly apparatus of footnotes, references, adjudication between conflicting research papers and the like. But you will find expertise. It is the expertise of those who have been through the psychiatric system, who have been on the receiving end of diagnosis, medication, sections, ward rounds, day hospitals, day centres, hostels and so on. Of course, such experiences are not usually thought to constitute any form of expertise at all—rather the reverse. Received wisdom has it that experts are what we *need*, not what we *are*. But in forming itself as a group, Consortium has enabled many of us to realize that we are not alone in what we think about our treatment, it has enabled us to reflect collectively on raw experience and turn it into judgement, and consequently to insist that the perspectives which we have on psychiatry are just as valid as the perspectives held by professionals. If users can persuade professionals that this is so, then we will be admitted as an essential voice in the debate about community care.

In a single chapter like this one we are forced to be selective. The remainder of this introduction will briefly consider the much-discussed 'crisis in community care'. The rest of the chapter falls into three sections—on crisis provision, on housing and on employment and alternatives to employment.

The crisis in community care

A rare consensus seems to exist amongst mental health workers from all disciplines and all shades of 'political' opinion that community care, as a policy and a practice, is in crisis. Most politicians, the mass media and large sections of the public agree. The 'crisis' finds its apotheosis in the figures of the bag lady sorting through her belongings or the dishevelled, homeless young man talking to himself on the streets. Less dramatically, professionals at all levels as well as relatives, friends and neighbours worry about those who have 'fallen through the net', who sit at home (wherever home may be) doing nothing, lacking social skills, locked in misery or fantasy and oblivious to that busy social world in which all 'normal' people participate as a matter of course.

The dream of deinstitutionalization has failed in the eyes of this consensus. But here the consensus begins to come apart. For one school of thought, the issue is to find the remedies which will make the dream come true: more money, better training, more staff. From another point of view, however, this is a doomed quest. For the dream of deinstitutionalization was always just that—a dream, an illusion. Mentally ill people can never be expected to cope in mainstream society and the crisis in community care is testimony to the truth of that argument. Better retain hospitals—improved ones, of course—where the chronically sick can be looked after. Usually this view is put a little more cautiously—better retain hospitals *until* proper community care is in place. But what counts as 'proper' is left unspecified and a very long wait is both acceptable and expected.

We agree that there is a crisis in community care. In the inner city where we live, community provision ranges from the non-existent through the patchy to the shambolic. This is despite the efforts of some dedicated mental health workers. But we do not believe that the problem lies with the inadequacies of psychiatric patients. Lack of resources is certainly an issue. Whether in hospital or in the community, mental health provision is at the bottom of the heap when it comes to the allocation of finances and this fact needs to be repeatedly rammed home to those who hold the purse strings.

However, there is more to it than this. The community provision that does exist is deeply unappealing to the majority of service recipients. For instance, people often do not attend the day centres to which they have been assigned and they are then usually saddled with the label 'lacks motivation'. But the real problem can be that the day centre is a fantastically boring place where there is either nothing at all to do or else there is an enforced regime of activities well-suited only to school children. There are therefore two quite different solutions to the 'problem' of non-attendance—motivate the individual or change the day centre.

The general point is that such community provision as exists is designed in all respects by professionals based on their understanding of what is wrong with users, what our needs are and how they should be met. We are not consulted at all, we have no control, we have no power. We suggest that those who conclude that community care has failed because psychiatric patients cannot cope in the community should ask themselves whether the kind of services they provide do not actually constitute a *barrier* to re-integration. We shall expand upon and illustrate this argument in other sections of this chapter.

Stigma

However, we do not say that the multifarious problems which beset care in the community are all to be laid at the door of mental health workers. There exists a profound obstacle in the 'community' itself and that obstacle is the one of negative attitudes, stereotypes and stigmatization. For a variety of reasons, the authors of this chapter have 'come out' about our psychiatric histories but in the past we have felt the compulsion to keep this is a deadly secret and experienced the terror lest even close friends find out. We know at first hand how the 'community' feels about people like us.

Stigmatization has reached new heights in the guise of supposedly concerned press coverage of the very crisis in community care discussed above. Were the media to be believed, the typical person discharged from a psychiatric hospital is living on the streets picking through rubbish bins for food, is very likely to be violent and dangerous, is probably addicted to alcohol or hard drugs or, at the very best, is totally pathetic and unable to manage even the most basic tasks of life. This is the hard face of the crisis, according to 'responsible' journalism. But these images are a myth—and a very damaging one.

Our argument is not that what is depicted in these media representations *never* happens. It is that these portrayals give an entirely skewed idea of the lives of most people with mental health problems. We are represented as utterly outide the boundaries of normal society. It is then not surprising if there is a deep ambivalence about letting us in. Whether the media reflects or shapes public opinion, this kind of coverage is damaging since it encourages the 'community' to think of us as pariahs and to see us as a threat.

In addition to the images which circulate in society, we have to contend with the consequences of the fact that for more than a century now, those who seem to be mad have been conveniently kept out of sight and out of mind—in hospitals. Some of us now try to remain socially invisible. Others do not or cannot. All of us are confined by the web of stigmatization. The solution most often proposed is to teach us the skills of being 'normal'. But integration into the community should not be a one-sided affair, something *we* must achieve. The community must learn some social skills, must learn to accept troubling distress and difference. The first step towards that objective is to break down the barriers that are built of ignorance, stereotypes and misplaced fear.

COPING WITH CRISES

Severe emotional distress can take many forms and provoke a range of reactions both from the person affected and those around them. Millions of people in our society turn to drink in times of crisis, stopping just short of the level that would get them into serious trouble. Others become abusive, verbally or physically, towards those closest to them. Yet others suppress and deny their distress, carry on as 'normal' and drive themselves to physical illness. It is only occasionally that reactions such as these result in interventions which exclude the person concerned from ordinary social life. Yet this is what happens when distress is manifest in a form that makes it recognizable, first to relatives and friends, possibly to the police, and finally to doctors, as 'mental illness'. When this happens, the odds are high that you will find yourself in a mental hospital.

Much is made in the psychiatric literature of the improvements that have taken place in mental hospitals over the past two decades—the move from huge Victorian institutions to small units in district general hospitals, changes in nursing training and practice, and so on. For the writers of this chapter, experience varies. For some, the old ways are as alive and kicking today as they were twenty years ago. For others, the nightmares of twenty years ago have given way to something that approaches good care. It depends on such contingencies as where you live, where the doctor has his or her beds, where and whether there is a bed to be had.

But whether specific hospitals are malign or benign is not the only point. They differ in *how* they do things but in large measure they share a basic framework of *what* they do. The real point is that you have no alternative but to be caught up in the psychiatric system. When mental distress is recognizable as mental illness, there is no other option. In times of crises, 'care in the community' offers no choice to the recipient.

What we would like to see, as part of community care, are places of refuge, of asylum in the original sense. They would be small, they would be local, they would take the problems you experience on your own terms and they would omit much of the paraphernalia that is intrinsic to the psychiatric system. We can expand on this by describing just two ways in which a 'crisis house' and a mental hospital would differ. These involve the initial interview and the help that is offered.

What happens first?

Typically, on admission to a psychiatric ward, you are interviewed by a doctor. Many people expect this to be an opportunity to tell all that is troubling them to an expert who will help. But much of the interview is wholly baffling. 'Count backwards from 100 in sevens.' 'Do you believe your thoughts are being controlled?' There appears to be no space to say on your own terms and in your own words, just what are the difficulties that have reduced you to this situation. Your understanding of your own situation has become irrelevant, seemingly the last thing the doctor wants to know about.

The interview is also extremely long. If you are depressed and feel worthless in the face of expertise, you are likely to feel that you 'ought' to go through with it. If you are restless you will be told to try to sit still and answer the questions. If you are confused or suspicious, the endless stream of questions and the doctor's compulsive writing behaviour just compounds the situation.

The initial interview is 'diagnostic' (not that the patient is informed of this) and, as we know, diagnosis is a prelude to treatment. We will deal with treatment in a moment.

Obviously, if 'crisis houses' were provided as part of community care, the user would have to have an initial talk with a worker. But we envisage that this would be radically different to the diagnostic interview just described. The major principle of the discussion would be to take completely seriously the nature of your emotional distress as defined by *you*, the person experiencing it. The agenda would be set not by a pre-given series of questions, but by the priorities of recipients. This means not least that certain issues could be raised which are simply ruled out by the diagnostic interview— economic issues, housing matters, social questions. These are vital since, if crisis provision is to be part of community care, it is imperative that a person's links with his or her community are not damaged because of the crisis and how it is handled. In the mental hospital these are matters for the social worker, a person of low status, secondary.

But more than this, the user's definition of his or her mental distress must be respected. This might sound far-fetched, but it is not. We do not deny that 'mental illness' involves the very extremes of feeling, mental confusion and the like. What we deny is that the person's explanation of what is going on is *meaningless*, mere babble, just symptoms. If I say that my father is planning to experiment on my brain, that is unlikely to be literally true. But he may yet represent a great threat to me. My fear can be dealt with by writing 'paranoid' in my notes or by taking my fear seriously and exploring it. In the first case we have two people talking at cross purposes, in the second two people trying to negotiate some common ground. This brings us to the question of treatment.

The help to be offered

The diagnostic interview is likely to conclude on the recipient's part with disappointment and on the doctor's part with a decision as to what kind of mental illness the person is suffering from and the prescription of medication. Both of these things will probably be secret. In particular, you are unlikely to be told about the prescription until you are called to the trolley at the next drugs round.

Come time, most people start to experience 'side effects' from their drugs that range from the unpleasant to the terrifying. What is totally unforgivable is that the majority of hospitals give people absolutely no information about these negative effects. What would you think if you suddenly experienced tremors, stiffness and inability to move your limbs or even your eyes? Many people think, literally, that they are dying.

The widespread lack of information about medication is linked to something broader. Apart from occupational therapy, largely regarded as a time-filler, medication is the *only* treatment the mental hospital has to offer. (Some units have nurses trained in counselling skills and this is welcome, but such places are rare.) The staff have total control over the drugs, they are the major source of their claim to expertise, and patients are expected to swallow them obediently and without question. The relationship that exists in the giving and taking of drugs is one of power.

Would a crisis house use medication? Some say 'no', vehemently. Drugs are nothing but poisons masquerading as cures. For others of us, the question of drugs is up to the individual user. It is a choice. However, what is vital is that this choice is an informed one, unlike the situation that usually pertains at present. Moreover, it is no good professionals complaining that recipients cannot understand the complexities at stake or that they will be 'put off' if told about side effects that are very unlikely to arise. The answer to this, tedious though it may be for mental health workers, is to repeat the information as often as necessary.

But whether or not a crisis house would use medication is not the central question because medication would certainly not be the only assistance offered. What would be offered would partly depend on the individual—emotional crises are not homogenous in their roots or their expression. For some people, help to untangle and resolve social and personal relationships might be of the first importance. For others, refuge from a world that has simply become too much and then help to return to it afterwards would do most good. People who had withdrawn from the world would be helped to understand why and then to slowly decide to what kind of world they would like to attach themselves, if any. Some people would need a great deal of time. So long as a person thinking of suicide stays in the house, they must be prevented from acting on these thoughts. Someone who is very disoriented must have company constantly.

We do not advocate intensive psychotherapy with people who are in deep emotional crises. We do advocate respect for the person's definition of his or her distress and as much, or as little, exploration of it as the person wants. We also insist that a crisis house, as part of community care, should prioritise the maintenance or the re-establishment of social, personal and economic links with the person's community of origin or, if that is not feasible, the establishment of links with a new one.

Space does not permit us to discuss the many issues relevant to crisis provision. We will make just one final point. Community care is not cheap. The kind of crisis care we envisage would not be cheap. A high level of staffing would be necessary since non-hospital care must be an option for everyone, no matter how disturbed initially. But we live in a rich society, millions of pounds are spent annually on psychiatric drugs, much more on high technology medicine. It is not too much to ask.

HOUSING

Problems arising from lack of housing, loss of a home, or depressing, noisy accommodation are often the reason for people's admission to a psychiatric hospital. Many also return to the wards following the difficulties experienced after discharge when necessary support often cannot be found. This destroys any benefits which may have been gained during treatment, and creates further heavy expense for administrators and tax-payers. Even the most resilient person can be worn down by living in desolate bed and breakfast accommodation. This is particularly so when you lack food and money because a GIRO has not arrived and find yourself surrounded by people who are desperate and hostile. No matter how reluctant, a person may be driven back to a mental hospital through the absence of someone to turn to out of office hours and at weekends. The inability to contact friends is even more crucial and in these circumstances one's return to a psychiatric hospital can happen in spite of personal condemnation of such places.

In preparing this chapter, we spoke to groups of recipients who had left a large institution to live in the 'community'. Many people felt that the public should be advised of plans to create housing for mentally distressed people in their area, believing that it is better to talk over any resentment and opposition before accommodation is secured than to become residents who are met with prejudice and ostracism later. They recognized an urgent need for public education on matters of mental health. This should happen in exactly the same way as the public is informed about physical wellbeing and how to maintain it, and how to respect and help physically ill people. We cannot exaggerate the keen sense of discomfort and isolation felt by most people upon being once again in the maelstrom of 'civilized society' with its stigmatizing attitudes, media-induced fear and ancient desire for a scapegoat on whom to pin the blame for its violence.

Recipients who have been consulted about housing arrangements (since planners began to seek their opinions) generally feel that a variety of accommodation should be made available for persons who have suffered and are suffering from mental distress. This variety should cater for our diverse needs and preferences and our progress or lack of it when living in the community. It is important that people can move on as they become more independent or receive more support if their ability to cope diminishes. It is also vitally important that people feel more secure and respected in their housing than it is ever possible to feel when living in an institution which often surrounds its users with threatening, degrading and humiliating situations.

Many recipients who have been hospitalized for lengthy periods feel that core and cluster-type arrangements should be organized with an adequate telephone system provided to link people up with their friends, families and support workers. A 24 hour service, with someone always available to talk, is an essential provision. Professionals who insist this is financially impractical should consider the rising costs of hospitalization. A friendly helpline would be an excellent preventative service. Lack of a means of communication is a prime reason for despair and suicide.

For people who move from hospital or more sheltered accommodation into new surroundings, the early novelty of a place of one's own can soon wear off. A feeling of isolation and inability to cope with all the new situations that arise can then set in and grossly undermine integration into community life. Obviously, this should be avoided at all costs. Recipients we spoke to felt that when people are placed in individual accommodation, expensive furnishings are of far less importance than easy access to a workscheme, leisure facilities and a phone. At the same time, it is important that group and residential homes are planned or modified to permit privacy. At times, people need to create a space around themselves away from other tenants, residents and staff, and be able to enjoy that space with invited visitors if they wish.

At this point, we should stress that *all* housing for people in mental distress needs to have easy access to suitable support. This should include a home visitor when a person cannot get out and about as easily as they might wish and would encourage and aid reintegration into the community and the development of greater independence. Befriending schemes too can be very valuable, and should be funded by Borough Councils and voluntary organizations in conjunction with any housing service. Planners must take into account how uncertain and anxious people may become about ordinary life after the confined and regulated life of a psychiatric hospital, or when a traumatic event has severed someone from their past and familiar surroundings. A befriending scheme can aid the use of social facilities when a person is reluctant to go out and having difficulty in making even short journeys and creating a new life and friendships. These points apply as much to the young person who finds they are having repeated admissions to an acute ward as they do to people being discharged after a long stay in a large institution.

Whatever accommodation is provided, planners must ask themselves how they would feel in the client's environment and bear this in mind continually. Staff should be of the kind who will unobtrusively assist people to value themselves, give help in seeking information on rights and welfare benefits, and show people how to budget and how to vote. They need to be prepared to help formulate a complaints procedure and make sure it is used. People should have the opportunity to contribute to the communities to which they belong and to help dissolve the myth that people who have suffered mental distress are second-class citizens with nothing to offer.

EMPLOYMENT AND LEISURE

Employment

In the 1960s and early 1970s there often seemed to be an underlying assumption among mental health workers that most short-term inpatients would sooner or later return to the world of employment albeit at a lower level than before. The current reality is substantially different. For most former recipients of inpatient psychiatric care, whether long term or short term, employment now will be quite unlikely if not completely impossible.

The barriers facing users who seek employment in the open market are formidable and have been well known for many years. Employers remain largely ignorant or misinformed on what 'mental illness' actually amounts to and how it will affect an individual's capacity to perform particular duties. As a result job applicants with a psychiatric record repeatedly face the agonizing choice of attempting to conceal their past or undertaking an open explanation of their lives to justify themselves in the eyes of their interviewers. Too often, even when the latter course is chosen, individuals will not receive fair treatment, will fail an interview and then discover that their medical and psychiatric references have not been pursued. In the light of such attitudes and the continuing reluctance of government to enact anti-discrimination legislation for people with psychiatric histories, it is hardly a surprise that so many of us are unemployed or working in jobs that barely reflect our true abilities.

Discussions at Camden Consortium underline the shortcomings in the system that gives advice and support to those seeking employment. Disablement Resettlement Officers (DROs) are normally not held in high regard. There appear to be too few of them to meet the real needs. They are often not adequately trained to deal with the problems particular to people with psychiatric records. As a result meetings with a DRO may proceed from the starting point of 'We can't really do much to help in your case . . .'

and may later reveal that the DRO has no specific knowledge of the implications of psychiatric diagnoses anyway. It is hard to avoid concluding that the way DROs are trained, the broad remit of their responsibilities to different groups, and their position within the employment-providing chain, frequently prevents them from acting assertively and effectively to meet the individual employment needs of people with psychiatric histories.

The situation with regard to the quota system for employing disabled people is also quite unsatisfactory. For a number of years there seems to have been a cynical acceptance that the quota system does not work. Many people who have been diagnosed as 'mentally ill' strongly resist the idea of registering as disabled and this is sometimes used as an argument to play down the importance of having a quota system at all and to condone the failure to make it work properly. But unless an effective quota system is devised and made to work, its relevance to people with psychiatric records may always be marginal. In the meantime, quotas may do more to reassure the establishment that 'something is being done' than to convince those seeking work that anything is seriously intended.

In light of the above problems, we are now looking for a new approach to meeting our employment needs: an approach that addresses our individual desires and needs and offers more sensitive and more intensive advice and support. Under current social and economic conditions, it actually seems unrealistic to expect many people coming out of psychiatric institutions to make a successful return to open employment without skilled and consistent personal support. People seeking work should be supported in small groups that have regular (more than once a week) access to a worker with special training in areas of employment. It would be better that these groups met and were focused around places where people choose to spend their time (drop-ins, day centres, community centres), than in Jobshops or council offices. Unless small-scale, local and ground-level initiatives of this kind are funded it is not likely that the particular needs of individuals will ever be met.

Our employment needs are extremely varied. In this sense as in so many others it is unhelpful to think of us as a single group—the so-called mentally ill. Not only are there differences in the desire for open or sheltered employment but also—and most crucially—for full-time and part-time employment. At present those who want part-time or flexible employment schemes which allow them to adjust to new routines or acquire or re-establish skills often find themselves falling into a benefits 'trap' which destroys all incentive to make permanent employment a goal. Although a number of schemes that provide imaginative ways around such barriers do now exist, they remain relatively isolated examples of good practice in an area where concerted attempts to reintegrate through employment are uncommon.

One way to avoid the inadequacies of present systems would be by recipients setting up their own employment schemes, employing themselves and each other. In other countries, notably Italy, worker cooperatives involving people who have been in psychiatric institutions have had some success. But even here there is a need for skilled support and whereas in Italy mental health professionals seem to have been ready to move out of institutional settings and get involved in such initiatives, in this country it is far from clear that the 'mental health business' really sees employment as part of their concern. Containment and treatment are essential. Employment is merely desirable.

Leisure

Poverty is a central feature in the lives of people who return from psychiatric hospital to live in the community. In this respect it is perhaps optimistic to speak of us as having real leisure opportunities, particularly if we have to rely on state benefits for our income. When adequate housing, food and transport become problems of day-to-day concern, the availability of leisure, in the sense that the majority of society would understand it, becomes very much a secondary issue.

Nevertheless if quality of life is seen as a measure of the success of community care initiatives, leisure opportunities are important. When existing facilities are being discussed there is a real need for clear thinking. Many day centres provide leisure opportunities. But in what sense are art therapy or social skills groups part of an ordinary perception of leisure? How much of the provision in day centres is leisure and how much something else altogether? When leisure opportunities are considered it would be helpful to begin by asking users what they would like to do in their leisure time and try to meet those desires rather than a series of needs that have been deemed to be relevant. If leisure is not going to be individual and person-centred then it is not going to be leisure.

Choice is vital. We should be supporting people to use the widest range of community leisure facilities rather than concentrating on creating a system of leisure provision only used by people with psychiatric histories. To achieve this it will be necessary to educate workers in adult education institutes and community centres to meet our particular problems more sensitively. At present it is evident that more people with psychiatric records are using ordinary community facilities and that workers are finding it increasingly difficult to cope with this demand. Coherent support strategies are now needed; both to encourage people to use the full range of opportunities and to enable workers to make their leisure facilities successful and open to all members of the community.

Day centres

Given the problems with employment and most kinds of leisure, many of us spend at least some time passing the day in day centres. For some, this is an active choice and for some it is a prescription with which we comply. Many people attend 'for something to do', to assuage boredom or at least be bored in company.

The chance to meet with others who have had similar experiences is important. No matter how dedicated and sensitive, a professional can never *empathize* with someone who has suffered severe emotional distress and been a recipient of the psychiatric system. Friendships and mutual support between users are nearly always beneficial yet they are often discouraged. The very existence of a hierarchy of 'helpers' and 'helped' can discourage recipients from seeing each other as a source of support in the ordinary sense. At the worst, mental health workers will label a relationship between users as 'pathological'. This is patronizing and damaging. It is also hypocritical since any relationship can be seen as pathological at some level.

At the same time as providing the opportunity to meet others, however, day centres run the risk of being psychiatric 'ghettoes'. In them the people nobody wants to know can be herded away and supervised all day. To avoid this, structures need to be changed. In some centres, users are encouraged to be there all day every day. But this defeats the object of assisting people to reintegrate into the community (always assuming that is the object). We should be allowed to use day centres flexibly and that would involve them being open in the evening and at weekends. Many users want the help and support it takes to live in the community but want it as and when it is necessary and convenient.

To avoid the ghetto phenomenon, it would also be ideal to open day centres to use by other community groups and the general public. It will, in the first instance, be very difficult to bring this about such is the stigma surrounding anything to do with mental illness. But much of what we advocate will be difficult for this and other reasons and difficulty is no excuse for not bothering.

In all aspects of day centre functioning, it is vital to ask recipients what it is they want to see provided at the centre and to discuss this fully. Some places have weekly meetings which any user or worker can attend and the structure and nature of activities at the centre can be negotiated there. Camden Consortium was involved with one centre where a management committee was set up and where centre users had guaranteed places on the committee. This was not without problems. Few people with a psychiatric history have extensive experience of how committees work or of the power and responsibility involved. However, with commitment these obstacles can be overcome and this is one concrete way of empowering people who are usually placed in a helpless position.

CONCLUSION

We object to that strand in much thinking about people with psychiatric histories which concentrate on the *deficits* of those returning to the community or trying to make their way in the community. Whether it be in the areas of housing, employment or leisure, it is time to move away from approaches that focus on deficits in the person with a psychiatric history. On the one hand, this stance renders invisible our strengths. On the other, it is blind to the fact that social responses, the responses of the community itself, are also deficient. Mental health workers should acknowledge these arguments and take action.

INDEX